Color Vision

Leo M. Hurvich
University of Pennsylvania

COLOR VISION

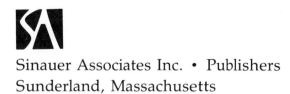

Sinauer Associates Inc. • Publishers
Sunderland, Massachusetts

to Dorothea

COLOR VISION

Copyright © 1981 by Sinauer Associates Inc.

Printed in U.S.A.

Library of Congress Cataloging in Publication Data

Hurvich, Leo M., 1910–
    Color vision.

    Bibliography: p.
    Includes index.
    1. Color vision. I. Title.
QP483.H87   599.01′823   80-19077
ISBN 0-87893-336-0
ISBN 0-87893-337-9 (pbk.)

5 4 3 2 1

Contents

Color Plates

Color plates appear following page 88.

Preface

Over the years I have had numerous requests to recommend a single book that gives a clear, simple picture of color vision and how it works. These inquiries have come from various sources: from undergraduate and graduate students; from colleagues whose professional interests—scientific and humanistic—lie elsewhere than in sensory psychology and physiology; as well as from personal friends curious about and interested in what Dorothea Jameson and I have been doing in our laboratory research. It has been difficult to comply with these requests. Having done research for so many years in color vision and having organized the material within a theoretical paradigm that has clarified the issues for me, it is not surprising that I have not found books written from the viewpoint of others that are congenial to me. There are excellent accounts of what is known about the physiology of color vision; there are many reviews of the quantitative data of psychophysics; there are interesting discussions of perceptual phenomena; and there are historically valid accounts of color vision theory. But none of these aims at what I have tried to do in this text: to present a systematic, comprehensive, scientifically rigorous development of the topic of color vision in the context of a unified, coherent theoretical model—an opponent–process theory of color vision. In this sense, I believe the book is unique among color vision texts.

In trying to present a coherent story line I have resisted breaking up the individual chapters into multiple subsections interrupted by topical headings. I believe that the continuity is more important than fragmented subtopics for the readers to whom the book is directed; that is, readers with a minimum of technical or scientific background. I have cross–referenced chapters profusely to emphasize the relatedness of individual topics. The Background Readings at the end of each chapter include books and articles that bear directly on the topic covered. It was, of course, necessary to be selective, and I trust that anyone who feels I have slighted his or her work will realize the problem I faced. Each chapter also has references to Further Readings to direct the interested reader to more advanced technical or mathematical treatments. These are fewer in number and either represent classics in the field or provide fuller coverage of certain selective topics discussed in the chapters. Illustration credits are given following the text. All references may be located from the author index.

Dorothea Jameson and I have pursued our research on color vision in the context of the opponent–process theoretical formulation. This book reflects my own understanding of color vision as it developed from that work; hence the many citations of our jointly published original journal and handbook articles. We are indebted to the National Science Foundation and the National Institutes of Health for many years of research support.

I should like to thank both Gerald Jacobs and Robert Sekular who read an early draft on the manuscript and made very helpful comments and suggestions. F. Dent Varner and Patti Gasper read the completed manuscript and pointed out some errors, some inconsistencies, and some infelicities in the text. I appreciate this and also want to thank Patti Gasper for her assistance with various computations.

Eleanor Faith Dixon watched me deface and erase her carefully typed manuscript pages without a complaint for longer than either of us cares to recall. I am deeply and forever grateful to her for this and for the many other tasks she assumed that helped in the preparation of this book.

Carlton Brose, my editor, worked on the book with an amazing attention and commitment to its every detail and Joseph Vesely supervised its production with an overriding concern that it come out the way I wanted it to. My thanks to them.

This book, for which I alone am responsible, would never have been possible if it were not for my collaboration of more than three decades with Dorothea Jameson. I am certain it would have been a better book had I been able to convince her to make it yet another collaborative effort. Her interests at the time of my writing this book took her in a different direction and she preferred to work on problems of art and perception which concern her deeply and on which she continues to work independently. Nevertheless, she suffered interruption after interruption in her own work in response to queries of every conceivable sort that I posed to her. This is a public apology and a public thanks.

North Truro, Massachusetts

1
Classification of
Visual Experience

LOOKING out from my study window in a cottage near the ocean's edge, I see clouds separated from sky, sky separated from the sea, the sea from the dune, beach grass and dusty miller from the dune, finches from the dusty miller, and the male finch from the female finch. I also see pitch pine as distinct from scrub oak, and wild roses as separate from bayberry and wild plum and locust bushes.

What makes it possible for me to distinguish these many forms and objects? Primarily, differences in color, for our visual world is made up only of differently formed colors. The objects I see are nothing but colors of different kinds and forms.

This is nicely demonstrated by insects, fish, and animals whose protective coloration enables them to escape the notice of predators. Moths and butterflies provide excellent examples. The dead-leaf butterfly of the Far East is said to be the most famous camouflaged insect in the world. These butterflies are very conspicuous on the wing, but in a position of repose, in the quaint phrasing of an early naturalist, "they so closely resemble a dead leaf attached to a twig as almost certainly to deceive the eye even when gazing full upon it." An equally dramatic example is shown in Plate 1-1, where a flower mantis sits on the red flowers of an orchid.

The first thing we have to get clear is the number and varieties of colors we experience. How many different colors are there? Answers to this question differ from one another by more than a factor of a million! For example, whereas some people have claimed that we can see more than a million different colors, others have proposed more modest figures—hundreds of thousands. But another answer differs drastically from all these: we see only six fundamentally different colors.*

_____

* Many introductory textbooks and popular accounts of color emphasize three so-called "primary" colors: red, green, and blue. These colors cannot fully describe what we see but refer to a theory of the color-vision mechanism that draws heavily on the results of light mixtures (see Chapters 9 and 11). Art teachers tend to emphasize three different "primary"

Suppose that I look at the sky through a small hole punched in a large piece of paper or cardboard. This arrangement allows me to examine in small patches what would otherwise appear as a wide expanse of sky, all of one color, say light blue. But looking through the peephole at one piece of sky after another, I can distinguish dozens—probably hundreds—of different colors. The "uniform" blue sky seems to be composed of a large number of different blues. The same is true of the wide expanse of the sea. And the sky and sea are only two natural "surfaces" among countless others. What about man-made products? There are perhaps one-half million commercially available colors, not all of which have names. There are many fewer color names than there are discriminable colors. Analogously, there are many fewer absolutely identifiable colors than there are discriminable ones. Only a dozen or so hues can be used in practical situations where absolute identification is required. Nevertheless, the number of color names is large enough to fill a small dictionary. *Color. Universal Language and Dictionary of Names* of the National Bureau of Standards lists some 7500 different individual color names, and the *Methuen Handbook of Colour* tells us that about 8000 color names are used in the United Kingdom (see Chapter 20). Many in these lists of names are fanciful products of advertising copywriters: Vamp, Wafted Feather, Heart's Desire, Stardew, Cinderella, Fancy Free, Angel Wing, Murmur—names that are chosen primarily for sales promotion. The names themselves, although they may arouse subjective feelings, bring no particular colors to mind.

Other names in these lists are more familiar to most of us and are of the sort that appear in *Webster's New International Dictionary,* 2nd ed. (1958), where we find listed 130 different colors. These colors are based on names of flowers, fruits, plants, minerals, metals, animals, and other natural and man-made objects. Among them we find rose, lavender, violet, wisteria, lilac, heliotrope, mauve, orange, lemon, citron, coffee, chestnut, olive, hazel, henna, ruby, emerald, amethyst, sapphire, turquoise, alabaster, copper red, cobalt blue, chrome malachite, aurora, sky blue, fire red, sea green, ultramarine blue, canary yellow, buff, purple, salmon, peach, taupe, brown, beaver, mouse gray, ivory, vermillion, claret red, chocolate, bottle green, crimson, peacock blue, auburn, indigo, magenta, scarlet, and cardinal.

One hundred and thirty is still a large number and, not surprisingly, very few people seem to know what colors the names cyan, magenta, taupe, or mauve represent. Can we systematize our color experiences in

---

colors: red, yellow, and blue. This set, too, is not adequate to describe what we see. It is essentially an instruction for mixing pigments, since appropriate combinations of three such primary colors enable us to produce a wide range of colors (see Chapters 8 and 21).

a simple way that makes us less dependent on a knowledge of objects (or dyes) and yet encompasses our total experience of the color world? The answer is yes. If pressed to the greatest possible economy of color terms we find that we can describe all the colors we discriminate by using only six terms and their various combinations. These are red, yellow, green, and blue, the four UNITARY HUES, and black and white, the two extremes of the series of hueless colors.* All other color names, both those we commonly use in everyday language, such as pink, violet, gray, and brown, and the more technical ones, such as cyan and magenta, can be described by referring to these six terms and combinations of them.

Let us see what the *perceptual* interrelations are among those colors that have hues, the reds, yellows, greens, and blues. All the hues that we see can be ordered in a closed circle, often called a HUE CIRCLE. If we place hues that are minimally different next to each other, we can form a continuous series that turns back on itself.

Ewald Hering, a famous nineteenth-century German physiologist, has described the complete color circle that results from such a procedure (Plate 1-2). If we take any color as the starting point on a color circle, for example a red (one associated with the long-wavelength end of the spectrum; see Chapter 4), then moving clockwise the colors become increasingly more yellowish; simultaneously, the redness of each color recedes until passing through orange and gold yellow we reach a yellow that has no trace of the redness that was obvious in the orange. Other yellow colors follow this yellow, tending more and more toward green (sulfur yellow, canary yellow); farther on, the yellow recedes more and more while greenness (as in sap green) becomes gradually more prominent, and we finally reach a green that looks completely free of yellow. Green colors following this green tend into blue (sea green); farther on, the blueness becomes continuously stronger and the greenness continuously weaker (sea blue), until we reach a blue that no longer shows any greenness. After this blue come blues of increasing redness and hence decreasing blueness (blue violet, red violet, purple red), until the last trace of blueness vanishes in a true red. Then red hues that begin to show yellowish traces follow this red until we return to the initial red from which we started.

This description of the hue circle makes it clear that there are four UNIQUE POINTS in the circle. There is a place where a yellow occurs in which we cannot detect any red or even any green. It is a transition point where we experience a hue that is uniquely yellow. The same is true of blue. As we move through the color circle we can find a blue that has not

* Black and white are often referred to as "colorless" ("achromatic" by the scientists), but since the word "hue" is limited to the reds, yellows, greens, blues, and their combinations, it is more accurate to describe blacks and whites as "hueless" rather than "colorless."

the slightest trace of either red or green: this we call a unique blue. We also see that in such a circle there are two other transition points, a red one and a green one. In these cases we can see a red without a trace of blue or yellow and the same is true of the green. It is neither a yellowish nor a bluish green. These four unique hues—red, yellow, green, and blue—are the four unitary hues.

Plate 1-2 illustrates such a color circle with a selected number of samples and shows the four unique hues located so that they divide the circle into four quadrants. At the 12, 3, 6, and 9 o'clock positions we have a red, a yellow, a green, and a blue selected so as to show no trace of each other's hue quality. If we consider the circle divided by a vertical diameter, all colors on the right-hand side of the uniquely red and green hues are yellowish to varying degrees; all colors on the left-hand side have blue in common. If we consider the circle divided by a horizontal diameter, all the colors in the upper half above the uniquely yellow and blue hues are red to some degree; in the bottom half they share a greenness property.

If we consider each quadrant, we see that the colors between two unitary hues are of intermediate hue: they are BINARY HUES. Thus in the first quadrant (12–3 o'clock) all the intermediate hues resemble red and yellow, but to different degrees. The intermediate orange is both reddish and yellowish, but as we move toward unique red the intermediate loses in yellow and as we move toward unique yellow the intermediate color loses in redness. The other quadrants contain hues intermediate between yellow and green, green and blue, and blue and red.

Plate 1-3 contains a simple geometric figure that shows the way the intermediate colors are related to two unitary or unique colors. If the two unitary colors are blue and red, a rectangle composed of an upper blue and lower red triangle enables us to show more precisely the similarity between different intermediate or binary hues and the two unitary colors (Plate 1-3a). For each intermediate color represented on the baseline we need only erect a vertical line and note the heights of the segments that lie in the blue and red triangles. The ratio of these two segments expresses the ratio of blue to red quality that characterizes the hue in question. Thus at position a the ratio of blue to red is 3:1, at position b the ratio is 1:1, and at position c it is 1:5. As the vertical line moves from left to right, the amount of blue decreases and red increases. Violet lies closer to a, and crimson lies closer to c. Plate 1-3b summarizes by means of two juxtaposed triangles all the hues and their variable proportions between the end points red and yellow. Orange, which partakes equally of red and yellow, lies at the midpoint position at b' and most people would agree that "signal red" lies at a' and "carrot red" at c'.

If we now move the two rectangles so that they abut at the full red position, we have a schematic representation of all hues ranging from blue through mixtures of blue and red, red, mixtures of red and yellow, and finally yellow. Except for the more exotic silver and grays now available on cosmetic counters, note that this color series encompasses the hues of all lipsticks regardless of manufacturer or the names they have chosen to identify their products. Any assembly of conventional "red" lipsticks can be sorted sequentially. Every lipstick will find a place along the baseline of our combined rectangles and we will have a series that starts at the reddish-blue end and moves through blue-reds (or red-blues) to bluish red to those that are exclusively red. Next to these we will find some with what seems to be a slightly yellowish tinge, then on to those that are orange, and with less and less redness we end up with increasingly yellow lipsticks.

This sort of schematic representation of the ratio of hue similarity can be extended to the remainder of the color circle. Plate 1-4 provides such a summary in circular form.

It is clear from such a representation that all the natural and man-made objects that we encounter—all the lights; pieces of color paper; advertisements; color photographs; yarns; labels; wrapping papers; clothing; textiles; paint pigments that we can examine in shops, art supply houses, and paint stores; and all other items that have a hue—are referable to the schematic representation of Plate 1-4.

The color or hue circle tells us nothing about the physics of light (which we will discuss in Chapter 3). It tells us nothing about the chemistry of dyes and pigments nor what painters should expect to get from mixing particular pigments on a palette. It is concerned only with color appearance and the way various colors are interrelated and grade into one another. The color circle makes it clear that however useful we may find the words aquamarine, orange, and violet, for example, they are reducible to green-blue, yellow-red, and red-blue and, depending on our estimate of the ratio of the two unitary hues (hue elements), we can find a place for each along the circumference of the color circle. The same is true of the color words tangerine, cyan, and magenta: red-yellow, blue-green, and blue-red, respectively. The hue elements are the same for both triads; for similar colors, for example orange and tangerine, only their relative proportions differ.

The summary diagram of the hue circle tells us something about hues that often goes unnoticed. In systematizing the perceived hues and relations, we express the fact that we experience yellow-greens and blue-greens, but nowhere do the green and red segments or crescents of the diagram overlap. No radial line intercepts red-green simultaneously. There are no red-greens or green-reds. Similarly, this systematic summary makes it clear that there are no yellow-blues or blue-yellows in our color experience. Blue and yellow, like red and green, fall on opposite sides of the hue circle, with no overlap. We can go from red to blue via a series of red-blue intermediates or from red to yellow via red-yellow intermediates; this is also true of green. Here, too, we can move to blue or yellow by way of intermediate green-blues and green-yellows. But there is no gradual transition of this sort between red and green. To move from red to green requires passing through a color that differs from each of them—yellow or blue. Similarly, to move from yellow to blue requires passing through red or green, two colors totally different from blue and yellow.

We know that every item that has a hue is referable to the schematic representation of Plate 1-4, but what about brown? Surely, this is a color that cannot be described simply as red or yellow or green or blue. Nor can it reasonably be described by a simple combination of terms, such as red-yellow, yellow-red, green-blue, or blue-red. Brown seems to be clearly distinctive from all four unitary hues or any imaginable combination of them. Nonetheless, brown is relatable to the unitary hues, as we shall soon see, but first we must extend our descriptive analysis.

Up to now, we have concentrated exclusively on the four unitary hues and the color circle, although we did note briefly that the totality of our color experience can be summarized by relating it to the four chromatic qualities, red, yellow, green and blue, and the two achromatic or hueless qualities, black and white. Yet it is only with the addition of the black/gray/white series of color, which ranges from the deepest black imaginable through grayish black, blackish gray, gray, whitish gray, grayish white, and the purest white imaginable, that we can extend the limited hue circle of four unitary colors and their combinations to encompass the vast multiplicity of all visible colors—the thousands upon thousands of colors that I mentioned at the beginning of the chapter.

It is easy to visualize a series of achromatic colors that ranges from black through midgray to white. Such an ordered series is presented in Figure 1. The steps between the separate chips are intended to be visually equal. (The perceived difference between chips 3 and 4 is the same as that between chips 4 and 5, and so on.) It is possible to characterize the intermediate grays as containing different proportions of midgray with the two end members, black and white. Different intermediate grays may be said to have white and midgray in the ratio of, say 3:1 or 1:1, or black and midgray in the same ratios. Here we are thinking only in perceptual

1 ACHROMATIC COLOR SERIES. This ordered series ranges from black through midgray to white. The steps between the individual items in the series are intended to be visually equal.

terms. We are not, for the moment, concerned with the physical stimuli that produce the grays. Our interest is only in the appearance of these grays and in how much "whiteness" relative to "grayness" and "blackness" relative to "grayness" we see in a given gray.

There is a fairly simple way to set up a graded series of achromatic colors that ranges from white to midgray to black. First, place a piece of white cardboard or paper flat on a table or desk near a window (Figure 2). Then hold a similar piece of white cardboard with a 1-inch cutout (square or circular) in its center just above the first one. The second sheet of paper is held horizontally about 10 inches or so above the lower one. Care has to be taken not to cast a shadow on the lower one. The hole then looks like a small field that is pretty much the same white as the top surface. If we then rotate the top cardboard about a horizontal axis and tilt its front edge downward toward the light from the window, the small center aperture becomes continuously grayer and even blackish gray. If the top cardboard is rotated in the opposite direction, the hole becomes increasingly white in appearance. Even though the position of the bottom sheet remains fixed and a fixed amount of physical light radiation (see Chapter 3) is coming through the hole, we can produce a series of colors that ranges from white through to darkish gray. A similar series of grays can, of course, be produced by mounting the upper white sheet in a fixed position and rotating the lower one toward and away from the light.

Just as part of the white paper can be made to appear very dark gray by surrounding it with a bright white surround, if we place a piece of orange paper on the table and rotate the same white paper with the cutout above the orange paper, we can make the orange color take on a brown appearance. Ewald Hering used a simple apparatus to make the point in a very dramatic and striking way.* Figure 3 depicts a perspective view of

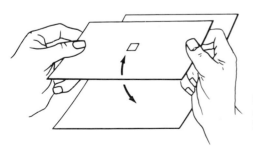

2 SIMPLE ARRANGEMENT to produce a graded series of achromatic colors. See text for procedure.

* Hering, who is now mainly known for his research on binocular vision, eye movements, and color vision, was, incidentally, the first person who correctly analyzed the cellular structure of the liver (1866) and first stated the interrelations between breathing and vasomotor control centers in the brain (1870).

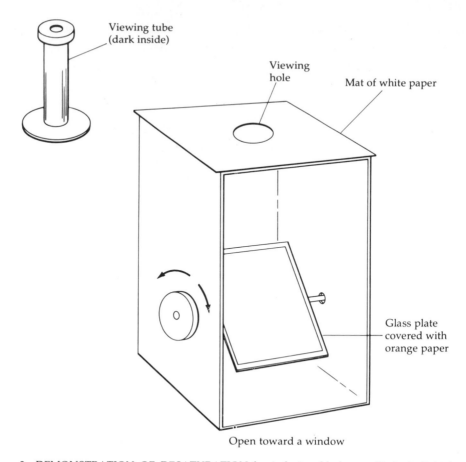

Viewing tube
(dark inside)

Viewing
hole

Mat of white paper

Glass plate
covered with
orange paper

Open toward a window

3 DEMONSTRATION OF DESATURATION by inducing blackness. Hering's light box enables one to vary the amount of light on a colored paper by rotating the glass plate about a horizontal axis. The paper can be viewed with or without a white surround. With the internally darkened viewing tube in position, we see an appropriately selected colored paper as orange at all positions of the rotatable plate. When relatively small amount of light is reflected toward the eye from the orange-appearing paper and the viewing tube is abruptly removed, thereby introducing the white surround, the colored paper is seen as brown. Paper of other colors may also be used. In all instances the introduction of the white surround induces a blackness quality.

the setup. "It is a box open toward the window so that sky light can fall on a glass plate contained in the box. The glass plate can be rotated about a horizontal axis and it is covered with colored, say, orange, paper. On the top panel of the box is a stiff, opaque sheet covered with mat white paper and containing a round hole on which, when needed, a dark viewing tube can be placed as shown in the figure. If the tube is removed and the glass plate placed as shown in the figure, then one sees from above a circular orange-colored field in the plane of the white paper. Now if the glass plate is rotated toward the back, then the orange is increasingly veiled with black, and becomes first light brown, then dark brown, and finally brownish black. If one replaces the viewing tube without changing anything else, then through the tube one immediately sees once more a glowing orange, which is transformed just as quickly again into brownish black when the viewing tube is again removed. . . ." Hering added that "This is a sight that surprises even those familiar with it." It must be emphasized that simply decreasing the amount of light that falls directly on a piece of orange paper will not produce a brown appearance. Lowering the illumination will make the orange appear more faded or gray, not brown.

Browns are mainly dark-grayish or blackish-orange and dark-grayish- or blackish-yellow colors. But there are also red browns and olive browns. There are many browns in our environment. The earth, wood, leather, human hair, and human skin appear to contain different proportions of yellow and red as well as different proportions of black and white. The other primary hues, red, green, and blue, can also be "veiled" or desaturated with black. We tend to call these dark or blackish reds, dark greens, and dark blues. We have no special word like "brown" for these other dark colors. And this may simply be so because they occur much less frequently than do the browns.

Chromatic colors (i.e., those that have hues), can also be veiled or desaturated with white as well as with black. The techniques are varied. It can be done, for example, by adding reflections from a white surface to a colored one. With these methods we get light blues, light greens, pinks, and so on—the pastel colors.

Schematically, Figure 4 represents the total gamut of colors of a single hue. Let the point labeled Y in this triangle represent an imaginary yellow that is free of any other qualities, that is, a yellow that has no red, green, black, gray, or white in it, and let the line W-Bk represent the series of colors that ranges from white through midgray to black. Let Gy be a point

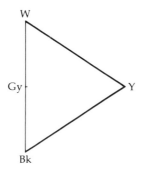

4 COLOR TRIANGLE that represents the total gamut of colors of a single hue (in this case, yellow).

that is an intermediate gray. All the possible visible yellows can be represented on the sides and within such a triangle. If we move along the side of the triangle Y-W in the direction of W, we have a series of yellows that become increasingly white and less yellow; we may think of these as yellows that are increasingly desaturated or veiled with whiteness. If we move along the side labeled Y-Bk toward black, we have a series of yellows that are increasingly desaturated with blackness. And if we move along the axis labeled Y-Gy toward the W-Bk axis, the yellows are increasingly grayer. Where will the browns be located in such a triangle?

We can, of course, construct a color triangle that represents the various combinations of any of the other unique hues with the white, gray, and black achromatic series. If we set up a blue triangle and place it so that it faces the yellow one, the resultant diamond shape is as shown in Figure 5. When we set up a pair of facing red and green color triangles and interlace them so that they are perpendicular to the plane of the yellow/blue pair, we obtain the diagram shown as Figure 6.

The horizontal plane that contains R, Y, G, and B is midway between white and black. It is the midgray (Gy) plane, which is the plane in which the hue circle of Plate 1-2 lies. We can select any intermediate or binary hue in the circle and construct a color triangle by linking it with white, midgray, and black. Thus color triangles exist for all hues, whether unitary or binary (i.e., red-yellow, green-yellow, etc.). When such triangles are placed adjacent to each other in the appropriate positions, they form the figure shown in Plate 1-5. Notice that hue circles could be drawn at any arbitrary whiteness, grayness, or blackness level we choose. Those in the upper part of the figure would contain hues that are seen to be desaturated with grayish white; those in the lower part of the circle would contain hues that appear to be desaturated with grayish black. Such a figure summarizes the totality of our color experiences and enables us to locate any color that we see somewhere along the surface or at some internal position (see Chapter 20).

There will, of course, be minor differences among normal observers

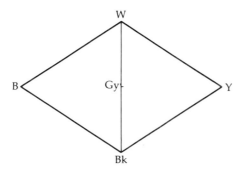

5 DUAL SET OF COLOR TRIANGLES that represents the total gamut of two colors (in this case, blue and yellow).

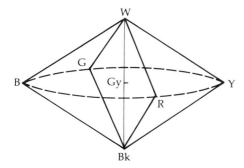

6 SET OF FOUR COLOR TRIANGLES placed so that the red/green triangle pair and the yellow/blue triangle pair are perpendicular to each other.

when they are asked to categorize colors in proportions of four hues and the achromatic colors. Certainly, if one is handed a single color and asked to specify it in these terms, the numerical proportions reported may differ markedly from another person's estimates. The end points of the system, the "purest" whites, black, reds, yellows, and so on, are conceptual and personal in the last analysis. But in relational terms (i.e., in comparing colors) there will be a high degree of agreement. Of two reds that differ appreciably from each other, two observers will almost always agree about their relative blueness or yellowness, or darkness or lightness (i.e., blackness, grayness, or whiteness). The same is true for yellows. There are many examples in the visual literature of consistent data obtained from different observers when colors are named in a way that permits numerical comparisons as well as when they are scaled in proportional terms.

At the beginning of this chapter it was noted that the first thing we must establish is the number and variety of colors that we experience. It must be first because, to explain how the nervous system (the visual aspect) interacts with light rays and certain object properties (such as reflectance) to generate color experiences, it is critical that we know how many basic colors we need to account for. Furthermore, the systematization of the perceived color world in terms of six colors and their various combinations has important implications for our ideas about the way the eye and the nervous system work to make it possible for us to see colors. We saw earlier that our classification of the perceived world of colors tells us that no red-green or green-red colors are ever seen, nor are there any yellow-blue or blue-yellow colors. That red and green are never seen simultaneously in a color and that the same is true of yellow and blue are perceptual facts that are saying something very important to us about the way our visual system is organized. The remaining chapters will tell us about this organization and the way it works in both normal and color-deficient individuals.

In Chapter 2 we will discuss a few general principles of neural organization and visual experience.

Background Readings

Bartleson, C. J. 1976. Brown. *Color Research and Application 1*: 181–191.

Halsey, R. M., and Chapanis, A. 1951. Number of absolutely identifiable spectral hues. *J. Opt. Soc. Amer. 41*: 1057–1058.

Hering, E. 1920. *Grundzüge der Lehre vom Lichtsinn.* Springer-Verlag, Berlin. (*Outlines of a Theory of the Light Sense*). Translated by L. M. Hurvich and D. Jameson. Harvard University Press, Cambridge, Mass., (1964).

Hurvich, L. M. 1969. Hering and the scientific establishment. *Amer. Psychol. 24*: 497–514.

Indow, T., and Stevens, S. S. 1966. Scaling of saturation and hue. *Percept. Psychophys. 1*: 253–271.

Ishak, I. G. H., Bouma, H., and van Bussell, H. J. J. 1970. Subjective estimates of colour attributes for surface colours. *Vision Res. 10*: 489–500.

Jameson, D., and Hurvich, L. M. 1959. Perceived color and its dependence on focal, surrounding, and preceding stimulus variables. *J. Opt. Soc. Amer. 49*: 890–898.

Judd, D. B., and Kelly, K. L. 1939. Method of designating colors. *J. Res. Natl. Bur. Stand. 23*: 355–385.

Kelly, K. L., and Judd, D. B. 1964. *Color. Universal Language and Dictionary of Names.* Natl. Bur. Stand. (U.S.) Spec. Publ. 440. Washington, D.C.

Kornerup, A., and Wanscher, J. H. 1967. *Methuen Handbook of Colour,* 2nd ed. Methuen, London.

Marks, L. E. 1974. *Sensory Processes.* Academic Press, New York.

Nickerson, D., and Newhall, S. M. 1943. A psychological color solid. *J. Opt. Soc. Amer. 33*: 419–422.

Teller, D. Y., Peeples, D. R., and Sekel, M. 1978. Discrimination of chromatic from white light by two-month old human infants. *Vision Res. 18*: 41–48.

Webster's New International Dictionary of the English Language. 1958. 2nd ed. unabridged. Merriam, Springfield, Mass.

Further Readings

Berlin, B., and Kay, P. 1969. *Basic Color Terms: Their Universality and Evolution.* University of California Press, Berkeley, Calif.

Boynton, R. M. 1975. Color, Hue and Wavelength. In E. C. Carterette and M. P. Friedman (eds.), *Handbook of Perception,* Vol. 5, *Seeing,* Chap. 9, pp. 301–347. Academic Press, New York.

Evans, R. M. 1974. *The Perception of Color.* Wiley, New York.

Troland, L. T. 1929. *The Principles of Psychophysiology,* Vol. 1, *The Problems of Psychology; and Perception.* D. Van Nostrand, New York.

2
Color Experience and the Nervous System

AS we have seen, colors can be systematically arranged in a way that simplifies their description. But what is color? Is color something that inheres in objects themselves? Are green leaves green because of their physical-chemical makeup? The mere fact that the green leaves of summer turn into brilliant reds and yellows and into many different kinds of browns as their chemical constitution changes with the coming of fall would seem to argue strongly that this is so. Yet the leaf that looks bluish green in outdoor daylight appears somewhat yellowish green when carefully looked at in incandescent room illumination. Could it be that the light that falls on the leaf constitutes its color? There are still other possibilities: light, as we shall see, is absorbed by photochemicals in the receptors at the back of the eye and different kinds of light are absorbed to different degrees. Is color therefore a photochemical event that occurs in the receptor layer of the eye? Or is it perhaps a neural brain-excitation process? Or a psychical event?

Color is all these things and we shall study most of them later in greater detail. But for the moment the main point to be made is that our perception of color ordinarily derives from an interaction between physical light rays and the visual system of the living organism. Both are involved in seeing objects and perceiving color.

To see colors, we ordinarily need an external light stimulus. To see the colors in any of the figures in this book or, for that matter, even to see the book or any other objects in the room, we need room illumination, from artificial or natural light radiation. If we turn out the lights (assuming the room to be windowless and the illumination artificial), the room is plunged into darkness and we fail to discriminate the colors in the figures, the book, or the objects. Essentially the same thing happens when the sun gradually sets and we are somewhere where there are no street lights—at the seashore, for example, or in the country on a moonless night. The variety of colors seen in daylight gradually disappear and we are left in a grayish darkness.

Even in the presence of light energy we can, of course, by simply closing our eyes, achieve the same result—a grayish darkness. Whether it is a child or an adult playing "blind," a hand or handkerchief over closed eyes blots out the normal world of colors. Occasionally, there are reports that some individuals can distinguish colors by touch or feel, but for most of us the fingertips, the back of the hands, or closed eyelids do not respond to light rays in such a way as to generate colored experiences. (The reddish light seen with closed eyelids in bright sunlight is simply the light that passes through the thin skin of the lids and is scattered on the retina.*)

Light energy is necessary to see colors, but an intact visual system (see Chapter 10) is also necessary and, in a certain sense, is even more important. Without an intact visual system, no amount of light energy will avail. But oddly enough, if the visual system is intact, we can "see" by using stimuli other than light. Such stimuli are called "inadequate," but a better word would be "inappropriate."

Pressure is one of the inappropriate stimuli that can arouse visual experiences. If we close our eyes and press very gently the side of one lid or rub the eye, we often see diffuse white patterns and sometimes pinpoint scintillating light patterns. These are called pressure-evoked PHOSPHENES. If a person is accidentally hit in the eye by a tennis ball or on the head in a bodily contact sport, or has the misfortune to fall or be hit on the head, he or she will see a colorful array of "stars." "I kept seeing these big red stars," said a reporter for a Detroit underground newspaper in recounting his attack by two of the Guru Majaraji Ji's zealots several years ago.

Magnetic field stimulation and electric currents of appropriate voltages flowing through the head also produce colored phosphenes. In the case of electrical stimulation, a change in the direction of current flow between electrodes placed on the skull surface will change the color that is seen from, say, a yellow to a blue. In more recent experiments electrodes have been implanted in the brains of blind persons. Pulsing electrical stimulation is used to generate visual effects, usually diffuse "flickering lights." The ultimate hope, apparently, is that by rigging television cameras to the electrodes, the external light patterns picked up by the television cameras will be converted directly into patterns of electrical stimulation, and blind people will be able to "see" the world about them. This goal is in the very distant future; many scientists are dubious that it will ever be realized and question the wisdom of electrical brain stimulation.

X-rays are known to produce visual effects and recently, astronauts in space have reported seeing flashes in the absence of light. This has

* The anatomy of the eye is discussed in Chapter 10.

raised the possibility that cosmic rays also produce visual experiences (see Figure 2 in Chapter 3). Much more widely known are the effects of drugs. Mescaline has long been known to induce colored phenomena and it is now fairly common knowledge that LSD and related psychedelic drugs may produce striking visual effects during a "trip." "Fantastic pictures of extraordinary plasticity and intensive color seemed to surge toward me," wrote Albert Hofmann, the discoverer of LSD.

It may seem odd at first that what we are calling the visual system can be set into action by such a variety of forces or energies. But there is an obvious analogy that makes it seem less startling.

Consider the primer that contains percussion powder to ignite an explosive charge. Igniting an explosive charge is its basic property. There are, however, a number of ways in which the primer can be set into action. The primer can itself be ignited by friction, by applying an electrical charge to it, or it can be set off by percussion (e.g., by the tripping of a hammer that strikes the priming cap in a gun). The latter is the most common technique. But given that the primer has the property of being able to ignite an explosive charge, it is immaterial what way we choose to set it into action; any one of a different number of forces or stimuli can be applied to achieve the end result of ignition.

And so it is with the visual mechanism, if we are concerned only with generating a visual experience and not with the particular nature of that experience or with its relation to illuminated objects in the environment. It is immaterial whether the physical stimuli that "agitate" the organism are light rays, mechanical stimulation on the eyeball, magnetic fields, electrical currents sent through the head, cosmic rays, or drugs. As long as the nervous tissue that is related to the visual process is excited, we will *see*.* The specific nature of the stimulus that excites the nervous tissue responsible for the visual experiences is relatively unimportant.

This is true not only of vision but also of the other senses: taste, smell, hearing, and touch. Thus the particular physical stimulus or stimulus event that sets the taste system into action may vary, but whatever the stimulus, it will lead to a taste sensation. For example, stimulation of the tongue with electrical impulses of different frequencies will produce sweet or bitter tastes even though the taste system is more appropriately set off by chemical solutions of salts and acids. And similarly for hearing; sound vibrations of certain amplitudes are the stimuli for hearing. But electrical stimulation or a blow on the head will produce buzzing and ringing sounds. The crux of the matter is that the neural auditory system is somehow activated by the inappropriate stimulation.

* Nervous tissue includes the cells in the retina, the optic nerve, the lateral geniculate, the striate visual cortex, and beyond (see Chapter 10).

The different qualitative experiences that we associate with the different senses—the experiences of light, sound, taste, smell, and touch—arise from the activation of different sets of nerves that terminate in different places in the cortex. However excited, the optic nerve gives visual experiences; the auditory nerve, sound experiences; and so on.* It is to the activation of different neural pathways and various brain loci that we owe the difference between taste and smell, between pain and sound, and between any one of these and visual experiences.

If each sense modality is related to a different neural system, it is logical to expect that within a given sense, say vision, each and every color experience will be associated with the activation of a different neural element. But if our color experiences run into the thousands upon thousands, or possibly even millions, we place an almost impossible burden on the optic nerve and the rest of the visual system. This was appreciated at least as long ago as the eighteenth century, and most color theorists have looked for a few, usually three, basic receptor-neural systems whose combined activation might produce the multiplicity of perceived visual effects. With the development of electrophysiology, which makes it possible to record directly neural-electrical events in nerve and brain tissue, it has been hoped that the NEURAL CODE for sensory qualities can be "cracked" or "broken." By neural code I mean the system by which neural events register, represent, and translate into sensory qualities and their magnitudes (see Chapter 12). By establishing precise correlations between perceived events and neural events, we would be able to specify the neural code. We would know, for example, that each time such and such a given neural event occurred, we experienced, say, "redness"; and similarly for the other qualities. Each hue quality would "go with" a specifiable neural excitation or neural organization, since perceptions or psychological qualities are thought to be in some way directly related to particular physiological or neural events. If every sensory event is based on a neural event, there is a direct correspondence between sensory and neural events. For every equality and similarity in sensory events, there is an equality and similarity in the physiological events, and vice versa. Furthermore, for every difference in the sensory events, there is a difference in the nature of the physiological events, and vice versa.

If assumptions of this sort are valid, then even in the complete absence of independent data from electrophysiological studies, we have some good clues to the general nature of the neural code for color.

If our visual experiences are ordered and schematized as outlined in Chapter 1, so that they can all be characterized in terms of only red,

* Sensory physiologists and sensory psychologists have long referred to this idea as the "doctrine of specific nerve energies."

yellow, green, blue, black, and white, the visual neural apparatus must be similarly constituted. Somewhere in the nervous system there must be a number of different processes or mechanisms (or substances) that relate to the whites, blacks, yellows, blues, reds, and greens of our perceived color world. When certain of these processes are set in motion—if the neural activity or patterning is of a sort that is specific to "yellow and white"—the experienced color will be a yellow-white; if the physiological excitation is of a "green-black" nature, the experienced color will be a blackish-green; if it is "yellow-green-black" nervous activity, we will experience an olive color; if the activity is of the "red-yellow-black" type, the color experience that correlates directly with it is a brown, and so on. How these NEURAL EVENTS are transformed into varieties of conscious awareness, or how conscious awareness might influence neural events, are very different issues and remain pretty much a mystery.

Once we accept the idea that there is a direct correspondence between sensory and neural events and that variations in the central neural mechanisms correspond to variations in our color experiences, it follows that our color perceptions can be regarded as a direct readout of what goes on in the nervous system. This enables us to go beyond the simple statement that there must be six differently coded chemical and electrical neural events that correspond to the six unitary colors.

A variety of perceptual facts—the mutual exclusiveness of certain colors, successive contrast effects (afterimages), simultaneous contrast phenomena, the peripheral color blindness of persons with normal foveal* color vision, and congenital color deficiencies—lead to the conclusion that the six unitary colors are organized as three paired antagonistic systems: red/green, yellow/blue, and white/black. The implications for the way neural response activity is organized are obvious. Let us examine these phenomena in turn.

In the discussion of the hue circle, and again at the end of Chapter 1, we noted that there are no red-green colors. We see red-yellows and red-blues, green-yellows and green-blues, but no red-greens. Nor do we ever see any color that is describable as a yellow-blue. We see yellow-reds and yellow-greens, blue-reds and blue-greens, but not yellow-blues. Red and green cannot be seen in the same place at the same time. The same is true of yellow and blue; both cannot be seen in the same place at the same time. Red and green are mutually exclusive; so are yellow and blue. In some basic way the members of each pair are opposite or antagonistic.

These OPPONENT-PROCESS aspects of the red/green, yellow/blue, and black/white colors become even more obvious if we consider the successive

* Center of eye used for fixation (see Chapter 10).

contrast effects, usually called AFTERIMAGES. Look first at the fixation point on the top left in the center of the white square in Plate 2-1. Now turn the eyes to the yellow area on the right and keep the eyes fixed on the small black fixation dot for 15 to 20 seconds. At the end of the count look back at the center of the white area. What color do you see now? The portion of the visual field that was previously excited by the yellow area now looks bluish compared to the remainder of the field. Now stare at the green square of the figure for 20 seconds or so. Note the color you see when you shift your gaze to the "white" field on the left. A slight variation of this procedure is sometimes even more striking. Take a 2-inch square of colored paper and place it at the top of a sheet of white writing or typewriter paper. Fixate the center of the piece of paper for 20 seconds or so and then, keeping the eyes fixed in position, flip the colored paper aside. (If the colored paper is prepared with a slightly raised corner, it will make this movement easier to execute.) In its place we see the opposite color of the opponent pair. (Repeat these demonstrations using one eye for viewing the colored stimuli and then alternately shut and open each eye when looking at the "white" background.) Colored papers that are red give green afterimages, greens give reds, yellows give blues, blues give yellows, white gives black, and black, white. Colored papers that appear of binary hue, say, reddish yellow, give greenish-blue afterimages; and so on. In general, the hue aftereffects can be summarized by referring to the hue circle. The seen afterimage usually lies about 180 degrees from the hue of the initially inspected stimulus on the opposite side of the hue circle. However, the situation is somewhat more complex than this because the kind of light used for the inspection stimulus and for the projection surface, as well as the adapted state of the observer, are all factors that affect the appearance of the afterimage (see Chapters 14 and 15).

These successive contrast effects express the antagonistic nature of the three color pairs, red/green, yellow/blue, and white/black, in the most direct fashion. Staring at any one of these colors evokes upon cessation the opposite member of the pair. If we stare first at a binary hue, we find upon cessation its binary opponent color.

The opponent nature of the color pairs (i.e., the reciprocal antagonism between the members of each of these three color pairs) is also seen when they are placed in juxtaposition to each other or when any one of them is placed next to, or surrounding, a gray stimulus. These are the phenomena of simultaneous color contrast, illustrated in Plate 2-2. The two gray strips in this figure are physically identical; they have the same reflectance (see Chapter 3 for a discussion of reflectance). If we fixate the center of the gray strip on the left, we note that it has a reddish appearance. After shutting our eyes for a few moments and returning our gaze to the center of the gray strip on the right, we note that it looks slightly yellowish. The effect can be increased appreciably if we first place a piece of thin tissue or tracing paper over the entire field.

There are many ways to produce simultaneous contrast effects (see Chapter 13) and a slight variant of the illustration in Plate 2-2 enables us to check the effects of many colored fields. A narrow strip of gray paper about ¼ inch in width and about 3 or 4 inches long with a tiny black fixation dot in its center is held above a sheet of white writing paper. (A paper clip can be used to hold the gray strip.) Then with the eyes fixed firmly on the fixation dot a sheet of colored paper is introduced behind the gray strip of paper. The gray strip takes on a hue opposite in appearance to each of the different colored papers used: greenish if the background paper is red, reddish if the background paper is green; yellowish for a blue background, blue for a yellowish background.

These facts—perceptual exclusiveness, successive and simultaneous contrast—make a convincing case for an opponent, mutual exclusiveness between members of the pairs red/green, yellow/blue, and white/black. The facts of color zones and color deficiencies also bear on the paired linkages between red/green, yellow/blue, and white/black.

For a simple demonstration, paste a small orange chip on a sheet of gray paper. Shut the left eye and look directly at this chip with the right eye. If you keep your head fixed and slowly move your fixation toward the right, a point will be reached where the somewhat blurred-looking test chip no longer looks orange but, rather, yellowish. If, with your head still, you continue to move your fixation even more to the right, the chip may become grayish in appearance. Since knowledge of the way the chip looks to start with interferes with making an unbiased judgment, a better way to do this experiment would be to select a naive person to report on what he sees. For example, ask the observer to close his left eye and to fixate with the right eye a small target point straight ahead. Then on the gray background hold the same yellowish-red chip (whose appearance is unknown to the observer) at eye level but way out to the observer's right, and ask him to state the appearance of the chip. The first reports, if the object is out far enough in the periphery, will be that the chip is grayish (or chance guesses). As the test chip is moved slowly toward the observer's fixation point he will report it to be yellow and finally orange as the central fixation point is approached. (It will pass for a moment through the observer's "blind spot"; see Chapter 10.) It is important to remember that this change in reported appearance takes place even though precisely the same test object of precisely the same wavelength distribution (see Chapter 4) is stimulating the eye.

If a bluish-green chip were used instead of an orange one, the first reports would probably be dark gray and then blue and finally blue-green as the chip is moved in and the center of the eye is finally stimulated. Again the light reflected from the stimulus object remains unchanged; only the locus of stimulation on the retina has changed.

Precisely controlled experiments of this sort can be carried out with careful specification of the colored targets, their sizes, the illumination level, the rate of target movement, the number of meridians or axes along which the test is made, and so on. Instruments especially designed for this kind of work are called VISUAL PERIMETERS and are used in clinical eye testing, since the "visual field" determinations play an important role in diagnosing various eye diseases.

The results of studies carried out on persons with normal vision show that the visual field can be divided into zones. In the most central portion of the eye, as shown in Figure 1, all the colors are seen: reds, greens, yellows, blues, whites, and blacks. As we move in either direction toward the sides, the eye loses its sensitivity to red and green hues; test targets reported to be reddish yellow and reddish blue in the center at average illuminations are now reported to look yellow or blue, respectively. The same is true of objects that are reported to be greenish yellow or greenish blue in the central portion of the eye. They start to lose their green quality as we move outward. With still further movement toward the periphery we reach an area where the stimuli that were seen as colored in the center are now reported to be white, gray, colorless, dark gray, and so on. Hues are no longer seen. (If the light energy, or target sizes, are increased, the zone limits will, of course, change.)

This experiment makes it clear that a particular physical stimulus does not always produce the same color experience. It also makes very clear the pairwise linkage between the hues that we have already noticed. When we reach an intermediate retinal zone where red hues of given strength (saturation) or vividness are missing, greens of similar strength are also lacking. Furthermore, at the extreme periphery, where yellows are no longer seen, neither are there any blue perceptions. Relative to the central region, the extreme periphery of the normal eye can therefore be said to be totally color deficient or totally color blind. In relative terms we can say that the intermediate zone of the normal eye is red/green-deficient or color blind, for we do continue to see yellows and blues in this intermediate region.

Perceptual data of this sort make it obvious that different parts of the retina and the organization of the neural tracts associated with them must differ from place to place. Otherwise, there would be no explanation for the different visual experiences produced by identical stimuli that are

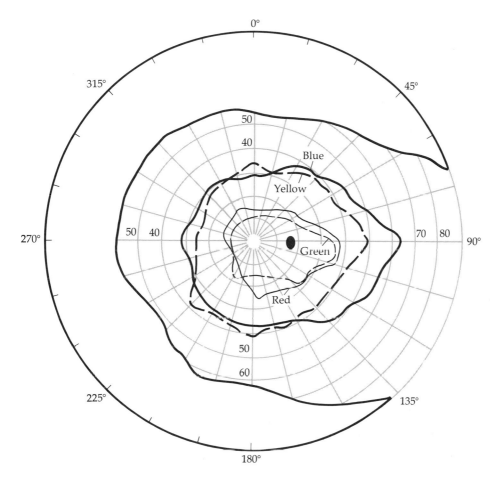

1 CHART OF THE RETINAL COLOR FIELDS. The limits of the visual field of the right eye are shown for a small blue, yellow, red, or green uniform spot of light of a moderate light level. Note that the blue and yellow "zones" have approximately the same size and shape and extend beyond the red and green "zones," which also have approximately the same size and shape.

simply imaged on different parts of the eye. There is, moreover, a paired loss of red/green and yellow/blue function.*

Additional support for the linkage of the reds and greens and yellows and blues as paired systems comes from what we know about the color vision of color-deficient individuals. These defects may be congenital or they may be acquired and related to diseases and toxins.

---

* Failure to equalize the colors for saturation will, of course, not reveal the paired losses. It is necessary to use equally saturated colors in these experiments.

Some individuals appear not to perceive red and green hues even when they are fixating centrally with the fovea. Since they see only yellows, blues, blacks, and whites and confuse what we discriminate easily as yellow-reds from yellow-greens or as reddish blues from greenish blues, they are called red/green deficient, red/green blind, or red/green confusers (see Chapter 17).

Plate 2-3 shows a reproduction of a painting by Georges Braque. We can deduce that to certain red/green blind individuals the grays and blacks would continue to look gray and black but the reds would have the hue of the yellow shown in the 3 o'clock position in Plate 1-2. Had Braque used a green like the one shown at about the 5 o'clock position in Plate 1-2 instead of yellowish-reds for the birds, the greens would look to these red/green blind individuals like the yellow at 3 o'clock. Since the poster paints and the illumination are the same for all observers and yet the perceived colors differ for various individuals, we must assume that something about the eye, its structure and workings, is responsible for the differences seen. Note again that red and green are paired. The individual who fails to make these color discriminations does not fail to see reds alone, or greens alone. He fails to see reds and greens. What he does see are yellows and blues, and blacks and whites.

It will come as no surprise at this point to learn that there is still another type of color deficiency, one in which there are confusions between yellows and blues. They occur less frequently than the red/green deficiencies and such individuals distinguish only red, green, black, and white. We have already noted that red/green confusions occur in the peripheral region of the normal eye. The rarer abnormal condition of yellow/blue confusion also occurs in normal vision with very tiny areas of stimulation, but it occurs in the very center of the eye as well as in the peripheral regions.

Comparable to the extreme periphery of normal eyes are individuals who see no hues whatsoever—the only colors they see are blacks, grays, and whites. Their world, it is often said, is like a black-and-white television screen. Even the picture on a color television screen appears to such people to be exclusively black and white (see Chapter 18).*

How can we be so confident about what color deficients see when it is known that their use of color words is erratic and often unreliable? Because in addition to inferring the color perceptions of color-blind persons from color confusions and color-matching behavior, we have two other good sources for understanding their color perceptions. One comes

---

* Still another type of color deficiency is known. It is called "anomalous trichromatic vision" and will be discussed at length in Chapter 16.

from those rare individuals whose color blindness is limited to one eye. Since they are normal in one eye and "know" all the colors and their appropriate names, these people are able to report accurately what colors they see with the defective eye. The other reliable source is the group of individuals whose color-vision deficiencies are acquired. Since their deficiencies may develop after many years of normal vision, such individuals have good memory standards against which to make statements about their present perceptions.

The various perceptual phenomena have been cited to provide us with some important but rather general notions about the way the color-vision mechanism is organized. If no green is seen simultaneously where there is a red, it implies that there is some sort of exclusion of one neural process by the other in that region of the nervous system where the events critical for the perception of color are occurring. There is a similar opponent process for yellow/blue and for white/black. In each instance we have a pairwise neural linkage of an opponent sort.

A precise account of the color-vision mechanisms, however, requires that we provide a rigorous underpinning for these general notions if we are to "explain" how color vision comes about. To do this we must first undertake an analysis of the adequate stimulus to vision and color vision— light energy—and relate it in turn to our varied color experiences. We turn first to a consideration of the physical stimulus, light energy.

Background Readings

Asher, H. 1961. *Experiments in Seeing,* Chap. 9. Basic Books, New York.

Baird, J. W. 1905. *The Color Sensitivity of the Peripheral Retina.* Carnegie Institution, Washington, D.C.

Barlow, H. B., Kohn, H. I., and Walsh, E. S. 1947. Visual sensations aroused by magnetic fields. *Amer. J. Physiol. 148*: 372–375.

Boring, E. G. 1950. *A History of Experimental Psychology,* 2nd ed., Chap. 5, pp. 80–95. Appleton-Century-Crofts, New York.

Burnham, R. W., Hanes, R. M., and Bartleson, C. J. 1963. *Color: A Guide to Basic Facts and Concepts.* Wiley, New York.

Dimmick, F. L. 1948. Color. In E. G. Boring, H. S. Langfeld, and H. P. Weld (eds.), *Foundations of Psychology,* Chap. 12, pp. 269–296. Wiley, New York.

Dobelle, W. H., Mladejovsky, M. G., and Girvin, J. P. 1974. Artificial vision for the blind: Electrical stimulation of visual cortex offers hope for a functional prosthesis. *Science 183*: 440–443.

Duke-Elder, S. (ed.). 1968. *System of Ophthalmology,* Vol. 4, *The Physiology of the Eye and Vision,* Chap. 10, pp. 465–468. Mosby, St. Louis, Mo.

Fernberger, S. W. 1931. Further observations on peyote intoxication. *J. Abn. Soc. Psychol. 26*: 367–378.

Hering, E. 1878. *Zur Lehre vom Lichtsinne,* Part 6. Gerolds Sohn, Vienna.

Hering, E. 1920. *Grundzüge der Lehre vom Lichtsinn.* Springer-Verlag, Berlin. (*Outlines of a Theory of the Light Sense.* Translated by L. M. Hurvich and D. Jameson, Harvard University Press, Cambridge, Mass., 1964.)

Hofmann, A. 1959. Psychotomimetic drugs: Chemical and pharmacological aspects. *Acta Physiol. Pharmacol. Neerl. 8*: 240–258.

Hurvich, L. M., and Jameson, D. 1970. In D. A. Hamburger and K. H. Pribram (eds.), *Perception and Its Disorders,* Vol. 48, Chap. 2, pp. 12–25. Williams & Wilkins, Baltimore, Md.

Hurvich, L. M. and Jameson, D. 1974. Opponent processes as a model of neural organization. *Amer. Psychol. 29*: 88–102.

Kravkov, S. V., and Galochkina, L. P. 1947. Effect of a constant current on vision. *J. Opt. Soc. Amer. 37*: 181–186.

McNulty, P. J., Pease, V. P., and Bond, V. P. 1978. Visual phenomena induced by relativistic carbon ions with and without Cerenkov radiation. *Science 201*: 341–343.

Moreland, J. D. 1974. Peripheral Colour Vision. In D. Jameson and L. M. Hurvich (eds.), *Handbook of Sensory Physiology,* Vol. 7/4, *Visual Psychophysics,* Chap. 20, pp. 517–536. Springer-Verlag, Berlin.

Pinsky, L. S., Osborne, W. Z., Hoffman, R. A., and Bailey, J. V. 1975. Light flashes observed by astronauts on Skylab 4, *Science 188*: 928–930.

Schober, H. 1964. Die Direktwahrnehmung von Röntgenstrahlen durch den menschlichen Gesichtssinn (The direct perception of X-rays in human vision). *Vision Res. 4*: 251–269.

Uttal, W. R. 1973. *The Psychobiology of Sensory Coding.* Harper & Row, New York.

Further Readings

Békésy, G. v. 1968. Problems relating psychological and electrophysiological observations in sensory perception. *Perspect. Biol. Med. 11,* 179–194.

Bullock, T. H. 1967. Introduction: Signals and Neuronal Coding. In G. C. Quarton, T. Melneschuk, and F. O. Schmitt (eds.), *The Neurosciences: A Study Program,* pp. 347–352. The Rockefeller University Press, New York.

Hubbard, J. I. 1975. *The Biological Basis of Mental Activity.* Addison-Wesley, Reading, Mass.

Hurvich, L. M. 1966. The Indispensibility of a Bimodal Black-White Color Vision Process. In *Internationale Farbtagung Luzern 1966,* Vol. 1, pp. 167–172. Musterschmidt-Verlag, Göttingen.

Mountcastle, V. B. 1967. The Problem of Sensing and the Neural Coding of Sensory Events. In G. C. Quarton, T. Melneschuk, and F. O. Schmitt (eds.), *The Neurosciences: A Study Program,* pp. 393–408. The Rockefeller University Press, New York.

Troland, L. T. 1921. The enigma of color vision. *Amer. J. Physiol. Opt. 2*: 23–48.

Uttal, W. R. 1967. Evoked brain potentials: Signs or codes. *Perspect. Biol. Med. 10*: 627–639.

3
The Stimulus:
Spectral Radiation

COLOR, as we have seen in Chapter 2, can be experienced by pressing on our eyeballs, by passing electric currents through the head, by taking drugs, or by having our heads jarred by blows. These forms of stimulation are, of course, inappropriate for vision, and although the phenomena emphasize the role of the nervous system in light and color perception, they are of interest mainly to the visual scientist. Ordinarily, we see objects and colors only when our eyes are open and light enters them. Light derives from the sun and from a variety of artificial sources such as candles, oil lamps, and luminescent and incandescent lamps. In this chapter we examine physical light radiation in greater detail.

One thing is clear: we do not have to know anything about light radiation in order to see, because most people are, in fact, totally ignorant about its physical properties. Most people have no need to go beyond the use of descriptive words and color names to talk about the visual environment and their interaction with it. Most people are not even concerned with knowing that their world of color experiences can be organized in the meaningful and coherent fashion described in Chapter 1.

The same sort of situation prevails as far as our other senses are concerned. In our everyday lives we have no need to know the "physics" of the stimulating situation. We hear ourselves and others talk, we hear all sorts of sounds and noises, we listen to music. If our neighbor's stereo plays on interminably into the night and is excessively loud, we do not have to know anything about the physics of sound production or the measurement of sound energy in technical terms to ask the neighbor (or landlord) to turn the volume down. We do not have to know anything about gaseous molecules, their dispersion in the air, and issues of osmotic pressure to think the young woman in the theater lobby is wearing a pleasant, fragrant, "exciting" perfume, or to find the same perfume oppressive and "heavy" in the close quarters of a small elevator. We do not have to know that acids are measured in terms of a chemical quantity referred to as pH to know that the salad dressing we are confronted with is too vinegary or too sour. We do not have to be trained in the physics of measuring force or pressure to know that we are not going to be able to stand the dentist's drill for another instant. That such knowledge about the physical and chemical aspects of stimulation of the senses is not critical for our everyday lives is clear from the fact that such knowledge is had by only a tiny fraction of the population, primarily scientists, chiefly sensory psychologists and physiologists.

Whatever the sense modality—hearing, taste, smell, or vision—and however ignorant of physics we are, we are responding in all instances to physical stimulation in the form of energy and energy changes. The scientist interested in these matters wants to establish the critical properties of these energy changes and their relations to the nature and qualities of the experiential event, that is, to the sounds, the tastes, the smells, and the colors. What he wants to know is how the physical energies are transformed (transduced) by the various sense organs to excite the nervous system and what particular nervous system changes correlate with which perceptual events.

The physical stimulus that initiates the visual process is LIGHT. Light is a small part of the totality of electromagnetic energy; it is a form of energy (particles of matter called photons) that is radiated or emitted from a source (the sun, for example) as an electromagnetic vibration (Figure 1).

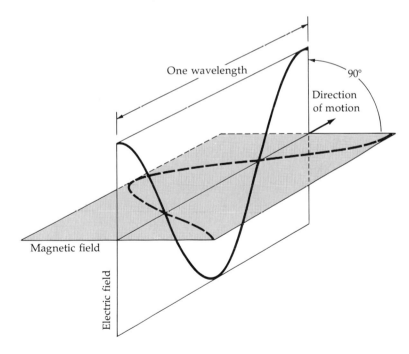

1 ELECTROMAGNETIC STRUCTURE OF LIGHT WAVES. The electric and magnetic fields of the sinusoidal electromagnetic wave are perpendicular to each other and to the direction of the wave motion.

The ELECTROMAGNETIC SPECTRUM ranges from cosmic rays through electrical power waves, and this complete spectrum is shown in diagrammatic form in Figure 2. As we see, the difference among the various rays—cosmic rays, gamma rays, X-rays, radio waves, and so on—is their vibration frequency. Different vibration frequencies occur naturally, but scientists and engineers have found ways to generate and precisely control electromagnetic energy. They have also devised instruments and detectors that are sensitive to these specific vibration frequencies. We need only note radar and its use of microwaves, and television and its use of ultra and very high frequencies from the electromagnetic spectrum, to make this point.

The human organism is affected by electromagnetic energy that comes from different parts of the frequency spectrum and, unless care is exercised, these effects may sometimes be harmful. We often respond to electrical currents as tingling shock, sometimes as painful shock, and on a rare occasion someone reacts to them as a lethal shock; microwaves emitted by radar ovens are now recognized as potentially hazardous; X-rays in overdosage amounts are ultimately lethal since they destroy tissue; ultraviolet radiation gives us our summer tans—as well as our painful sunburns; and infrared rays generate warmth and heat as well as pain. Imaged on the retina these can, in large amounts, "cook" it. Ultraviolet rays can also damage the cornea and lens of the eye and produce cataracts (see Chapter 10). Sitting between these potentially damaging vibration frequencies are the electromagnetic vibrations between about 4.3×10^{14} and 7.5×10^{14} cycles per second* (or hertz, abbreviated Hz)—the LIGHT RAYS, to which the normal eye reacts with a color response (see Chapter 4). If we occlude or stop these rays or close our eyes to exclude them, we do not see objects in the external world.

Light radiation of all vibration frequencies travels in waves in all media—air, gas, water. Figure 3 shows an oscillating wave of low frequency and one of high frequency. The peak-to-peak (or trough-to-trough) distance in each instance represents a WAVELENGTH. For the high-frequency wave the wavelength is relatively shorter than in the low-frequency case. In fact, frequency is reciprocally related to wavelength ($\lambda = c/\nu$)† and in Figure 2 we see on the bottom horizontal line that the different types of radiation can be given in wavelength values just as we give them in frequency terms on the top horizontal line. Because it is easier to measure wavelength than to measure frequency, light radiation is more commonly given in wavelength measures. Corresponding to the frequency range 4.3×10^{14} to 7.5×10^{14} Hz, the visual spectrum varies in wavelength

* 430,000,000,000,000 to 750,000,000,000,000 Hz!

† λ = wavelength, ν = frequency, and c = light velocity (about 3×10^8 meters/sec).

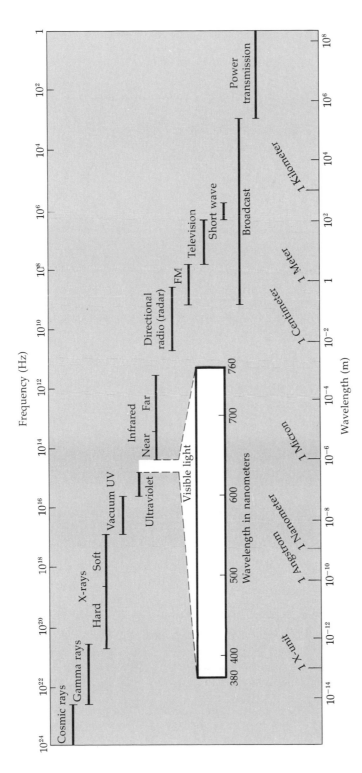

2 THE RADIANT ENERGY (ELECTROMAGNETIC) SPECTRUM.

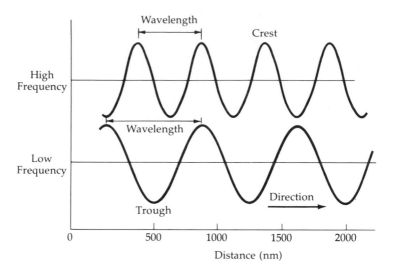

3 OSCILLATING LIGHT WAVES of two different wavelengths (and hence different frequencies). The amplitude of the wave motion (peak to baseline) is the same in the two instances.

between 400 and 700 nanometers. The nanometer is abbreviated nm and is equal to 1 millimicron, which is one billionth of a meter.

Electromagnetic radiation has ENERGY—the capacity to do work—and all the frequencies (or wavelengths) of light emit their energy in the form of large numbers of small particles called PHOTONS or LIGHT QUANTA. From physics we learn that the energy of a particle or quantum of light is directly related to the vibration frequency. Thus a short-wavelength light quantum (say at 400 nm) has more energy than a quantum at a higher wavelength (say at 700 nm), since the short-wave quantum is of higher frequency. But what is important to us at the moment is not the energy of a single light quantum but the fact that every source of light, whether it be the sun, a candle, an incandescent lamp, a mercury arc lamp, a fluorescent bulb, or a laser beam, usually radiates huge numbers of light quanta simultaneously at the different spectral frequencies or wavelengths.

The energy charges of the various light sources are released by the jumping about of electrons within the atomic structures. In different sources of light this occurs because of temperature increases (incandescent lights) or because of electric discharges in gases (neon or krypton glow tubes).* In the former instances the light quanta are emitted at all wave-

* Light emission not caused by heat is called luminescence. There are several varieties. Light produced by physiological processes in the firefly is called bioluminescence, that produced by chemical reactions, chemiluminescence. Other forms of luminescence are fluorescence, phosphorescence, and electroluminescence.

lengths and the number released in any one wavelength region depends on the temperature of the heated object. In the case of electric lights, as we know, the heated object is usually a tungsten wire.

The amount of energy released at different wavelengths in the spectrum can be measured wavelength by wavelength with a physical instrument called a SPECTRORADIOMETER (Figure 4a). These instruments, which are commercially available, depend on a discovery by Newton (see Chapter

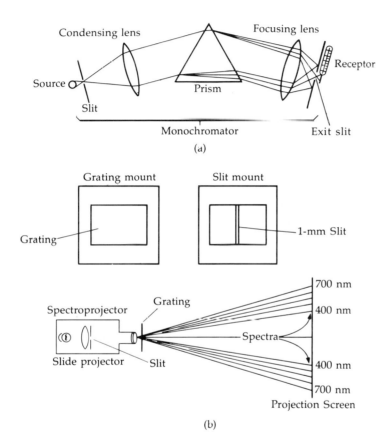

(a)

(b)

4 TWO INSTRUMENTS. (a) Spectroradiometer for the measurement of light energy. The light from the source that is to be measured enters the instrument through a narrow slit. A lens directs the light from the illuminated slit to the prism, which disperses the light. The different wavelengths of light imaged in the plane of the exit slit are measured with various detectors, some of which record the temperature of the emission as shown in the figure. (b) Spectroprojector to demonstrate the formation of a spectrum. The inexpensive grating (obtainable from Edmund Scientific Co., Barrington, N.J.) is mounted in a 2-inch by 2-inch Kodak Ready-Mount. A narrow (1 mm or so) slit made with black tape or cardboard is also mounted in a Ready-Mount. The slide with the slit is mounted vertically in the projector and the grating is held in front of the lens. In addition to a white image of the slit, two spectra are projected, as indicated.

4). If sunlight or light from any incandescent source is passed through a prism, the rays of light of different wavelengths are dispersed or spread out (Figure 4a). A narrow exit slit in the instrument permits only a narrow band of wavelengths to pass through to a sensitive detector that measures their energy. For the purposes of this type of measurement, the appearance of the different rays is irrelevant. Instruments of this sort are now highly automated and it is possible to get numerical printouts of the relative spectral energies of a light source in a few minutes. Our concern here is with those radiations that make up visible light, but it should also be noted that many instruments of similar type, used to measure energies in other regions of the electromagnetic spectrum, are now widely used in science, industry, and medicine, particularly to identify chemical solutions.

Most modern instruments use ruled diffraction gratings rather than prisms to disperse the light from a broad-band source into a spectrum. The gratings either have alternate bars and openings where as many as 30,000 fine grooves per inch are ruled on a reflecting metal surface or—more often now—are of the replica type, in which the grating has ridges instead of grooves, and a transparent surface. An inexpensive "spectro-projector" of a grating type can be set up quickly and inexpensively by anyone who has a slide projector available (Figure 4b).

Each light source has a characteristic energy versus wavelength distribution. Figure 5 contains the relative energy distributions of both sunlight and typical daylight illumination. Wavelength is represented along the x-axis (abscissa) and at each wavelength the spectral energy of the

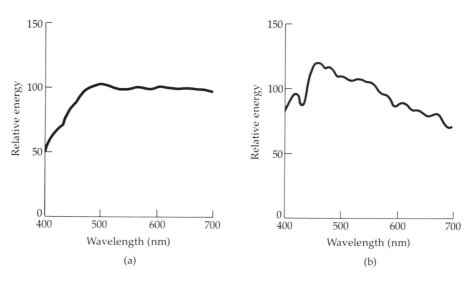

5 RELATIVE SPECTRAL ENERGY DISTRIBUTION of (a) sunlight and (b) typical daylight illumination.

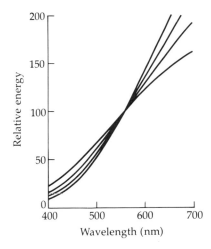

6　RELATIVE SPECTRAL ENERGY DIS-
TRIBUTION of several standard tungsten
incandescent lamps.

light as measured with a spectroradiometer is plotted on the y-axis (ordinate). These energy distributions are relative ones. The energy output
at 560 nm is taken to be 100 percent and all other energy measures are
shown relative to this value. Figure 6 shows the spectral-energy distribution curves in the visible region of the spectrum of several standard
tungsten incandescent lamps of the sort commonly used in home lighting.

The standard sources of radiation used by physicists are heated BLACK
BODIES. The spectral distribution of the radiation they emit depends only
on the temperature to which the black bodies are heated. These temperatures are stated in the Kelvin (°K) or absolute temperature scale (0°K =

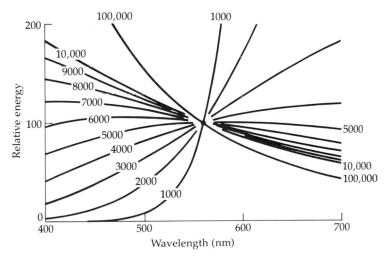

7　RELATIVE SPECTRAL ENERGY DISTRIBUTION of a black body heated to different
temperatures.

−273.16° Celsius). Figure 7 shows the relative energy distributions of a black body heated to different temperatures.

A convenient way of specifying spectral-energy distributions of light sources is to assign them the temperatures of black bodies that have similar distribution curves. These assigned temperature values (which often have no relation to the actual temperatures of the light source) are called COR-RELATED COLOR TEMPERATURES. The curves shown for the incandescent lamps in Figure 6 have color temperatures that vary from about 2700°K to 3000°K. The curves of four standardized light sources and their color temperatures are shown in Figure 8.

In the case of luminescent light sources, gaseous vapors are excited by an electrical charge and the spectrum is not continuous as it is in the case of the hot sun and heated tungsten filaments, where energy is radiated at all wavelengths. Energy is emitted only at certain discrete wavelengths by luminescent light sources, depending on the atoms in the given gaseous material. This is true of the emission spectrum of the mercury arc lamp and of the xenon arc now widely used in visual experimentation. Other gases have different LINE SPECTRA. The spectral energy distributions of fluorescent lamps vary with the types of chemical powders used in their construction. These lamps have continuous spectral-energy distributions on which line spectra are imposed. Several examples are given in Figure 9.

New sources of light are being developed and one of these, the electroluminescent crystal (gallium phosphide) has the relative energy

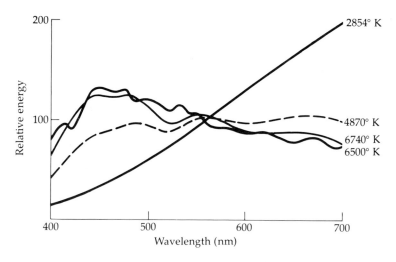

8 RELATIVE SPECTRAL ENERGY DISTRIBUTIONS of four standardized light sources and their color temperatures.

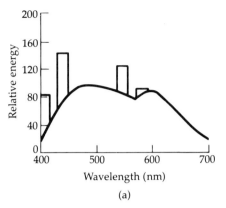

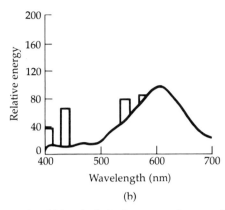

9 RELATIVE SPECTRAL ENERGY DISTRIBUTION of (a) a daylight fluorescent lamp and (b) a white fluorescent lamp.

distribution shown in Figure 10a. The outputs of the helium neon laser and ruby laser beams are shown in Figure 10b and c.

The light quanta or packets of light energy travel in straight lines when emitted by various sources and they travel at the very high speed of 186,282 miles/sec in air. (This is about 3×10^8 meters/sec.) When the

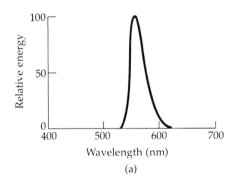

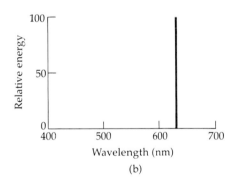

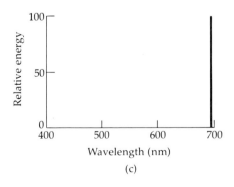

10 RELATIVE SPECTRAL ENERGY DISTRIBUTION of (a) a gallium phosphide electroluminescent crystal, (b) a helium neon laser, and (c) a ruby laser.

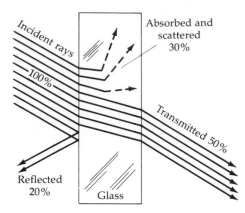

11 LIGHT QUANTA reflected, absorbed, and transmitted when a beam of light strikes a transparent piece of glass.

light quanta strike the surface of an object in their path, a variety of outcomes are possible. The light quanta may be reflected or bounced back from the surface, they may be absorbed by the surface, or they may be transmitted by it, depending on the surface's nature (Figure 11). When the light quanta pass through water, glass, or the various eye media, they are slowed down somewhat.

It is fairly easy with a spectroradiometer to determine the way transparent objects—a piece of clear glass, a piece of colored glass, or a gelatin filter*—transmit (and absorb) spectral light. In Figure 4 the spectroradiometer is in position to measure the output of a light source. Once we have measured the output, we can insert a piece of colored glass or a

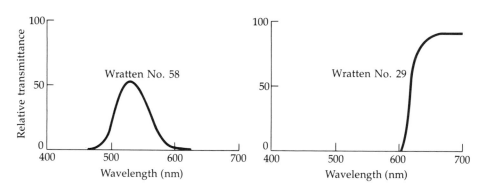

12 SPECTRAL TRANSMISSION CURVES for two broad-band Wratten filters.

* Gelatin filters are made by impregnating a gelatin base with various organic dyes and then sandwiching it between two pieces of clear glass or clear plastic. Colored filters are in common use in traffic signals, tail lights, directional signals, railroad signals, hazard indicators, advertising signs, plastic materials, and theatrical lighting.

LIGHT FILTER, as it is commonly called, in the path of the light rays on their way to the sensitive detector. A different record will be made by the spectroradiometer and it will vary with the nature of the filter material. The filter, depending on its composition, will be found to absorb light energies to different degrees at the various wavelengths.

By comparing the energy measures originally made without the filter in the light beam with the second set of energy measurements made with the filter in position between the light beam and the detector, we can learn the relative transmission of the filter material in question. Figure 12 shows the wavelength-distribution curves of the light transmitted by two different filters, Wratten filters nos. 58 and 29.* Narrow-passband filters are now widely used, particularly filters based on the property of optical interference between different wavelengths of light in thin films. They provide very restricted wavelength passbands at relatively low cost.

Spectroradiometers are used in essentially the same way to measure the spectral-light-ray distributions that are reflected or bounced off object surfaces. As in the light-transmission case, a comparison of energy measurements reflected throughout the spectrum with the energy distribution of the original light source measured directly gives us the surface reflectance. Figure 13 shows the reflectance curves of some typical natural objects. When the reflectance curve is flat, as in the case of fresh snow, the surface is said to be NONSELECTIVE. For laboratory work a smoked magnesium oxide surface is the standard. Its reflectance is set, by convention, as equal to 1.0 at all wavelengths. Spectral reflectance curves measured against this standard (since it is nonselective it does not affect the

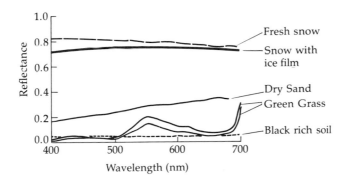

13 SPECTRAL REFLECTANCE CURVES of some typical natural objects.

* The transmission curves for several hundred commercially available filters have been summarized in graphic form in the book *Color Science* (Wyszecki and Stiles, 1967).

light distribution of the source) are available not only for natural objects but for many kinds of building materials, paints, metals, and so on.

Spectral transmittances, absorbances, and reflectances are physical properties of objects and do not change under normal conditions that do not alter their physical properties. But the physical properties alone tell us little about what we see.

How do lights of different wavelengths appear to an observer? How do broad-band spectral-energy distributions of different light sources look to an observer, and how do filters with different relative transmissions in the visible spectrum affect their appearance? What about objects with different relative reflectances? These questions are addressed in the next chapter.

Background Readings

Evans, R. M. 1948. *An Introduction to Color,* Chaps. 2–4, pp. 7–57. Wiley, New York.

Judd, D. B. 1952. *Color in Business, Science, and Industry.* Wiley, New York.

Kaufman, J. E. (ed.). 1972. *IES Lighting Handbook,* 5th ed. Illuminating Engineering Society, New York.

Kodak Filters for Scientific and Technical Uses, Publ. B-3. Eastman Kodak Company, Rochester, N.Y.

Rainwater, C. 1971. *Light and Color.* Golden Press, New York.

Riggs, L. A. Light as a Stimulus for Vision. In C. H. Graham (ed.), *Vision and Visual Perception,* Chap. 1, pp. 1–28. Wiley, New York.

Wyszecki, G., and Stiles, W. S. 1967. *Color Science.* Wiley, New York.

Yule, J. A. C. 1967. *Principles of Color Reproduction.* Wiley, New York.

Further Readings

Bragg, W. H. 1959. *The Universe of Light.* Dover, New York.

Henderson, S. T. 1970. *Daylight and Its Spectrum.* American Elsevier, New York.

Minnaert, M. 1954. *The Nature of Light and Color in the Open Air.* Dover, New York.

4

Spectral Radiation and Color Appearance

I SAAC NEWTON first established that when sunlight coming through a hole in a shutter is passed through a prism in a darkened room, the sunlight is "decomposed" into its constituent rays and forms a spectrum of colors spread out on a surface that reflects all rays uniformly (Figure 1). The prism, which is a wedge of glass, slows down the light quanta as they pass through it and bends the different wavelengths of light, all of which are contained in the white-appearing beam of sunlight, to different degrees; the series of different hues that are seen are associated with the different wavelengths of light. Newton described this as follows: ". . . the Spectrum . . . did . . . appear tinged with this Series of Colours, violet, indigo, blue, green, yellow, orange, red, together with all their intermediate Degrees in a continual succession perpetually varying. So that there appeared as many Degrees of Colours, as there were sorts of Rays differing in Refrangibility." Such a spectrum is shown in Plate 4-1.

A similar spectrum is produced with the single-prism monochromator shown in Figure 4a in Chapter 3. To obtain the precise relation between wavelength and the colors of the spectrum, we can use the setup shown there. Instead of placing a physical detector at the exit slit of the instrument, the observer places his eye at this position. He will see a uniformly illuminated circular disc filled with colored light. By rotating the prism in the horizontal plane, the spectrum is displaced laterally by known amounts and the exit slit intercepts and isolates the different spectral regions in turn. When the wavelengths are between 400 and 470 nm, the field is reported to look violet for an average light level; around 475 nm it is seen as mostly blue (Figure 2a). Blue-greens are seen at wavelengths between 480 and 490 nm; 500 to 510 nm looks mostly green (Figure 2b), then green-yellows and yellow-greens are seen all the way to about 580 nm, which looks yellow (Figure 2c). From 580 nm or so to 640 nm the hues are increasingly red (orange) and from there to 700 nm (Figure 2d), the end of the spectrum, the hues are redder still.*

* The hues associated with wavelengths are also dependent on the energy of the stimulus. The relations described here are for an average light level. The way appearance changes with changes in light energy is described more fully in Chapter 6.

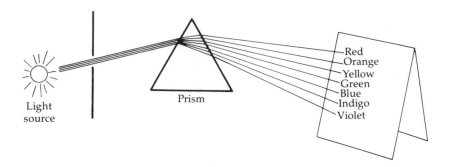

1 NEWTON'S EXPERIMENT to show the dispersion of light to form a spectrum.

A summary diagram is shown in Figure 2e. The three light sources shown in Figure 10 in Chapter 3, with radiation emitted in the narrow-band regions, 540 to 610 nm, 633 nm, and 694 nm, look greenish yellow, reddish yellow, and yellowish red, respectively, to the normal eye.

If a second set of prisms and lenses is used to reverse and recombine the dispersed radiation and the recombined rays are all imaged on the same part of the retina (whether viewed directly or after being reflected

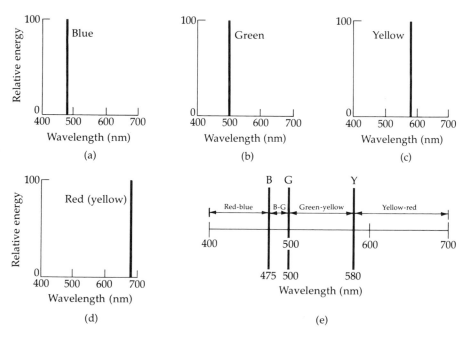

2 SPECTRAL LINES (a) 475 nm, blue; (b) 500 nm, green; (c) 580 nm, yellow; and (d) 700 nm, red (yellow) and their hues at an average light level for one observer. (e) Average locations of unique hues in the spectrum.

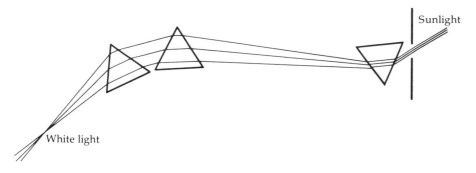

Sunlight

White light

3 RECOMBINATION OF SPECTRUM COLORS reverses the dispersion to produce a uniform white appearing light.

from a nonselective surface), we are, as Newton showed, right back to where we started. When all the rays of the dispersed spectrum are recombined and mixed simultaneously to fall on the same retinal area, we see a patch of uniform "white" light (Figure 3). For any set of viewing conditions we can state precisely the relations between wavelength and perceived color: individual wavelengths produce the hues we have listed and with all the wavelengths present, and intermixed on the retina as is the case with the broad-band sunlight stimulus (See Figure 5a in Chapter 3), we see a yellowish white. As Newton pointed out, the visible light rays themselves are not colored. They are no more colored than are any of the other rays in the electromagnetic spectrum. We perceive color only when the different rays fall on the retina to be transformed into some kind of neural signal.

The color appearances of other broad-band spectral-light distributions that are imaged on the retina depend on the form of the distribution curve. The incandescent-type light distributions (see Figure 6 in Chapter 3) all look slightly reddish yellow.* (The state of adaptation of the eye, as well as light level and stimulus size, affect color appearance. We assume here that the adaptation level is what we are calling "neutral." We will discuss this more fully in Chapter 15 and will see there why, if the eyes are adapted to the incandescent light, which is the more likely situation, the appearance of the light will be white and not reddish yellow.) The light from a mercury arc, which combines a continuous distribution of energy with a series of discrete high-intensity energy emissions at certain wavelengths—404.7, 435.8, 491.6, 546.1, 578.0, and 693.8—looks yellowish green. A simple setup like the one shown in Figure 4 can be used to compare directly the colors of different illuminants.

* See the preceding footnote.

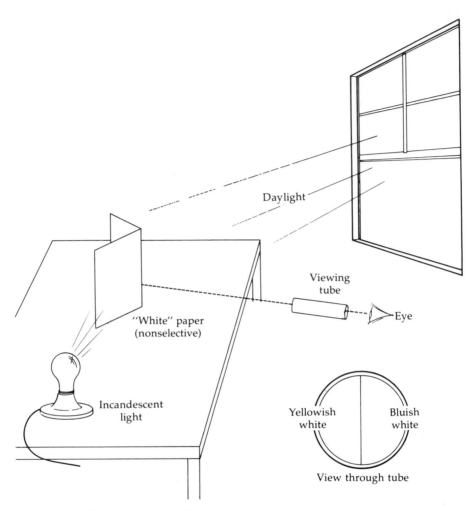

4 COLOR APPEARANCE of different light sources can be compared with this simple arrangement. A piece of "white" paper is folded as shown and set on a table. The two surfaces are illuminated by the lights to be compared. The observer looking through a small tube (made by rolling up a sheet of paper) directs it so that he looks at the edge of the wedge on the table. The inset shows the field of view. If daylight strikes one side of the reflecting surface and incandescent light the other, an astonishing difference is seen. One "white" light is bluish, the other "white" light looks yellowish.

If the stimulus-light distribution described by the curve of Figure 5a is focused on the eye, we are likely to say that it looks blue. If the distribution is like that in Figure 5b, we probably will agree that it looks green. If it is that of Figure 5c, we are likely to report that it looks yellow, and if it is that of Figure 5d, red (yellowish). And finally, if the distribution is that of Figure 5e, where only short and long wavelengths of light stimulate the eye, the report will be "purple."

Light distributions that are relatively broad and that are weighted preponderately with energy in the long wavelengths are seen as reds and yellows, those that are weighted in the medium wavelengths as greens, and those that are weighted in the shorter wavelengths as blues. Thus the hues of these broad-band stimuli tend to approximate the hues produced by narrow bands of spectral light.

The colors evoked by narrow-band spectral stimuli and the broad-band distributions differ. Broad-band stimuli are all seen as less saturated

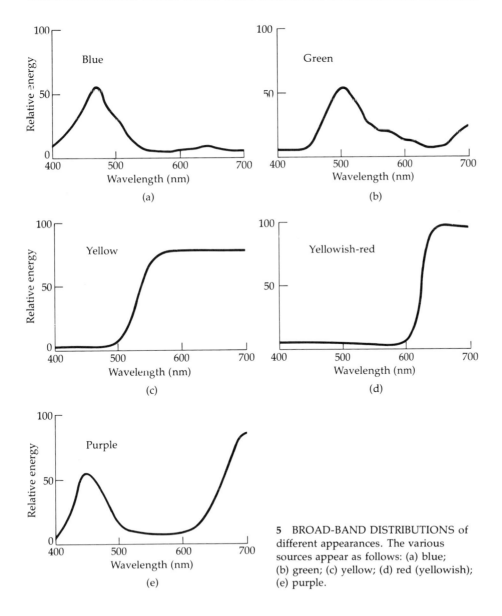

5 BROAD-BAND DISTRIBUTIONS of different appearances. The various sources appear as follows: (a) blue; (b) green; (c) yellow; (d) red (yellowish); (e) purple.

than spectral-line stimuli and in Chapter 7 we will see why this is so. Nevertheless, the hues generated by the stimuli shown in Figure 2a and Figure 5a are very similar: both are blue. The same is true of the stimuli shown in Figure 2b and Figure 5b: both are green. The hue generated by the spectral stimulus shown in Figure 2c is yellow, as is that generated by the broad-band stimulus shown in Figure 5c. The stimuli represented in Figure 2d and Figure 5d are both seen as reds.

The set of stimuli of varying band widths shown in Figure 6 also illustrates that different physical light distributions can produce the same hue. Although not precisely of the same color, the three different stimuli all appear close to unique yellow if the light level is the same for all. Figure 7 shows a pair of relatively broad-band light distributions that differ, but now both are weighted maximally at about the same spectral locus, 535 nm. The perceived color becomes somewhat more desaturated (paler) as the stimulus distribution becomes broader (less peaked) but, for equal light levels, the hue is the same in both instances: a yellow-green.

We shall see in Chapter 9 that it is also possible to produce exactly the same color (same hue, same saturation, same brightness) with physically different light distributions, but here we restrict the discussion to the hue dimension.

The distribution curves have just been described as if they were emissions from different types of light sources being viewed directly by the observer (or being completely and nonselectively reflected toward the

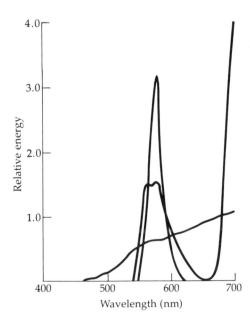

6 THREE DIFFERENT PHYSICAL LIGHT DISTRIBUTIONS that look yellow when seen at the same light level.

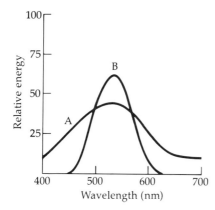

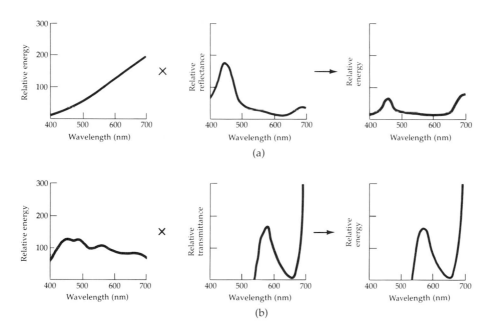

7 TWO DIFFERENT PHYSICAL LIGHT DISTRIBUTIONS that look yellow-green when seen at the same light level.

observer's eye). It would be virtually impossible, however, to find light sources with spectral distributions of the sort shown in Figures 5, 6 and 7. The distributions shown there are more likely to be representations of light-energy distributions that reach the eye after they have been reflected from the surfaces of objects with different reflectance properties, or following transmission through selective filters, or both (Figures 8 and 9).

8 RELATIVE LIGHT-ENERGY DISTRIBUTION that impinges on the eye is shown in the right-hand side of the figure. It is the wavelength X wavelength product of the object's spectral reflectance multiplied by the light distribution. (a) Light source is incandescent and (b) light source is illuminant C (daylight).

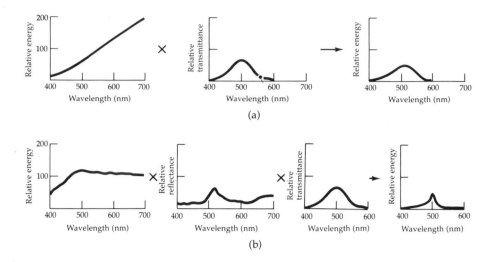

9 RELATIVE LIGHT-ENERGY DISTRIBUTION that impinges on the eye is shown in the right-hand side of the figure. (a) The light source is an incandescent light, used in conjunction with a filter that peaks at about 510 nm. (b) The light source is sunlight, which first falls on a surface whose reflectance is given in the second graph. This reflected light then passes through the same filter specified in (a).

Knowledge of an object's reflectance or a filter's transmittance does not itself permit us to infer their appearance. The relative transmittances and reflectances of filters and objects are physical properties, and the wavelengths of light transmitted or reflected by them will vary depending on the light sources with which they are used. Therefore, until we know the energy distribution of the light source used together with them, and thus the light-energy distribution that finally impinges on the eye, we cannot generalize about the probable appearance of the filter or object in question.

To make this point clearer, consider an admittedly extreme example. Suppose that we have a filter with the transmittance shown in Figure 10a. Suppose that the light source is the gallium phosphide electroluminescent crystal mentioned in Chapter 3, with the relative energy distribution shown in Figure 10b, and that in a darkened room the filter is placed between the light source and the observer's eye. What light rays will be imaged on the eye? Very few wavelengths with any appreciable energy. The filter transmits minimally in the midwave region of the spectrum, where the light source emits most of its energy, and above the midspectral region, where the filter begins to pass light, there is almost no source energy (Figure 10c). We have already noted that in normal vision, unless radiant energy impinges on the retina of the eye, we do not see object colors, and a nonselective surface would reflect a trivial amount of light under the circumstances described.

An object with a broad-band reflectance curve like that of snow (see Figure 13 in Chapter 3) may look "white" in incandescent light or in daylight. Can this object of fixed uniform reflectance throughout the spectrum be made to look blue? or green? or orange? How?

In any event, whether the distribution of light energy reaches the eye directly from a light source, or after it is reflected from the surfaces of objects, or after passing through a colored filter, light distributions that *differ* physically one from the other are capable of producing the same hues. What is the meaning of this?

In the previous discussion of the mechanisms of color vision (Chapter 2), the existence of three paired opponent-process systems—red/green, yellow/blue, and white/black—was emphasized. If we experience a green color, it can only mean that the neurophysiological process that is responsible for the green perception has been activated by the light stimulation. Since the two different light distributions shown in Figure 7 are seen as having the same yellow-green hue, we have to assume that the same basic neurophysiological processes (something correlated with "greenness" and "yellowness") are excited in the same way by the different stimulus distributions. Any other light distribution that evokes the same green and yellow experiences must also be assumed to excite both the "green" and "yellow" processes in the same way.

But have we not run into a serious paradox? If it is true that the perceived hues are correlated with the activation of the various types of neural processes, the hues we see as we move stepwise through the spectrum must be interpreted as the result of the activation of the different relevant neural processes. Thus we would list the processes activated by the various wavelengths of light as follows: 440 nm, blue and red proc-

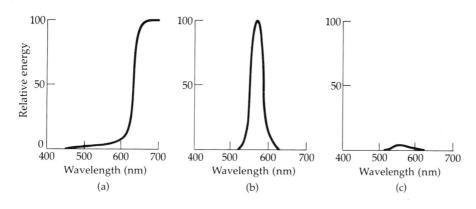

10 RELATIVE LIGHT-ENERGY DISTRIBUTION. When a filter with the relative spectral transmittance shown in (a) is used with a gallium phosphide crystal light source as (b) the relative light energy that reaches the eye is (c).

esses; 475 nm, blue; 495 nm, blue and green; 500 nm, green; 540 nm, yellow and green: 580 nm, yellow; 670 nm, red and yellow; and so on. If the 580-nm stimulus evokes the yellow process and looks yellow, how is it that the light distributions of Figure 6—distributions that include wavelengths that individually evoke the green and red processes in addition to the yellow one—evoke only a yellow sensation? How is it that neither of the other hues is seen?

The same issue is raised in the simpler examples presented in Figures 11 through 13. If a yellow experience is produced by the narrow-band stimulus centered at 580 nm in Figure 11, how does it happen that precisely the same yellow hue can be evoked by a mixture on the retina of two stimuli whose wavelengths are 540 nm and 670 nm? This is particularly puzzling since we have seen in the wavelength and sensation correlation series (above) that 540 nm alone evokes a greenish-yellow hue and 670 nm alone produces a yellowish-red hue.

If a green experience is produced by a narrow wavelength band centered on 500 nm (Figure 12), how does it come about that a hue that matches it precisely can be produced by a mixture on the retina of wavelengths 490 nm (which looks blue-green) and 540 nm (which looks yellow-green)? If a blue experience is produced by a wavelength band at 475 nm (Figure 13), how does it come about that we can evoke the identical blue hue with a mixture of 440 nm and 490 nm—two stimuli that looked at individually appear to be reddish blue and greenish blue?

Precisely the same sort of paradox seems inherent in the facts of Newton's experiments cited above. Individual wavelengths from different spectral regions evoke very different hue experiences. Yet as we saw, when all these wavelengths simultaneously impinge on the same retinal area, the visual experience is hueless and we see what are called "whites."

Newton also demonstrated that many pairs of wavelengths when

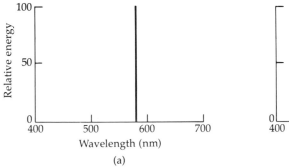 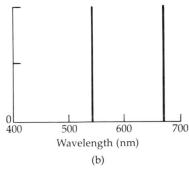

11 YELLOW IS SEEN when either (a) a 580-nm spectral stimulus or (b) a combination of 540-nm and 670-nm stimuli is used.

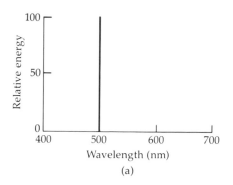
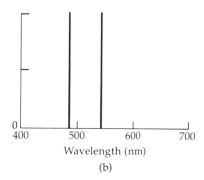

12 GREEN IS SEEN when either (a) a 500-nm spectral stimulus or (b) a combination of 490-nm and 540-nm stimuli is used.

*appropriately** mixed generate precisely the same white appearance as does the recombination of all wavelengths. If long-wavelength 670-nm light that looks yellowish red is superimposed on a screen that is reflecting 490-nm radiation and looks bluish green, the region where both stimuli overlap and that is imaged on the same part of the retina looks white (Plate 4-2a). If 580 nm, a yellow, is intermixed as in Plate 4-2b with a 475-nm blue-appearing area (in appropriate amounts), we again see a white-appearing area where the two-colored fields overlap in our visual field.

Pairs of wavelengths that behave this way, that is, pairs of wavelengths that generate a white experience when intermixed, are known as COMPLEMENTARY WAVELENGTHS.† The 670, 490 nm the 580, 475 nm

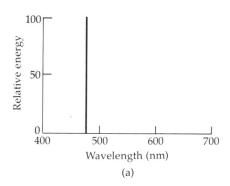
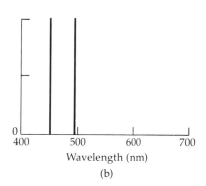

13 BLUE IS SEEN when either (a) a 475-nm spectral stimulus or (b) a combination of 440-nm and 490-nm stimuli is used.

* Discussed further in Chapter 6.
† In an alternative procedure, a "standard white" comparison light may be used. The relative energies of the selected stimulus pairs are varied until a match is made to the standard (see Chapters 8 and 9).

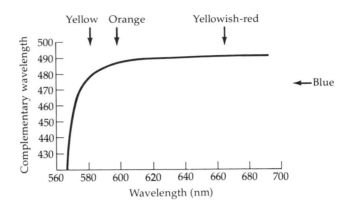

14 WAVELENGTHS OF COMPLEMENTARY HUES, lights that when mixed in appropriate ratio produce a white-appearing stimulus.

pairs are only two of an indefinite number that behave in this way. Figure 14 is a summary graph of experiments in which complementary stimuli were determined. It permits us to read off from it those pairs of stimuli that are complementary. If we take some one wavelength on the ordinate on the left, for example 465 nm, and project a horizontal line from it to intersect the curve to the right, then drop a perpendicular to the wavelength baseline, we obtain the value of the wavelength that is complementary to 465 nm, in this case 573 nm. Other pairs of stimuli that are represented in this graph are 440 and 568 nm, 490 and 640 nm, and so on.

Figure 14 is a graphical restatement of the empirical facts. It simply summarizes which wavelength pairs are complementary. It provides very little insight, however, into why the particular pairs of wavelengths represented in the curve (a rectangular hyperbola) evoke a white (or gray) experience.

To obtain this insight and gain a clear understanding of why different physical light stimuli can and often do evoke the same perceived colors requires that we take a closer look at the three paired neural functions, particularly the way they are affected by different wavelengths of light.

Background Readings

Boynton, R. M. 1975. Color, Hue, and Wavelength. In E. C. Carterette and M. P. Friedman (eds.), *Handbook of Perception*, Vol. 5, *Seeing*, Chap. 9, pp. 301–347. Academic Press, New York.

Hering, E. 1920. *Grundzüge der Lehre vom Lichtsinn.* Springer-Verlag, Berlin. (Outlines of a Theory of the Light Sense, Chap. 10. Translated by L.

M. Hurvich and D. Jameson. Harvard University Press, Cambridge, Mass., 1964.)

Hurvich, L. M., and Jameson, D. 1951. The binocular fusion of yellow in relation to color theories. *Science 114*: 199–202.

Newton, I. 1730. *Opticks,* 4th ed. London. (Reprinted 1952, Dover, New York.)

Purdy, D. McL. 1931. Spectral hue as a function of intensity. *Amer. J. Psychol. 43*: 541–559.

Troland, L. T. 1930. *The Principles of Psychophysiology,* Vol. 2, *Sensation,* pp. 140–156. D. Van Nostrand, New York.

5
Chromatic and Achromatic Response Functions

I T should be clear by now that object color is not physical light radiation itself, that it is not something that inheres in objects, having to do exclusively with the chemical makeup of the object, nor is it only the nervous excitation that occurs in the eye and brain of an observer. In our perception of object color all these elements are involved: there is light radiation, which is selectively absorbed and reflected in different ways by objects that differ physically and chemically; when the light rays coming from objects are imaged on the retina, they set off a complex series of neural events that are associated with the visual experience of color.

As we noted in Chapter 2, color perceptions are assumed to provide a direct readout of the net effect of particular activities in the nervous system. Thus the appearance of the spectrum at different wavelength regions is related to the activation of the different relevant neural processes. For example, if the region at 440 nm looks bluish red, we assume that two different neural processes, one related to blueness, the other related to redness, have been activated; if at 550 nm the spectrum looks yellowish green, two still different neural processes, one related to yellowness, the other related to greenness, have been activated; and so on. Furthermore, since the different regions of the spectrum do not appear equally bright or white, we must also look for different degrees of excitation of whiteness-related neural processes by different spectral lights, in addition to the excitation of the various neural processes associated with the hues. For example, the 440-nm region has very little perceived whiteness along with the bluish-red appearance, as compared with the 550-nm region, which is seen as a very whitish yellow-green. Thus according to our assumptions, the "white/black" neural process is excited less by a 440-nm spectral light than it is by a 550-nm spectral light.

But a 410-nm spectral stimulus, like the 440-nm one, looks bluish red; and a 530-nm spectral stimulus, like the 550-nm stimulus, looks yellowish green. Thus the 410-nm and 530-nm stimuli must also excite the same neural processes as do the 440-nm and 550-nm stimuli, respectively. In fact, very many spectral stimuli excite the same neural processes. For example, all wavelengths from 400 nm to about 470 nm appear to be made up of blues and reds. If we look closely, however, the perceived proportions of blue and red differ; the 400-nm stimulus is redder than the 470-nm stimulus.

Is there some way we can *measure* how much of each "hue response" is present at each spectral position? Precisely how much blueness and redness does a unit of stimulus energy (measured at the front of the eye, the corneal surface; see Chapter 10) produce at 400 nm? at 420 nm? at 470 nm? How much greenness and yellowness at 520 nm? at 540 nm? at 560 nm? The same question can be raised about whiteness (and blackness).* Can we measure how much whiteness the various wavelengths in the visible spectrum produce? More generally stated, can we measure the relative magnitudes of the chromatic and achromatic processes throughout the spectrum? The answer is yes, and the experimental procedure used to measure the chromatic processes is based on a fact we called attention to in Chapter 2: that the hue pair red/green and the hue pair yellow/blue are opponent or antagonistic. Both members of any one pair are not seen simultaneously in the same place.

If we consider a short-wavelength stimulus, say, 420 nm, we know that it is seen as having a certain amount of blueness. If we increase the amount of energy of this stimulus, the amount of blueness increases. The same is true of a different short-wavelength stimulus, say 440 nm. It, too, has a bluish appearance, and the amount of blueness increases with an increase in energy. But if we take a unit of energy of each of these two short-wavelength stimuli, we find that the amount of blueness differs. How shall we measure the amount of blueness there is in each instance? Since we know that a long-wavelength stimulus, say 580 nm, has a certain yellowness at an arbitrary energy value and that the yellowness increases as the energy increases (just as blueness does with an increase in energy), and since we know that yellowness is opposite to blueness, it is possible to intermix the 580-nm stimulus with fixed amounts of short-wavelength stimuli and, by varying the energy of the 580-nm yellow-appearing stimulus, cancel the blueness seen in the short-wavelength stimuli.

The procedure is a NULL METHOD. It might also be called a CANCELLATION (or "bucking") TECHNIQUE. The measure of a given chromatic response is obtained by determining how much of the antagonistic response is necessary to "zero" or "null" the system to an equilibrium position.

Null methods are very common in physics; the simplest example is

* Black is placed in parentheses here to indicate that there is no direct measurement of this function.

the balance scale. To determine the weight of an unknown object placed in one of the scale pans, weights of known values are added to the other scale pan until a balance or null position is reached. Once equilibrium is reached, the unknown can be precisely specified in terms of the known. The principle also finds wide application in electrical measures. To measure voltages, for example, potentiometers are used whereby the unknown voltage to be measured is evaluated by the amount of known specified voltage required to balance the current flow to zero. Similarly, with a Wheatstone bridge, resistance can be adjusted in the circuit to evaluate one of unknown value (Figure 1).

These analogies only illustrate the null principle, since physical quantities balance physical quantities. In the perceptual situation, physical quantities (wavelengths, light energies) are used and measured, but the balancing or nulling is done in the visual system, with the perceptual response serving as the meter.

Let us be more specific. I have described several times the appearance of the spectrum, in which the hues normally range from a violet (reddish blue) at one end, through blue, blue-green, green, yellow-green, yellow, reddish yellow, and slightly yellowish red at the other end (see Plate 4-1). We first restrict ourselves to the long-wavelength end of the spectrum, where we see red-yellows, yellows, and green-yellows, and set ourselves the task of measuring the amount of yellow chromatic response in this region. By means of a monochromator, which permits us to isolate narrow spectral bands, we will isolate the region centered on 510 nm and look at it through the eyepiece of a short-focus "telescope." What we see is a small field that looks roughly like the full moon on the horizon but is uniform in color; it is mainly green with a slight tinge of yellow. By means of a transparent mirror standing at 45 degrees to the beam of light coming

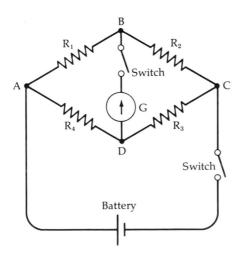

1 THE WHEATSTONE BRIDGE provides a way to measure an unknown electrical resistance. When there is no current flowing through bridge wire BD and the galvanometer registers a zero or null response, the arms of the two bridges are in balance: $R_1/R_4 = R_2/R_3$. If R_1 is an unknown resistance, R_2, R_3, and R_4 are adjusted by known amounts to balance the current to zero, and thus R_1 can be determined in accordance with the equation given.

from the first monochromator (I), we introduce and intermix with this beam the light that comes from a second monochromator (II) to the right of the observer (Figure 2; monochromator III is not used in these experiments). The wavelength drum of this second instrument is fixed in one wavelength position. It is fixed at, say, 475 nm, which appears to the observer to be a blue that is neither reddish nor greenish (i.e., what I am calling a "unique" blue). To measure the amount of yellow process produced by the 510-nm stimulus of monochromator I, the observer is asked to adjust a light-absorbing wedge that varies only the energy of the fixed-wavelength (475 nm) blue-appearing light until he reports that the yellow originally seen in the yellow-green field is canceled. If too much energy of the 475-nm stimulus is introduced, the observer will see a bluish-green field, if too little is introduced, he will see a yellowish-green one. We now record the amount of 475-nm light that is used to just balance the small amount of yellow seen in the 510-nm stimulus. When the blue just cancels the yellow, what is the appearance of the test field?

Now we replace the 510-nm stimulus of monochromator I with an equally bright 520-nm stimulus. The latter appears slightly more yellowish green than the 510-nm field did. We again intermix the 475-nm blue stimulus coming from monochromator I with the 520-nm stimulus and determine (by adjusting the energy) how much of 475 nm is now needed to cancel or "null out" the yellow in the 520-nm stimulus. It turns out that we need a little more of the 475-nm stimulus than we used for the 510-nm situation. We can proceed to make measurements of the amount of 475 nm needed to null out the yellow in 530 nm, 540 nm, 550 nm, 560 nm, 570 nm, and so on, to the end of the spectrum at 700 nm. (We could, of course, make our measurements at any wavelengths in this part of the spectrum—510 nm, 511 nm, 514 nm, 541 nm, and so on—but our interest is in the form of the spectral yellow-response curve and measurements made at equal 10-nm steps are convenient and not too widely separated to trace out the form of the curve.) Note that with the 580-nm stimulus, which evokes a whitish-yellow appearance that is neither reddish nor greenish, the intermixture with it of 475 nm (a blue) leaves as a perceptual remainder a whitish- or grayish-appearing field. Beyond 580 nm, to the end of the spectrum at 700 nm, the initial stimulus fields coming from monochromator I look reddish yellow, red-yellow, then yellowish red. When the amount of 475 nm that is needed to just balance or cancel yellow has been added at these wavelengths, the observer finds himself or herself looking at test fields that are slightly reddish in hue. For all wavelengths where the amount of yellow response is measured by canceling it with blue, the end point is a test field that is neither yellow nor blue in appearance.

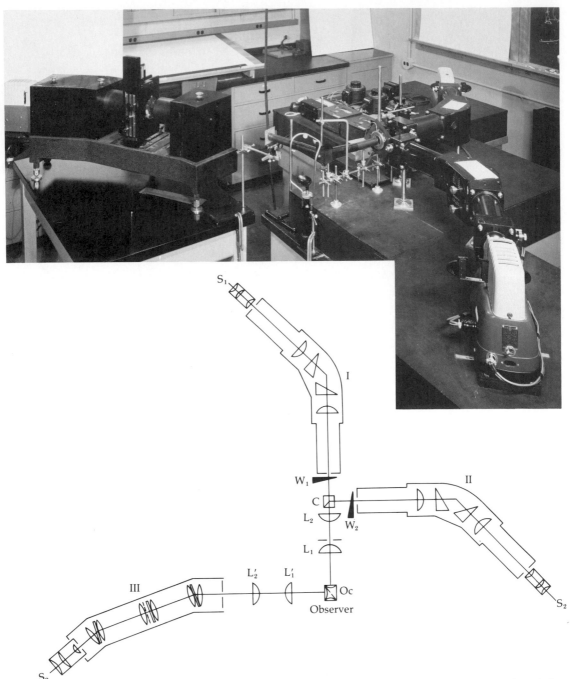

2 OPTICAL SYSTEM with three monochromators is depicted in the photograph and diagram above. Monochromators I and II mix lights in cancellation or nulling experiment; monochromator III is not used in these experiments. S = sources; W = wedges to vary light energies; L = lenses; C = mixing cube; Oc = ocular.

In Figure 3 a graphical representation is given of the amount of yellow response in the spectrum between the wavelengths 510 nm and 700 nm. The curve shown is, of course, a plot of the amount of the 475-nm stimulus required to produce the equilibrium state: the state that is neither yellow nor blue. We are simply assuming that the amount of yellow response that was canceled at each wavelength is proportional to the amount of the opponent stimulus (the blue-appearing 475-nm stimulus) necessary to cancel the yellow.

We now carry out a similar set of observations, but this time place in the viewing field wavelengths that range from 490 nm down to 400 nm. This series of stimuli is provided by monochromator I. Each stimulus is adjusted to look equally bright to the observer. They will vary in appearance from bluish-green hues to bluish-red ones.

For example, let us place a 490-nm stimulus in the field. We then add a 580-nm stimulus from monochromator II to the field. The 580-nm stimulus by itself looks uniquely yellow (i.e., it has no red or green) and we intermix it with the 490-nm bluish-green-appearing wavelength. The amount of the 580-nm light is then varied until the test field is judged to look neither blue nor yellow. What will the test field look like?

We then place a 480-nm stimulus in the field and repeat the canceling procedure, recording the amount of the 580-nm stimulus used for balancing. Then 470 nm, 460 nm, 450 nm, and so on, are used in turn. When the mixed field in each instance looks neither yellow nor blue, we have a measure of the blue chromatic response as given by the amount of the yellow-appearing 580 nm used for balancing it out. This curve looks as shown in Figure 4.

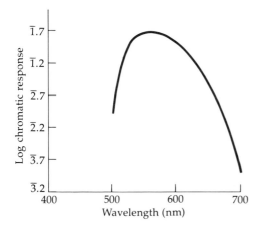

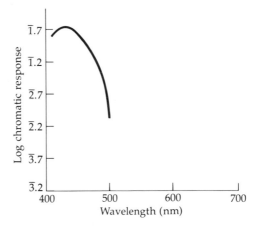

3 AMOUNT OF YELLOW RESPONSE in the spectrum between wavelengths 510 and 700 nm. Logarithmic representation.

4 AMOUNT OF BLUE RESPONSE in the spectrum between wavelengths 400 and 490 nm. Logarithmic representation.

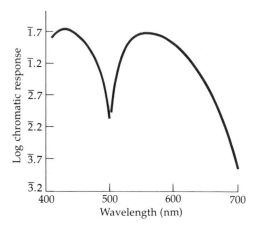

$\overline{1}.7$
$\overline{1}.2$
$\overline{2}.7$
$\overline{2}.2$
$\overline{3}.7$
$\overline{3}.2$

Log chromatic response

400   500   600   700
Wavelength (nm)

5 AMOUNTS OF YELLOW AND BLUE RESPONSES throughout the visible spectrum. Logarithmic representation.

Since both the 475-nm and 580-nm stimuli are common to each set of the chromatic functions shown in Figures 3 and 4, the separate "yellow" and "blue" curves can be combined in one graph as in Figure 5 by an appropriate adjustment of their relative heights.

The relative response values are plotted in logarithmic steps in Figures 3, 4, and 5. Logarithmic steps are geometric steps progressing as do the numbers 1, 2, 4, 8, 16, . . . , or 1, 10, 100, 1000, ... We can convert the logarithmic steps to simple arithmetic ones, as in the progression 1, 2, 3, 4, 5, 6, . . . , and we have done this in Figure 6. One of the two chromatic response curves can, at the same time, be represented as having negative values and the other one as having positive ones. The plus and minus values express the opposition between the paired response systems and the fact that when lights that would separately excite both processes are mixed, their simultaneous action is a subtractive one. Plotted in this

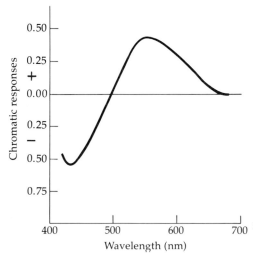

0.50
0.25
+
0.00
−
0.25
0.50
0.75

Chromatic responses

400   500   600   700
Wavelength (nm)

6 AMOUNTS OF YELLOW AND BLUE RESPONSES throughout the visible spectrum. Arithmetic representation. Yellow is arbitrarily assigned plus values and blue negative values to indicate their opposition.

way, the yellow and blue hue responses are distributed in the visual spectrum at each measured wavelength, as shown in Figure 6.

The fact that "blue" is shown here as negative is strictly arbitrary and has no particular significance. We could, if we chose, reverse the signs of the two curves and treat the yellow portion as negative and the blue as positive. The important point is that blue and yellow are opposite or antagonistic, and this is expressed by assigning negative values to one limb and positive values to the other limb of the combined curve. The nervous-system processes are in each instance real and represent some sort of electrochemical activities of the nervous system—activities, however, whose natures are opposite in their physiological properties (see Chapter 12).

The wavelengths between 500 and 700 nm are not only yellow-appearing; they look greenish yellow from about 500 to 570 nm and reddish yellow from about 590 to 700 nm. The spectrum at the short-wavelength end from 400 to about 470 nm or so looks reddish as well as blue. To measure the amount of red there is at these various wavelengths we simply use the cancellation principle already outlined. We repeat the presentation, one at a time, of individual wavelengths that look reddish blue or reddish yellow and intermix with them a green-appearing stimulus of, say, 500 nm, whose energy is varied until cancellation is achieved. Figure 7 shows how the redness response or process is distributed in the spectrum.

We proceed in similar fashion to measure the green response. For the cancellation stimulus a long-wavelength stimulus, say 700 nm, is used.*

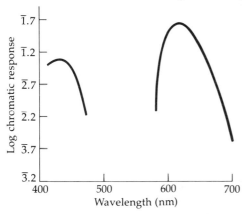

7 AMOUNT OF RED RESPONSE in the spectrum between 590 and 700 nm and between 400 and 470 nm. Logarithmic representation.

* There is a small amount of yellow in the 700-nm stimulus, but this does not affect the cancellation procedure. The observer's task is to produce a field that looks neither red nor green. The yellow associated with the 700-nm stimulus is simply part of the "remainder" perceived when red and green are balanced. It is, in fact, not necessary to use unique stimuli to obtain any of the chromatic response functions.

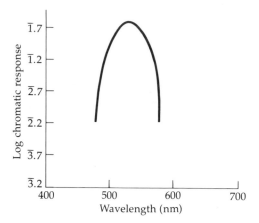

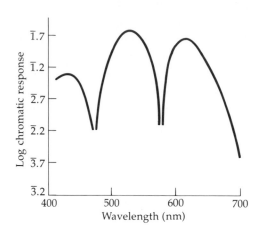

8 AMOUNT OF GREEN RESPONSE in the spectrum between 480 and 580 nm. Logarithmic representation.

9 AMOUNTS OF RED AND GREEN RESPONSES throughout the visible spectrum. Logarithmic representation.

This response function is shown in Figure 8 and the combined red/green function is shown in Figure 9. In Figure 10 the red/green function is converted to arithmetic values and red is arbitrarily labeled positive and green negative.

Let us now combine the separate graphs of Figures 6 and 10 in a

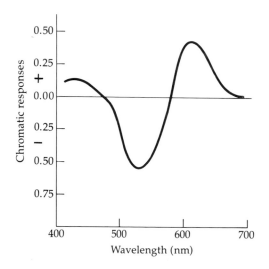

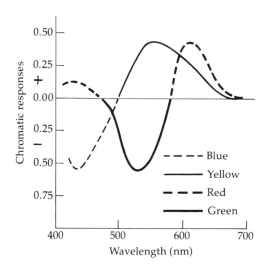

10 AMOUNTS OF RED AND GREEN RESPONSES throughout the visible spectrum. Arithmetic representation. Red is arbitrarily assigned plus values and green negative values to indicate their opposition.

11 YELLOW/BLUE AND RED/GREEN RESPONSE FUNCTIONS throughout the visible spectrum combined in a single graph. Arithmetic representation.

single graph. The two sets, the yellow/blue chromatic response function and the red/green chromatic response function, are shown in Figure 11. Their relative heights are adjusted at that wavelength where redness and yellowness are judged to be equal.

What about the achromatic aspect of the spectral stimuli? How does it vary across the spectrum? We learned in Chapter 1 that most objects are characterized as having both chromatic and achromatic aspects; in addition to their hue qualities, all objects are also seen as having some degree of whiteness, grayness, or blackness. In referring to spectral stimuli we have also noted that they can be seen to contain various degrees of whiteness. For example, when I referred to a stimulus at 580 nm, I called it a whitish yellow. It is also true that the yellowish-green and greenish-yellow mid-spectral stimuli seem relatively whitish when compared to the extreme violets (reddish blues) and yellow-reds of the two spectral extremes. In this respect, then, the spectral hues are very much like some object colors.

What about the blackness of spectral stimuli? When spectral lights or, for that matter, broad-band light distributions are seen in insolation, they look like glowing lights and contain no blackness.

The blackness response *cannot* be produced by direct light stimulation applied on a given retinal locus. Blackness responses are obtained indirectly, as it were. We could see an isolated spectral light go black if we surrounded it with very intense illumination. One way to produce a black response in a given part of the visual field is to stimulate a neighboring region with a stimulus that looks white. Another way is to stimulate the eye with the white-appearing stimulus and then remove it or block it out. In Chapter 1, in the discussion of the "brown" problem, we saw that we could produce blackness in the small center field by rotating the upper stimulus field toward the incoming light and thus increase the relative amount of light on the area surrounding the small field. Similarly, when afterimages are produced, it is the sudden cessation of "white" light stimulation that produces a black afterimage (see Chapters 2 and 14). Blackness is not evoked by the direct action of light from any particular portion of the spectrum; blackness does result indirectly from the contrast between stimuli (one of which is "white") presented side by side to different places on the retina. It also results at the same place on the retina when "white" stimulation is terminated.

The whiteness response of spectral stimuli is approximately equivalent to spectral brightness.* I have already said that we can measure the way

* Some investigators have recently resurrected the notion that brightness is not equivalent to whiteness. They reserve the term "brightness" for a response that combines whiteness plus a component from the chromatic responses. This is a complex issue that is not fully resolved. In the interests of simplicity we shall consider whiteness as equivalent to brightness.

whiteness is distributed in the spectrum, separately from the chromatic components, red/green and yellow/blue, and there are a number of ways to do this. We cannot use the null procedure to do this because, as we have just seen, there is no way of directly varying a stimulus to generate blackness. Other techniques have to be used to measure the whiteness response.

One way to obtain a measure of the whiteness distribution for the bright-adapted state of the eye is to measure the light threshold at various wavelengths throughout the spectrum, for example at every 10 nm.* A light-threshold measure is simply a measure of the amount of energy necessary at a given wavelength for the observer to *first* detect the stimulus. In the actual experiment one common procedure is to expose briefly the stimulus at a level of energy at which it is not visible and to gradually increase the light energy until the observer reports a flash of light. When the stimuli are first seen, they tend to be reported as without hue, or as achromatic (i.e., gray or white). It has therefore been assumed that when the stimulus is first seen at the threshold, the white (black) system has been tapped to the exclusion of the chromatic system. What does a "whiteness" curve measured in this way look like? The answer is given in Figure 12, where the reciprocal of the threshold energy is plotted against wavelength. This reciprocal measure is a measure of sensitivity and thus indicates that there is relatively more "whiteness" response in the midspectral region than at the spectral extremes. But more than that, the form of the curve shows precisely how "whiteness" is distributed throughout the spectrum: it is low at the spectral extremes and relatively high in the midspectral region.

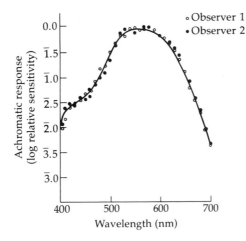

12 WHITENESS RESPONSE in the visible spectrum for two observers. Reciprocal of energy necessary to first perceive light represents the achromatic or whiteness response. This is sometimes referred to as a measure of spectral light sensitivity and is also called the luminosity function.

* We are not concerned here with the light threshold measured in a dark-adapted state, in which the rods are relatively more sensitive than the cones (see Chapter 10).

Another way in which the whiteness curve can be measured is by making what are called HETEROCHROMATIC BRIGHTNESS MATCHES. This method, which involves making brightness matches between fields that differ in hue, is not an easy one. One half of a circular test field contains a standard that looks, say, yellowish green. The other half contains one of a series of violets, blue-greens, oranges, and so on, and, as we just saw, the amount of hue varies from one wavelength to the next. Whiteness must be abstracted from these other qualities in order for the observer to make the match between the yellowish-green standard and the other stimuli. This can be done, and probably the best approach to making the abstraction is to minimize the clarity of the apparent border between the two fields.

In addition to threshold measures and heterochromatic brightness matching, other indices have been used to measure the LUMINOSITY FUNCTION, as this curve is now most frequently called. For example, measures of pupillary size, visual acuity, and flicker perception have also been used to specify this curve. The general form of the curve remains approximately the same for all criteria (Figure 13).*

The spectral luminosity function, shown in logarithms of energy, can also be plotted in arithmetic values. This curve appears in Figure 14.

If this is the way whiteness is distributed in the spectrum, we can superimpose this curve on the chromatic response curves of Figure 11. Combined in a single figure, the chromatic and achromatic (whiteness) functions then look as shown in Figure 15.

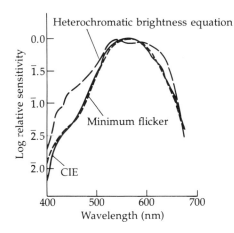

13 WHITENESS RESPONSE in the visible spectrum obtained with alternative techniques. (a) Heterochromatic brightness matches. (b) Flicker. The standardized curve labeled CIE (Commission International d'Éclairage) was obtained with yet a different method, called step-by-step brightness matching.

* If one is interested in expressing light energies in relation to the eye's sensitivity, light-energy distributions would have to be weighted by the luminosity curve. This procedure gives us stimulus intensities in photometric terms called luminance units. Unfortunately, there are many differently defined luminance units in use. Fortunately, however, they are not needed in order to understand the principles of color and color perception as developed in this book.

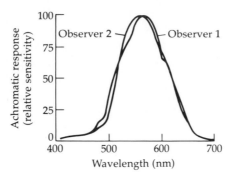

14 WHITENESS RESPONSE in the visible spectrum for two observers. Arithmetic representation.

One final point: all the measurements referred to in this chapter are made with the observer in a "neutral equilibrium state of adaptation." The observer usually sees the test fields after remaining in the dark for a short time, say 10 minutes. We shall see in our discussion of adaptation in Chapter 15 that spectral lights change their appearance when the observer is first "adapted" or exposed to various chromatic background fields. Under these conditions it becomes impossible to obtain meaningful measures of the chromatic response functions.

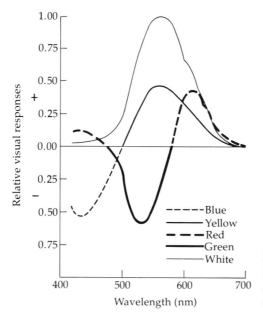

15 CHROMATIC (YELLOW/BLUE AND RED/GREEN) and achromatic responses (whiteness) throughout the visible spectrum. One observer. Arithmetic representation.

Background Readings

Donnell, M. L. 1977. Individual Red/Green and Yellow/Blue Opponent-Isocancellation Functions: Their Measurement and Prediction. Michigan Mathematical Psychology Program, Technical Report MMPP 77–9. Ann Arbor, Mich.

Hurvich, L. M., and Jameson, D. 1953. Spectral sensitivity of the fovea. I. Neutral adaptation. *J. Opt. Soc. Amer. 43*: 485–494.

Hurvich, L. M., and Jameson, D. 1954. Spectral sensitivity of the fovea. III. Heterochromatic brightness and chromatic adaptation. *J. Opt. Soc. Amer. 44*: 213–222.

Ives, H. E. 1912. Heterochromatic photometry. *Phil. Mag. 24*: 845–883.

Jameson, D. and Hurvich, L. M. 1955. Some quantitative aspects of an opponent-colors theory. I. Chromatic responses and spectral saturation. *J. Opt. Soc. Amer. 45*: 546–552.

Romeskie, M. 1978. Chromatic opponent-response functions of anomalous trichromats. *Vision Res. 18*: 1521–1532.

Sloan, L. L. 1928. The effect of intensity of light, state of adaptation of the eye, and size of photometric field on the visibility curve. *Psychol. Monogr. 38* (173).

Wagner, G., and Boynton, R. M. 1972. Comparison of four methods of heterochromatic photometry. *J. Opt. Soc. Amer. 62*: 1508–1515.

Werner, J. S., and Wooten, B. R. 1979. Opponent chromatic mechanisms: Relation to photopigments and hue naming. *J. Opt. Soc. Amer. 69*: 422–434.

Further Readings

Boynton, R. M. 1973. Implications of the minimally distinct border. *J. Opt. Soc. Amer. 63*: 1037–1043.

Werner, J. S., and Wooten, B. R. 1979. Opponent chromatic response functions for an average observer. *Percept. Psychophys. 25*: 371–374.

6
Chromatic and Achromatic Response Functions and Appearance of Spectral Lights

K NOWLEDGE of the precise forms and spectral distributions of the red/green, yellow/blue, and white/(black)* response functions enable us to understand the appearance of the variety of narrow- and broad-band stimuli discussed in Chapter 4. We need only assume that these functions represent the way the physiological neural mechanisms respond to spectral light stimulation, that they correlate directly with perception, and that the response effects produced by individual wavelengths sum in algebraic fashion when more than single wavelengths make up the stimulus.

On inspection these functions tell us what color is associated with any given wavelength. For example, at 450 nm in Figure 1, the value for red is +0.08, blue −0.44, and white +0.04; the response at 450 nm is thus a reddish blue that contains more blue than red and is also a little whitish. At 520 nm, to take another example, the responses evoked are yellow, +0.23; green, −0.58; and white, +0.65. This is a whitish, yellowish-green-appearing stimulus that contains more green than yellow and more white than the 450-nm stimulus. At 640 nm we have red equal to +0.23, yellow equal to +0.12, and white equal to +0.26. This is slightly yellowish red and less white than the 520-nm stimulus. The chromatic and achromatic values can, of course, be read off these curves at any wavelength of interest.

We have discussed the unique hues several times earlier and noted their use in measuring the chromatic response functions. The individual wavelengths that evoke unique hues are given directly in Figure 1. Look at wavelength 475 nm. Notice that here the red/green chromatic response function intersects the ordinate at the value zero. At this red/green balance position the blue response equals −0.30; thus the 475-nm stimulus sets

* Black is placed in parentheses here to indicate that there is no direct measurement of this function.

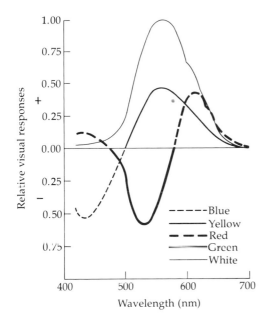

1 CHROMATIC (YELLOW/BLUE AND RED/GREEN) and achromatic (whiteness) responses throughout the spectrum. One observer. Arithmetic representation.

off a blue response that is neither red nor green, although we see that it does have some whiteness (about +0.08). At 500 nm on the wavelength scale we find that the yellow/blue response function is in balance at the zero ordinate value and green equals −0.24 and white equals +0.22; at 580 nm the/red green function again intercepts the zero baseline, and here yellow equals +0.40 and white equals +0.95. There is no single wavelength in this graphical representation of the response functions that evoke a redness response alone in the complete absence of either a blueness or yellowness response. Thus there is no single spectral stimulus that evokes a unique red response. This fact was known to Newton and to Goethe, the German poet, dramatist, and naturalist, whose scientific interests took him into problems of color and color vision. Even the most extreme long wavelength used, say 700 nm, stimulates some yellow (and white) response, however small, along with the red process.

Mixtures of pairs of spectral stimuli can also evoke the unique hues blue, green, and yellow. As noted earlier (Figure 13 in Chapter 4), the unique blue hue evoked by 475 nm (for an average standardized observer) can be matched by mixing on the retina two wavelengths, say 440 nm and 490 nm; unique green evoked by 500 nm can be matched by intermixing two wavelengths, 490 nm and 540 nm (Figure 12 in Chapter 4), and unique yellow produced by 580 nm can also be matched by intermixing two wavelengths, 540 nm and 670 nm (Figure 11 in Chapter 4).

The intermixing of the different stimuli is a simple matter (see, e.g.,

Plate 4-2). The superposition or additive light mixture of the different spectral stimuli can be efficiently done with an apparatus such as that shown in Figure 2 of Chapter 5. The individual wavelengths used for the mixture come from the two monochromators I and II and are simply imaged on the same retinal area as in the experiments described for the measurement of the chromatic response functions. By introducing the third monochromator (Figure 2 in Chapter 5) we can compare the mixture of two spectral lights with lights from monochromator III, which is used to provide a surround field for the intermixed stimulus pair. The principle underlying the generation of unique hues by mixing pairs of wavelengths is precisely the same as that of the cancellation experiments described at length in the previous chapter.

If we look at the response functions in Figure 1, we see that wavelength 440 nm excites the blue, red, and white processes; 490 nm excites the blue, green, and white processes. By manipulating the relative energies of wavelengths 440 and 490 nm, the red and green opponent systems can be brought to a balanced state of equality. When this is achieved we are left with a net excitation of blue (and white). If we consider two wavelengths, one on the shorter side of 500 nm—490 nm—and one on the longer side of 500 nm—540 nm—we see in Figure 1 that the latter excites the green, yellow, and white processes. Here, too, then, by appropriately varying the relative energies of the 490-nm and 540-nm stimuli, and precisely balancing the blue and yellow excitations to equality, we are left with a remainder that corresponds to the unique green hue, but one that is somewhat whiter than that produced by the single wavelength 500 nm. (A unit of energy at 500 nm has a white response of 0.22; unit energies at 490 and 540 nm sum to 1.04 of white response. The 1.04 comes from a 490 nm value of +0.13 and a 540 value of +0.9l.) Finally, the two wavelengths 540 and 670 nm, located one on the shorter side of 580 nm, the other on the longer side of 580 nm, evoke yellow, green and white, and yellow, red and white responses, respectively. When the green and red processes are balanced by adjusting the relative intensities of 540 and 670 nm, the outcome is a unique yellow hue.

Many combinations of two different wavelengths will generate a unique hue just as long as one member of the wavelength pair lies on the shorter-wavelength side and the other on the longer-wavelength side of the single wavelength that evokes the unique hue. The proportions of the components entering into the mixture will, of course, differ for different wavelength pairs.

If, for example, we were to mix 670 nm and 540 nm to evoke a unique yellow, it would be necessary to balance the red and green responses.

Since

$$1 \text{ unit of energy of } 670 \text{ nm} \rightarrow 0.06 \text{ red}$$
$$1 \text{ unit of energy of } 540 \text{ nm} \rightarrow 0.55 \text{ green}$$

we would have to increase the 670-nm stimulus by a factor of about 10 to balance red and green. If instead of 540 nm we were to use 560 nm and mix it with 670 nm, then since

$$1 \text{ unit of energy of } 670 \text{ nm} \rightarrow 0.06 \text{ red}$$
$$1 \text{ unit of energy of } 560 \text{ nm} \rightarrow 0.30 \text{ green}$$

then we would need to increase the 670-nm stimulus energy only by a factor of about 5.0 instead of 10.

The proportions of any other stimulus pairs, say, 620 nm and 540 nm or 610 nm and 560 nm, can be determined in the same way. The fact that different stimulus pairs when mixed evoke different amounts of yellow and white is, of course, a matter of indifference. In all cases the outcome will be a unique yellow since neither red nor green will be visible in any instance.

As we noted on page 67, there is no single spectral stimulus that gives a unique red hue: extremely long wavelengths are yellowish red, and extremely short ones are bluish red. How would one go about generating a unique red hue?

At the end of Chapter 4, we discussed the fact that many pairs of spectral stimuli are complementary (i.e., when mixed in a proper energy ratio, many pairs of wavelengths lead to an achromatic or white appearance). We are now in a position to examine the chromatic and achromatic response curves to see how this comes about.

The most obvious wavelengths to start with are 475 nm and 580 nm. As we have seen, only blueness and whiteness are stimulated by 475 nm, and 580 nm is the wavelength associated with the unique yellow sensation, a yellow that is somewhat whitish in appearance. By intermixing these two wavelengths on the retina and adjusting the relative energies of the two stimuli, we balance the blue excitation with an equal amount of yellow, and the remainder, or NET EXCITATION, is the sum of the two white excitations produced by each of these wavelengths. Thus 475 nm and 580 nm are complementary wavelengths. If we were to intermix 470 nm (a red, blue, white) with 580 nm, there is no greenness in 580 nm necessary to balance the red evoked by 470 nm. Similarly, if we move to 480 nm (a green, blue, white), there is no redness in 580 nm necessary to balance the green in 480 nm. Many other pairs of spectral stimuli that do not evoke unique hues are also complementary.

Thus if the wavelength 460 nm evokes a red response for unit energy equal to +0.05 a blue response equal to −0.35, and a white response equal to +0.05 unit, the wavelength that is complementary to it will have to evoke a green response of −0.05, and a yellow response of +0.35. Since red and green responses are opponent, they are represented by plus and minus values, respectively, and the same is true of yellow and blue. The situation can be represented in algebraic form as follows:

For 460 nm:	+0.05 red;	−0.35 blue;	+0.05 white
Complementary wavelength:	−0.05 green;	+0.35 yellow;	$+x^*$ white
Sum:	0.0;	0.0;	$+0.05 + x$

In short, the redness response evoked by 460 nm is exactly canceled by the greenness evoked by an appropriately selected stimulus, and the blueness also evoked by 460 nm is also exactly canceled by the yellowness evoked by this same stimulus. Since both stimuli excite a whiteness response that is not balanced by an antagonistic response, these excitations sum and remain effective in generating the white perception.

Precisely the same reasoning applies to all other complementary wavelength pairs. Calculations show that all complementary wavelengths are simply those that evoke equal amounts of opponent chromatic responses. In all cases the net effective response is the whiteness excitation that is common to each wavelength. It should be clear from the discussion of cancellation experiments in Chapter 5 that when the opponent chromatic responses are not in precise balance, the hue of the relatively more energetic stimulus is seen.

Once we realize that the whiteness aspect is simply the uncanceled excitation produced by both stimuli of the complementary pair, we need only seek out two stimuli in the spectrum whose chromatic excitations are opposite and equal in order to find stimuli properly characterizeable as complementary. A simple way of presenting the complementary light situation is therefore to restrict ourselves to the hue responses of the various wavelengths, knowing as we now do that the whiteness response is always evoked by the individual stimuli and is not canceled.

The relations between perceived hues and the chromatic response functions in the spectrum are given in "absolute terms" in Figure 1. That is, the amount of chromatic response at each wavelength is specified per unit of light energy. We can alternatively set up a direct expression of the relation between perceived hue and spectral wavelength in ratio or percentage terms. At any given wavelength we can state the ratio of each

* x represents a variable amount of white that changes as the energy of the complementary wavelength is adjusted to balance the two opponent chromatic processes. As in the case of the unique hues, its amount is a matter of indifference.

separate chromatic response to the sum of the total chromatic responses. This ratio or percentage value has been given the name HUE COEFFICIENT. Graphical representation of the spectral hue coefficients is given in Figure 2 for an average standardized observer. The blue curve represents the hue coefficient values for the blues (B/B + R and B/B + G) as a function of wavelength; yellow represents the yellow ratios (Y/Y + G and Y/Y + R); reds are the values for the reds (R/R + B and R/R + Y); and green represents the green ratios (G/G + B and G/G + Y). These coefficients have been calculated for an equal whiteness or brightness level throughout the spectrum. The light level is moderate.

The numerical ratios at any given wavelength are taken to correlate directly with our hue perceptions in the spectrum. Thus for the average observer "blue" has a value of 100 percent or 1.0 at about 475 nm, where the red and green values are zero; green has a value of 1.0 at about 500 nm and yellow a value of 1.0 at about 580 nm. At the wavelength 500 nm, both blue and yellow are zero, and at 580 nm, green and red are zero. Blue-green, green-yellow, and yellow-red are equally strong at a hue coefficient value of 0.50, and these three wavelength loci are 485, 560, and 595 nm, respectively. Other hue coefficient values are taken to represent the relative amounts of the two hues seen at the wavelength in question. At least a half-dozen experiments in which observers scale hues directly in percentage terms or estimate them in some related fashion confirm the essential correctness of the derived hue coefficient measure.

Using the hue coefficient functions, we can now determine comple-

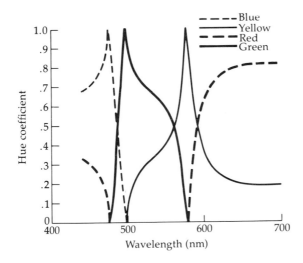

2 SPECTRAL HUE COEFFICIENTS represent the relative amounts of paired hues seen at each wavelength. These are values for an average observer at a moderate light level.

mentary color pairs directly and simply. We can, for a given wavelength, say 640 nm, read off on the hue coefficient graph the percentage of red as 80 percent and yellow as 20 percent. To find the wavelength that is complementary to it, we need only locate the wavelength for which the opponent green value is 80 percent and the opponent blue value is 20 percent. A horizontal straightedge shows that this wavelength intercept lies at 492 nm. This can be repeated for all long-wavelength positions, and the result is that when we plot the pairs of wavelengths that are complementary, we obtain a rectangular hyperbola. The intermediate yellow-green-appearing wavelengths do not have spectral complementaries. The wavelength 560 nm, for example, is 50 percent green and 50 percent yellow. Inspection of the hue coefficient function makes it instantly clear why there is no single spectral wavelength complementary to 560 nm. Why is this true?

When describing the hues associated with given wavelengths, I have pointed out that the discussion was being limited to a moderate level of illumination. The reason for this is simple: it is a well-known fact that a physical object changes its perceived hue as the light energy or intensity level changes. Therefore, unless we restricted our discussion initially to a single moderate fixed level of illumination, it would be impossible to discuss the connection between wavelength and hue.

Now that we have this association in hand for an average moderate level, we must look at the way perceived hue varies with illumination changes. For the same light distribution, red and green hues tend to predominate over yellows and blues at relatively low light levels, and the reverse is true at relatively high light levels. Blues and yellows tend to become relatively "stronger" at higher light levels. For example, a yellow-ish-green object will tend to look relatively greener when we see it at a low light level than when it is illuminated by the same light at a relatively high light level: at the higher level, it looks yellower.

This phenomenon, called the BEZOLD-BRÜCKE PHENOMENON (after two nineteenth-century vision investigators), has been the subject of considerable experimental work. These experiments vary in detail, but a simple type involves asking an observer to match two halves of a split field in hue appearance when the two light levels differ. One half-field is first set at a fixed wavelength and low energy, and the other at the same fixed wavelength and high energy. If the wavelength is 610 nm and looks yellow-red at the low energy, the high-energy 610 nm field will look much yellower. If the two fields are to be equated in hue, the observer must change the wavelength of the brighter field to make it appear redder. To make it redder requires that the wavelength be adjusted to 630 nm. Thus the increased yellowness of 610 at high energy is offset by a wavelength change.

A related change occurs at the short-wavelength end of the spectrum. Here the high-energy stimulation for a fixed wavelength produces a relatively "bluer" appearance than for the low-energy stimulus. Again the wavelength of the high-energy stimulus has to be adjusted but this time to offset the increased blueness that takes place with an energy increase. To do this means that the short-wavelength stimulus used initially at the higher energy level must be moved to shorter wavelengths, thereby increasing the redness of the stimulus to reestablish a hue match.

Figure 3 summarizes the results of one such experiment. The lines connecting the different wavelengths at the different energy levels used are called CONSTANT HUE CONTOURS. If the adaptation is neutral (i.e., if we start with a balanced equilibrium state; see Chapter 15), we find that there are three places in the spectrum where the appearance of a spectral light does not change as the light level changes. These INVARIANT HUES, as they are called, correspond to the three unique spectral hues, blue, green, and yellow.

If the hues associated with given wavelengths change in appearance with energy changes, what about the hue coefficient functions, which supposedly represent the way the hues look at different spectral positions? Not surprisingly, they change. In principle, raising the energy level means that the yellow/blue chromatic response function must increase its values relative to the red/green chromatic response function. Figure 4 summarizes the way the paired functions behave as stimulus energy increases. If we apply this principle to the curves of the average standard observer, we find that for a spectrum at a high level, the hue coefficient functions look

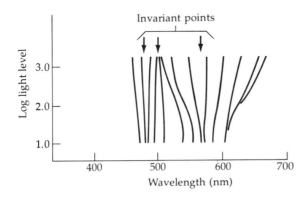

3 CONSTANT HUE CONTOURS. Except for the three wavelengths labeled invariant points, which are wavelengths that continue to look uniquely blue, uniquely green, and uniquely yellow (for a neutral adaptation condition) as light energy is increased, at all other spectral positions, the hue associated with a fixed wavelength changes as the light level is varied. The various curved lines link the wavelength/light intensity combinations that have the same hue.

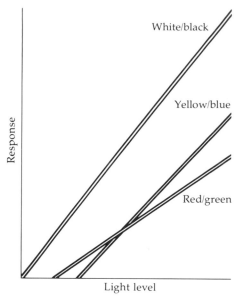

4 RELATIVE RATES OF RISE of paired chromatic and achromatic responses with an increase in the light level. This schematic representation shows that the white/black system has the lowest threshold (it is activated at a lower light level than either of the other paired systems) and that its response increases faster than either the red/green or yellow/blue paired systems. The red/green system has a lower threshold than the yellow/blue one, but its rate of rise is slower than that of the yellow/blue system.

as shown in Figure 5. It is important to note that although there is a relative increase in the blue and yellow hue coefficients, and a relative decrease in the red and green ones, the unique blue, green, and yellow spectral loci remain unchanged. We see, however, that the loci of the intermediate binary hues, those with 50 percent of each hue component, shift. The wavelength 485 nm, which was equally blue and green for the standard moderate light level, is now more strongly blue than green, and the hue that is equally blue and green occurs at about 490 nm. At 560 nm, where the hue for the standard light level was equally yellow and green, the hue is now more strongly yellow, and the equally yellow-green hue is found at about 553 nm. The wavelength that formerly elicited the equal red-yellow sensation, 595 nm, now elicits a more strongly yellow sensation and the wavelength for equal yellow and red hue coefficients has moved closer to 600 nm.

It might at first glance seem that the complementary wavelength function as derived from the hue coefficient function at a moderate level of illumination would change its form. But this is not true, as we see if we use the high-light-level coefficient function (or, say, one that is calculated for an illumination lower than the standard illumination). The form of the complementary function does not change because the percentage increase (or decrease) in the opponent hue coefficient values remains the same at the higher level for the complementary wavelengths selected at the moderate light level.

The discussion in this chapter of the appearance of individual spectral

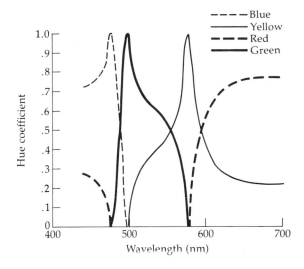

5 SPECTRAL HUE COEFFICIENTS for a high light level. Comparison with Figure 2 shows that a given wavelength has more yellow (or blue) at this light level than at the moderate light level.

lights, those that are unique (blue, green, yellow) as well as those that have a binary hue (i.e., red-yellow, green-blue, etc.); how the unique appearance of individual spectral lights can be duplicated by mixtures of pairs of spectral stimuli; and how mixtures of pairs of spectral stimuli can produce whites, should help clarify some of the puzzles referred to at the end of Chapter 5. Once we understand how the opponent principle operates, these puzzles are solved. We can now extend the discussion to include the appearances of stimuli with broad-band spectral light distributions.

Background Readings

Cohen, J. D. 1975. Temporal independence of the Bezold-Brücke hue shift. *Vision Res. 15*: 341–351.

Dimmick, F. L., and Hubbard, M. R. 1939. The spectral location of psychological unique yellow, green, and blue. *Amer. J. Psychol. 52*: 242–254.

Helmholtz, H. v. 1896. *Handbuch der physiologischen Optik,* 2nd ed., p. 456. Voss, Hamburg.

Hurvich, L. M., and Jameson, D. 1955. Some quantitative aspects of an opponent-colors theory. II. Brightness, saturation, and hue in normal and dichromatic vision. *J. Opt. Soc. Amer. 45*: 602–616.

Hurvich, L. M., and Jameson, D. 1958. Further developments of a quantified opponent-colours theory. In *Visual Problems of Colour II*, Chap. 22, pp. 691–723. Her Majesty's Stationery Office, London.

Hurvich, L. M., Jameson, D., and Cohen, J. D. 1968. The experimental determination of unique green in the spectrum. *Percept. Psychophys.* 4: 65–68.

Indow, T., and Takagi, C. 1968. Hue-discrimination thresholds and hue-coefficients. *J. Psychol. Res. 10*: 179–190.

Purdy, D. McL. 1931. Spectral hue as a function of intensity. *Amer. J. Psychol. 43*: 541–559.

Purdy, D. McL. 1937. The Bezold-Brücke phenomenon and contours for constant hue. *Amer. J. Psychol. 49*: 313–315.

Sternheim, C., and Boynton, R. M. 1966. Uniqueness of perceived hues investigated with a continuous judgmental technique. *J. Exp. Psychol. 72*: 770–776.

Further Readings

Larimer, J., Krantz, D. H., and Cicerone, C. M. 1974. Opponent-process additivity. I. Red/green equilibria. *Vision Res. 14*: 1127–1140.

Larimer, J., Krantz, D. H., and Cicerone, C. M. 1975. Opponent process additivity. II. Yellow/blue equilibria and nonlinear models. *Vision Res. 15*: 723–731.

7

Chromatic and Achromatic Response Functions and Appearance of Broad-Band Spectral-Light Distributions

IN Chapter 6 we saw that the appearances of relatively simple stimuli can be analyzed and explained in conjunction with the chromatic and achromatic response functions. However, few people ever get into a laboratory and see isolated patches of spectral light or mixtures of pairs of spectral lights. In our daily lives we see isolated colors produced by restricted wavelength ranges only when we look at such things as neon glow lamps, sodium-type street lights, rainbows, the colored rings produced by oil spills, soap bubbles, or when light is dispersed at the edge of a glass or vase, or by the facets of a diamond. In all these instances we are dealing with relatively narrow-band spectral stimuli. Almost all colored objects of our everyday experience, however, reflect many different wavelengths over a broad spectral region rather than isolated narrow wavebands of light. Can the appearances of the various broad-band stimuli diagrammed in Figures 5 through 9 in Chapter 4 be accounted for in the same way as are the appearances of relatively simple spectral stimuli?

Let us examine first the various light distributions shown in Figure 1, which are all weighted maximally in energy at the spectral locus 500 nm. We know that a narrow-band spectral stimulus at 500 nm looks uniquely green (i.e., it is neither yellowish nor bluish green). In Chapter 6 we discussed the fact that many different pairs of spectral stimuli, one on each side of a spectral stimulus that evokes a unique hue, will, when mixed in proper proportions, also produce a unique hue. To produce unique green, for example, we saw that if one stimulus evokes green, yellow, and white responses and a second stimulus evokes green, blue, and white responses, we need only vary the energy ratios of the two stimuli to precisely balance blue and yellow. When we have done this, we are left with a unique green (whitish). Thus the narrow-band stimulus

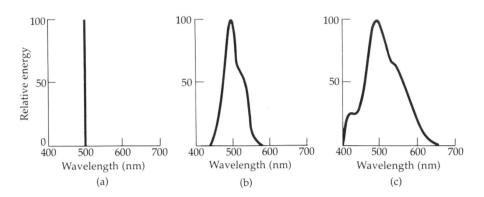

1 A UNIQUE GREEN HUE is produced by each of these three different spectral-light-energy distributions.

shown in Figure 1a evokes unique green and the broader one represented in Figure 1b does the same. A unique green hue is also seen when the broad-band distribution is that shown in Figure 1c. Simply put, many pairs of additional spectral lights on both sides of 500 nm are involved in the light distributions shown in parts (b) and (c).

But there is a difference among the colors evoked by the stimuli shown in parts (a), (b), and (c). As the stimulus distribution gets wider (and flatter) and energies of spectral stimuli are added on both sides of the central 500-nm wavelength, the whiteness excitation produced by these adjacent wavelengths increases. Thus although the hue (i.e., the green) remains unchanged because of the action of the cancellation principle, the perceived color becomes increasingly desaturated or paler as the width of the broad-band stimulus increases and more "whiteness" is added.

The two different broad-band light distributions in Figure 7 in Chapter 4 were said to have the same hue, yellow-green, but not the same color. By this we mean that they are of different saturations. We know this by looking at the two stimuli in the laboratory. It is possible, however, with the use of the chromatic and achromatic response functions to calculate both the hues and saturations of such stimuli as they would appear to the average observer. We can calculate a hue coefficient value for broad-band stimuli just as we did for individual spectral lights in Chapter 6. As we shall see in a moment, we can also calculate a saturation coefficient for individual spectral lights as well as for broad-band stimuli. With both hue and saturation specified in coefficient or percentage terms, we can get a good idea of what different stimuli, narrow or broad band, will look like.

As we have seen, the hue coefficient value of a given spectral light is determined by taking the value of any one chromatic response, say yellow, at a given wavelength and expressing it as a ratio relative to the sum of chromatic values at that wavelength, say yellow plus green (Y/Y + G). (Absolute values are used in calculating the total chromatic response.) To determine the hue coefficient value of a broad-band stimulus, a similar computation is made, but instead of limiting ourselves to a single wavelength the computation extends over the entire spectral range covered by the broad-band stimulus.

First, the relative energy at the eye of the broad-band stimulus at each wavelength is multiplied by the values of each of the chromatic responses (per unit energy) at the same wavelengths (Figure 1 in Chapter 6). Then we sum the values of these cross products algebraically throughout the spectrum. This is illustrated in Table I for the two light stimuli labeled A and B in Figure 7 in Chapter 4. For convenience and an approximate answer, the cross multiplication of relative energy and chromatic responses can be carried out for 10-nm steps. The result of such a computation gives us an integrated or total value for the chromatic responses. The hue coefficient value of the broad-band stimulus is then specified in precisely the same way that it is for a single spectral line—by taking the ratio of one of the chromatic responses to the sum of all chromatic responses. For the two stimuli that peak at about 535 nm in Figure 7 in Chapter 4, the hue coefficient values are 62 percent green and 38 percent yellow, and 68 percent green and 32 percent yellow. These calculated values are in close agreement with the way observers would respond if asked to characterize the hue of such stimuli directly in percentage terms.

How do we specify perceived saturation, the color variation that goes, for example, from strong red to whitish pink, or to grayish rose?

To calculate the saturation coefficient of a narrow-band spectral light of moderate light level, we have to relate it to both the chromatic and achromatic response at that wavelength. Consider the wavelength 570 nm in Figure 1 in Chapter 6. For one observer the yellow response = +0.45, the green response = −0.18, and the white response = +1.00 for a unit of energy. The total chromatic response without regard to sign = +0.63. (Absolute values are used in calculating the total responses.) The ratio of the chromatic to the total chromatic plus achromatic response is 0.63/0.63 + 1.00 = 0.38. At yet another wavelength, such as 440 nm, the blue response = −0.52, the red response = +0.12 and the white response = +0.04. The total chromatic response = +0.64. The ratio of chromatic to achromatic plus chromatic is 0.64/0.64 + 0.04 = +0.94. As our calculation shows, the saturation coefficient is relatively small, +0.38, at 570 nm, and relatively large, +0.94, at 440 nm. The calculated saturation coefficients for these two wavelengths agree in a general way with the appearance of these two spectral lights—the yellow of 570 nm is pale and the "deep" violet of 440 nm is very colorful.

We can, of course, calculate the saturation coefficients for a moderate

Table I Hue coefficient calculations for broad-band stimuli

(a) Light Stimulus A

(1) Wave-length	(2) Relative Energy	(3) Chromatic Response (R/G)	(4) Product (2) × (3)	(5) Chromatic Response (Y/B)	(6) Product (2) × (5)
400	8.90	+0.01*	+0.09*	−0.03*	−0.27*
410	11.76	+0.04*	+0.47*	−0.08*	−0.94*
420	15.23	+0.13*	+1.98*	−0.26*	−3.96*
430	18.58	+0.27*	+5.02*	−0.55*	−10.22*
440	21.87	+0.33	+7.22	−0.69	−15.09
450	25.73	+0.30	+7.72	−0.69	−17.75
460	27.92	+0.23	+6.42	−0.64	−17.87
470	31.47	+0.10	+3.15	−0.48	−15.11
480	34.55	−0.04	−1.38	−0.27	−9.33
490	37.47	−0.18	−6.74	−0.10	−3.75
500	39.93	−0.32	−12.78	+0.02	+0.80
510	42.21	−0.49	−20.68	+0.14	+5.91
520	44.08	−0.65	−28.65	+0.25	+11.02
530	45.10	−0.70	−31.57	+0.33	+14.88
540	45.21	−0.66	−29.84	+0.37	+16.73
550	44.60	−0.56	−24.98	+0.39	+17.39
560	42.80	−0.40	−17.12	+0.40	+17.12
570	39.66	−0.19	−7.54	+0.38	+15.07
580	35.02	+0.05	+1.75	+0.35	+12.26
590	31.04	+0.27	+8.38	+0.30	+9.31
600	26.97	+0.43	+11.60	+0.25	+6.74
610	22.89	+0.50	+11.45	+0.20	+4.58
620	18.58	+0.47	+8.71	+0.15	+2.78
630	15.08	+0.38	+5.73	+0.11	+1.66
640	12.31	+0.27	+3.32	+0.07	+0.86
650	11.02	+0.18	+1.98	+0.04	+0.44
660	10.66	+0.10	+1.07	+0.02	+0.16
670	10.57	+0.06	+0.63	+0.01	+0.06
680	10.03	+0.03	+0.30	+0.01	+0.05
690	9.40	+0.02	+0.19	+0.003	+0.01
700	9.91	+0.01	+0.10	+0.002	+0.01

$$\Sigma + = \ \ 87.28 \qquad\qquad \Sigma + = \ 137.85$$
$$\Sigma - = \underline{181.28} \qquad\qquad \Sigma - = \underline{\ 94.29}$$
$$\Delta \quad = -94.00 = \text{green} \qquad \Delta \quad = +43.56 = \text{yellow}$$

Hue coefficient $= \dfrac{G}{Y + G}$ and $\dfrac{Y}{Y + G}$; $\dfrac{|-94.00|}{|43.56| + |-94.00|} = \dfrac{94.00}{137.56} = 68\%$ green

$$\dfrac{|43.56|}{|43.56| + |-94.00|} = \dfrac{43.56}{137.56} = 32\% \text{ yellow}$$

* There is considerable variability in the short-wavelength region of the spectrum and the values marked by asterisks are only approximate.

(b) Light Stimulus B

(1) Wave-length	(2) Relative Energy	(3) Chromatic Response (R/G)	(4) Product (2) × (3)	(5) Chromatic Response (Y/B)	(6) Product (2) × (5)
400	—				
410	—				
420	—				
430	—				
440	—				
450	—				
460	1.66	+0.23	−0.04	−0.64	−0.10
470	1.33	+0.10	−0.13	−0.48	−0.64
480	6.31	−0.04	−0.25	−0.27	−1.70
490	17.20	−0.18	−3.09	−0.10	−1.72
500	30.30	−0.32	−9.66	+0.02	+0.60
510	40.10	−0.49	−19.60	+0.14	+5.60
520	46.10	−0.65	−29.97	+0.25	+11.53
530	48.30	−0.70	−33.74	+0.33	+15.94
540	47.30	−0.66	−31.22	+0.37	+17.50
550	43.80	−0.56	−24.47	+0.39	+17.08
560	37.30	−0.40	−14.92	+0.40	+14.92
570	28.40	−0.19	−5.40	+0.38	+10.79
580	18.90	+0.05	+0.95	+0.35	+6.62
590	10.60	+0.27	+2.86	+0.30	+3.18
600	4.80	+0.43	+2.05	+0.25	+1.19
610	2.20	+0.50	+1.09	+0.20	+0.44
620	0.70	+0.47	+0.33	+0.15	+0.11
630	—				
640	—				
650	—				
660	—				
670	—				
680	—				
690	—				
700	—				

$$\Sigma + = \quad 7.28 \qquad\qquad \Sigma + = \quad 105.50$$
$$\Sigma - = \quad 172.49 \qquad\qquad \Sigma - = \quad 4.16$$
$$\Delta \quad = -165.21 = \text{green} \qquad \Delta \quad = +101.34 = \text{yellow}$$

$$\text{Hue coefficient} = \frac{G}{Y + G} \text{ and } \frac{Y}{Y + G} \; ; \; \frac{|-165.21|}{|101.34| + |-165.21|} = \frac{165.21}{266.55} = 62\% \text{ green}$$

$$\frac{|101.34|}{|101.34| + |-165.21|} = 38\% \text{ yellow}$$

energy light level throughout the spectrum in wavelength-by-wavelength steps, and such a function is shown in Figure 2a. It shows that for the average observer spectral saturation is at a minimum at about 580 nm and that the spectral extremes are relatively more saturated. How well do these calculations, based on the measured chromatic and achromatic response functions, compare with more direct estimates of the appearance of the spectrum? The experimental results shown in Figure 2b give the answer. The experimenters determined the number of just noticeably different changes between a given spectral color and a stimulus that appears white. They assumed that a high degree of saturation corresponded to a large

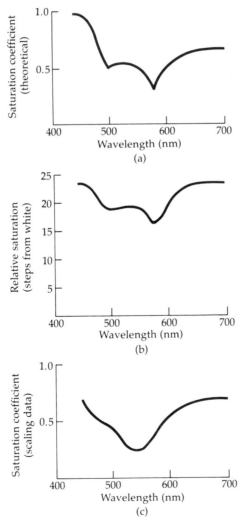

2 SPECTRAL SATURATION MEASURES. (a) Saturation coefficients calculated for the average observer at a moderate light level. (b) Saturation scaling data. The ordinate value of relative saturation specifies at each wavelength tested the number of just-noticeable color steps between a spectral light and white. (c) Saturation scaling data. In these experiments the subject made a direct estimate at each wavelength of the percentage of hue seen relative to the hue and whiteness combined. The surround in this case was a desaturated bluish green.

number of just-noticeably different steps between some spectral stimulus and a stimulus that appears white.

The experimenters began with a spectral light alone and intermixed a small amount of white-appearing broad-band light until the mixture looked just noticeably paler than the spectral light alone. This procedure was repeated progressively until no hue was seen. We see in Figure 2b that there are very few steps between the yellow at 580 nm and white, compared with the number of steps between the spectral stimuli at the extremes and white. Since 580 nm is very nearly white to start with, this is not at all surprising. Since 440 nm and 670 nm are highly saturated to begin with, many more just-noticeable steps of desaturation are necessary in order to reach a white-appearing condition. The results of still another experiment, wherein the observers were asked to state directly in percentage terms how much hue they saw relative to hue and whiteness combined, is shown in Figure 2c. The agreement between these more direct determinations and the theoretically calculated coefficient values is remarkably close.

Just as we can calculate hue coefficients for object colors seen under different illuminants, we can also calculate the saturation coefficients for object colors. For a given broad-band light-stimulus distribution we need only sum the chromatic and achromatic responses weighted by the stimulus distribution across the entire spectrum and calculate the saturation coefficient by expressing these summed values as the ratio of chromatic/chromatic + achromatic.*

The specification of the spectral colors both in hue and saturation coefficient values can be summarized in a color diagram. This is done in Figure 3. The hue coefficients are expressed in percentage terms around the circumference of the hue circle in each quadrant and the saturation coefficients are expressed along the radii. Zero saturation lies at the center of the circle, and full or 100% saturation lies on the circumference.

The same form of representation can be used for broad-band stimuli and Figure 4 shows in diagrammatic form how the three light-stimulus distributions of Figure 6 in Chapter 4 and the two shown in Figure 7 of Chapter 4 compare in hue coefficient and saturation coefficient terms.

Calculated hue and saturation coefficients for the five stimulus distributions shown in Figure 5 in Chapter 4 are plotted in Figure 5. The hue and saturation coefficients of the "blue" object are 5 percent green and 95 percent blue and 37 percent saturation; of the "green" object 32 percent yellow and 68 percent green and 37 percent saturation; of the "yellow"

* For the average achromatic function or "whiteness" function, the values of the average photopic luminosity curve are used. See Figure 13 in Chapter 5.

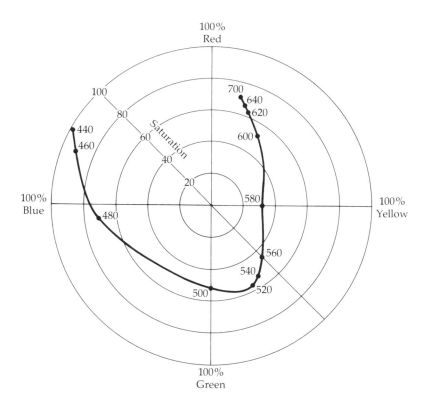

3 HUE AND SATURATION COEFFICIENTS of spectral stimuli represented in a polar coordinate diagram. Hue is plotted circumferentially and saturation along the radius. This is a perceptual space.

object 28 percent red and 72 percent yellow and 30 percent saturation; of the "red" object 99 percent red and 1 percent blue and 43 percent saturation; and of the "purple" object 75 percent blue and 25 percent red and 47 percent saturation. The coefficients for the spectral stimuli 475, 500 and 580 nm are also shown in Figure 5. Notice that the spectral stimuli are more saturated than the broad-band stimuli of the same hue, reflecting the fact that a single spectral stimulus stimulates proportionately much less of the achromatic system than a relatively broad-band stimulus does.*

If we were to calculate the hue and saturation coefficients for the stimulus distributions of Figures 5a and 6 in Chapter 3, we would conclude that the stimuli are nearly white in the first case and slightly reddish-yellow in the second. If we were to analyze a mercury arc source in the

* Approximately the same light levels are assumed. Almost any spectral stimulus can be made to look white or completely desaturated if the energy level is sufficiently high (See Figure 4 in Chapter 6).

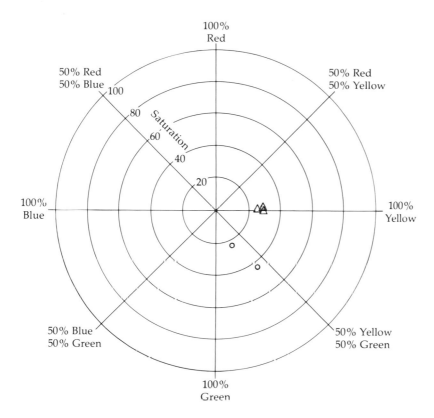

4 HUE AND SATURATION COEFFICIENTS calculated for the three stimulus-light distributions shown in Figure 6 in Chapter 4 and the two stimuli shown in Figure 7 in Chapter 4.

same way it would turn out to be a greenish-blue. For the "white" outcome for the stimulus of Figure 5a in Chapter 3 the sums of the weighted red and green chromatic responses are approximately equal and opposite and thus sum algebraically to nearly zero. The same is true of the sums of the weighted yellow and blue chromatic responses. This, as we saw earlier, is precisely the situation for pairs of spectral stimuli that are complementary: the net chromatic excitations are all equal to zero.

We should not be surprised that the broad-band stimulus of Figure 5a in Chapter 3 produces a net chromatic response that is approximately equal to zero, since a broad-band stimulus of this form can be regarded as made up largely of many pairs of complementary stimuli. The two wavelengths 580 and 475 nm in Figure 6a produce a white experience, as we have already seen. If we add wavelengths 575 nm and 470 nm in Figure 6b, the stimulus continues to look white, since the added wavelengths are also complementary ones. Let us add two additional wave-

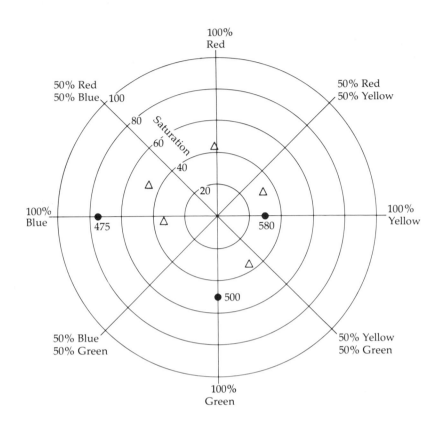

5 HUE AND SATURATION COEFFICIENTS calculated for the five stimulus-light distributions shown in Figure 5 in Chapter 4 and for three spectral stimuli—475, 500, and 580 nm—for an individual observer.

lengths, 570 nm and 452 nm, shown in Figure 6c. The white result is unchanged (except for an increase in brightness). We can continue in this fashion and add all the wavelength pairs shown in Figure 14 in Chapter 4 to be complementary pairs. We will still see a white. If we continue to add wavelengths from the midspectral region between 560 nm and 520 nm for which there are no single complementary wavelengths in the spectrum, the broad-band stimulus will begin to take on a slight greenish-yellowish tinge. How would we have to go about canceling these hues to maintain the whiteness of the broad-band stimulus?

We have had many examples of the fact that different stimulus distributions may look alike or match. For example, many different pairs of spectral lights can be adjusted to match one another in whiteness. The last example emphasizes that any one of a number of different pairs of complementary stimuli can be equated to a broad-band white-appearing stimulus.

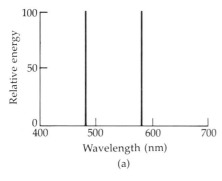

(a)

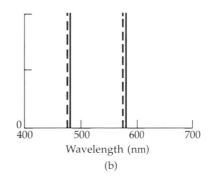

(b)

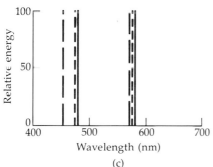

(c)

6 PAIR OF COMPLEMENTARY LIGHTS evokes whiteness. Adding additional pairs of lights that have this same property simply maintains the whiteness aspect of the stimulus appearance and we continue to see white.

This equality of appearance of different physical stimuli comes about, of course, because the same physiological state of excitation underlies the experienced sameness of the perceptual event "whiteness." Different physical stimuli can effect the same physiological excitation because the individual wavelength components can be manipulated as necessary to both excite the whiteness mechanism and to excite and cancel the opponent chromatic mechanisms.

We have been discussing color mixture throughout the last three chapters. The time has come, however, to treat the facts of color mixture in a more systematic fashion. This will lead us to consider the early stages of light absorption in the retina that precede the neural achromatic and chromatic responses and extend our understanding of the visual system. Later (Chapter 20) we shall see that the facts of color mixture are basic for precise color stimulus specification.

Background Readings

Evans, R. M. 1948. *An Introduction to Color,* Chap. 5, pp. 58–76. Wiley, New York.

Hurvich, L. M., and Jameson, D. 1955. Some quantitative aspects of an opponent-colors theory. II. Brightness, saturation, and hue in normal and dichromatic vision. *J. Opt. Soc. Amer.* *45*: 602–616.

Hurvich, L. M., and Jameson, D. 1956. Some quantitative aspects of an opponent-colors theory. IV. A psychological color specification system. *J. Opt. Soc. Amer.* *46*: 416–421.

Jacobs, G. H. 1967. Saturation estimates and chromatic adaptation. *Percept. Psychophys.* *2*: 271–274.

Jameson, D., and Hurvich, L. M. 1959. Perceived color and its dependence on focal, surrounding, and preceding stimulus variables. *J. Opt. Soc. Amer.* *49*: 890–898.

Jones, L. A., and Lowry, E. M. 1926. Retinal sensibility to saturation differences. *J. Opt. Soc. Amer.* *13*: 25–34.

Martin, L. C., Warburton, F. N., and Morgan, W. J. 1933. *Determination of the Sensitiveness of the Eye to Differences and the Saturation of Colours.* Med. Res. Council Spec. Rep. Ser. 188.

Color Plates

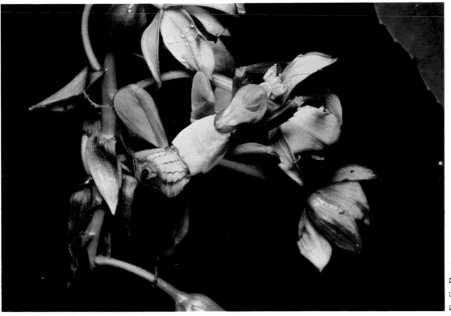

PLATE 1-1   PROTECTIVE COLORATION. The flower mantis (*Hymenopus coronatus*) of Malaya on the blossom of an orchid.

E. S. Ross

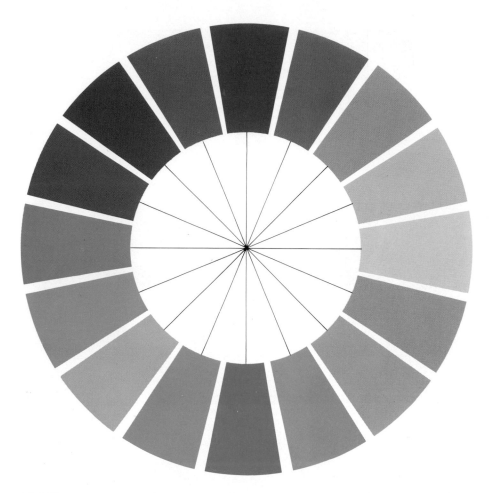

PLATE 1-2 HUE CIRCLE. A series of colors ordered in a circle according to hue. Unique red (neither yellowish nor bluish) is located at the 12 o'clock position, unique yellow (neither reddish nor greenish) at the 3 o'clock position, unique green (neither yellowish nor bluish) at the 6 o'clock position, and unique blue (neither greenish nor reddish) at the 9 o'clock position.

PLATE 1-3 SCHEMATIC REPRESENTATION OF RATIOS OF HUE SIMILARITY (facing page, top). (a) The intermediate or binary hues are related to the two unique or unitary colors, blue and red. (b) The intermediate or binary hues are related here to the two unique or unitary colors, red and yellow.

PLATE 1-4 FOUR-CRESCENT HUE CIRCLE (facing page, bottom). This schematic representation is an extension of Plate 1-3 to include all the hues we see. Red-yellow, red-blue, green-yellow, and green-blue hue combinations (or their inverses) occur in various proportions. We never see red-greens or yellow-blues (or their inverses).

(a)

a　　　b　　　　c

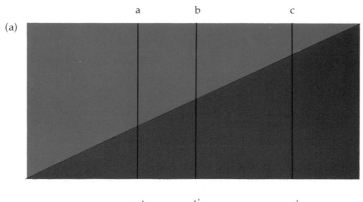

(b)

a'　　　b'　　　　c'

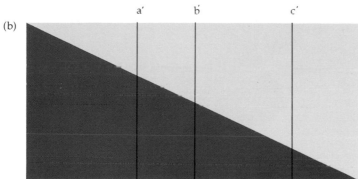

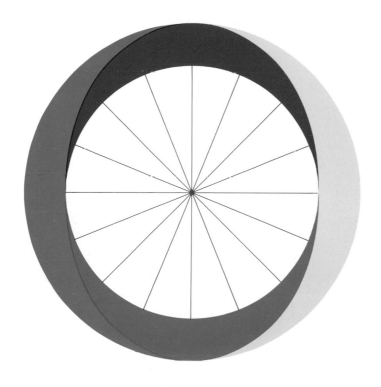

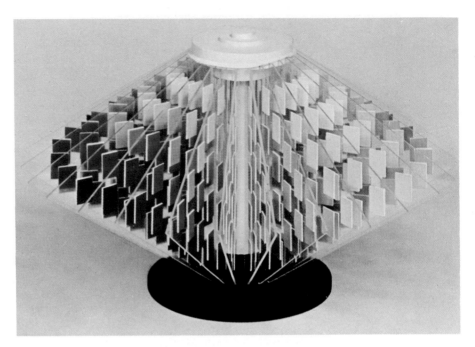

PLATE 1-5 MULTIPLICATION OF COLOR TRIANGLES to encompass the entire color gamut. Hue circles can be drawn at any whiteness or blackness level.

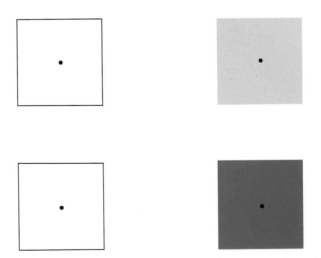

PLATE 2-1 AFTERIMAGE DEMONSTRATION. Look first at the white square at the top left. Then fixate for 20 to 30 seconds on the small black dot in the center of the yellow square. At the end of this period look back at the center of the white area. It will now appear bluish compared to the rest of the visual field. After a short pause, repeat this procedure with the two bottom squares.

PLATE 2-2 SIMULTANEOUS CONTRAST DEMONSTRATION. Each gray strip in the figure is physically identical. They have the same reflectance (see Chapter 3). If we continue to look at the center of the strip on the left, after a short time it will begin to take on a slightly reddish appearance; if after a brief pause we look at the right-hand gray strip, it will begin to look yellowish.

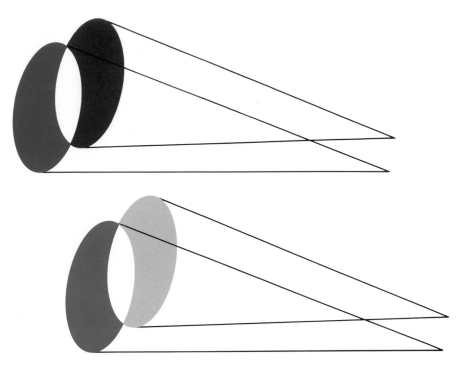

PLATE 4-2 MIXTURE OF LIGHTS of two wavelengths in appropriate ratio produces a white appearance: (top) 670 nm (yellowish red) mixed with 490 nm (bluish green); (bottom) 580 nm (yellow) mixed with 480 nm (blue).

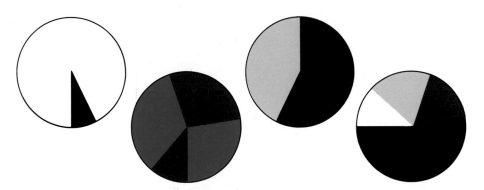

PLATE 8-1 VARIABLE PROPORTIONS of differently colored sectors can be presented on the color wheel.

PLATE 8-2 EXAMPLE OF POINTILLIST COLOR MIXTURE (facing page). The colored elements in the top part of the figure differ from the color reproduced in the bottom part. When viewed from a distance of 10 to 12 feet, the small colored elements are too small to be resolved by the retinal grain and we get fusion or color mixture, and top and bottom fields match.

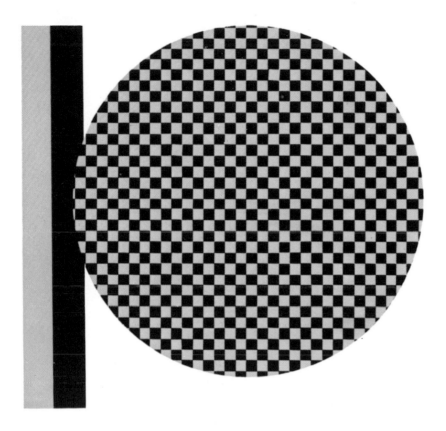

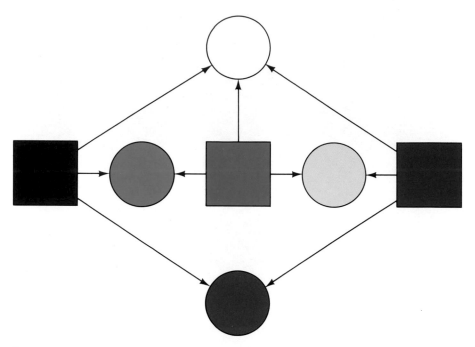

PLATE 8-3 ADDITIVE COLOR MIXTURE. The color that results from the additive mixture of two (or three) components is located at the position of the arrowheads.

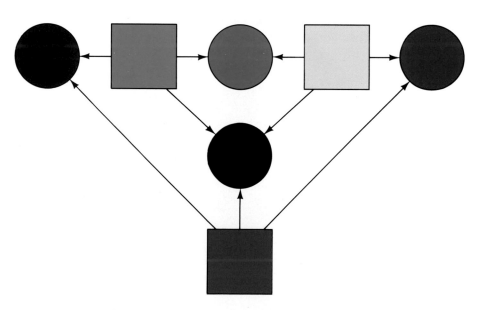

PLATE 8-4 SUBTRACTIVE COLOR MIXTURE. The color that results from the subtractive mixture of two (or three) components is located at the position of the arrowheads.

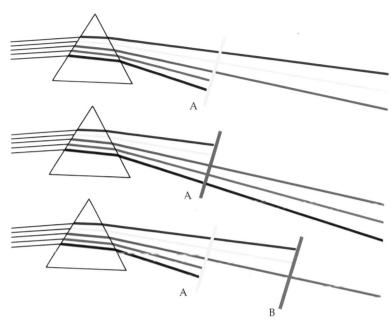

PLATE 8-5 SELECTIVE ABSORPTION OF SPECTRAL LIGHT to illustrate that the combination of appropriate yellow- and blue-appearing filters produces a green color experience. This is an example of subtractive color mixing.

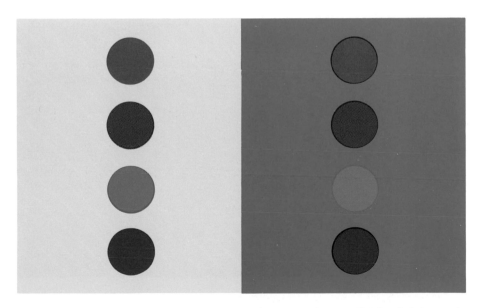

PLATE 13-1 SIMULTANEOUS CONTRAST EFFECT. The four small colored disks are the same on both the right and left sides of the figure. Only the surround colors differ in the two instances.

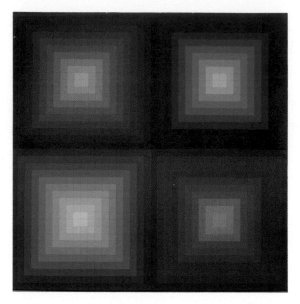

PLATE 13-2 "GLOWING" AXES in this Vasarely composition, *Arcturus* (1970), are generated by physiological contrast mechanisms of the visual system. The artist has painted square frames of ever-decreasing light levels from the center outward in each quadrant. The light level of each frame is uniform and equal.

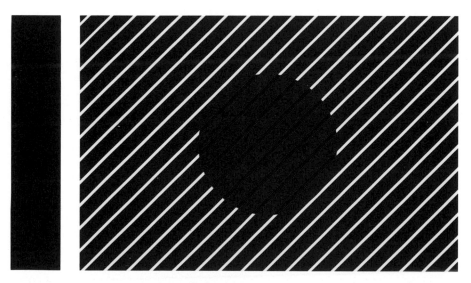

PLATE 13-3 ASSIMILATION EFFECT. The background has the same spectral distribution throughout the figure. It is also shown in the large rectangle at the left of the figure. The central disc surrounded by bluish stripes takes on a bluish-red appearance. Conventional contrast would lead us to expect an increase in yellowness.

PLATE 14-1 DECREASE IN PERCEIVED SATURATION with continued stimulation. Place a piece of white paper over the right half of the yellow rectangle. Stare at the fixation cross for about 30 seconds. Then quickly remove the white mask while continuing to stare at the fixation cross. Note the relative saturations of the left and right halves of the yellow rectangle.

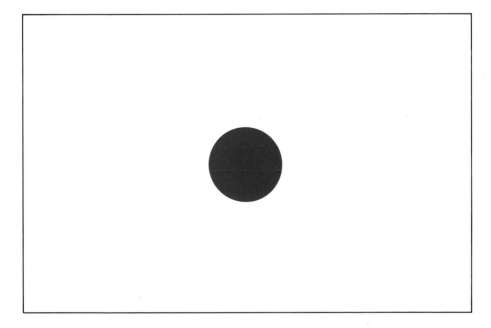

PLATE 14-2 GREEN FOCAL AFTERIMAGE is seen after viewing a small reddish stimulus on a white surround. The afterimage of the white surround is seen as pinkish.

PLATE 14-3 RED FOCAL AFTERIMAGE is seen after viewing a small white stimulus on a red surround. The afterimage of the red surround is seen as greenish.

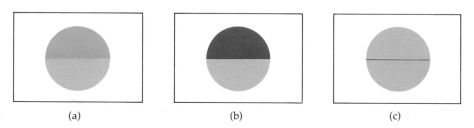

(a) (b) (c)

PLATE 16-1 TEST STIMULI seen in a bipartite field of an optical instrument used to detect color deficiencies. (a) 535-nm stimulus on top, 589-nm stimulus on bottom. (b) 670-nm stimulus on top, 589-nm stimulus on bottom. (c) Mixture proportions of 535 nm/670 nm adjusted to be indistinguishable from appearance of 589-nm stimulus on the bottom.

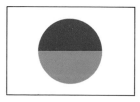

PLATE 16-2 NORMAL MATCH between 535 nm/670 nm and 589 nm as it apparently looks to a shifted deuteranomalous observer.

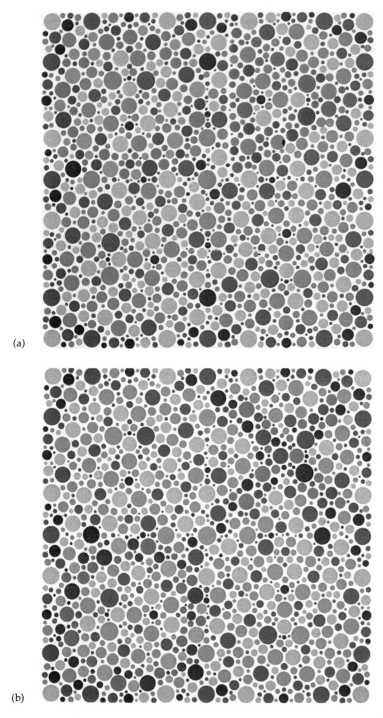

(a)

(b)

PLATE 17-1 TWO EXAMPLES OF TEST PLATES from the Hardy-Rand-Rittler series of test plates.

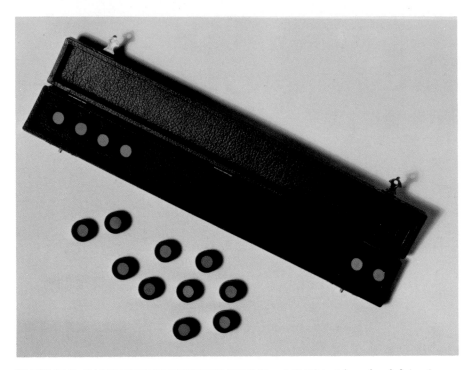

PLATE 17-2 FARNSWORTH DICHOTOMOUS (Panel D-15) test for color deficiencies.

8
Color Mixture:
Hue Matches

ADDITIVE light mixture is essentially the physical superposition of different wavelengths of light on the same point or points of the retinal surface to produce a pooling of the individual light effects of the different wavelengths. We discussed this phenomenon several times earlier in the book. In Chapter 4 we saw that sunlight that is dispersed on refraction will produce "whiteness" when all the rays are recombined both in external space and on the retina, that pairs of spectral stimuli can be mixed to produce the same hue that single spectral stimuli produce, and that selected pairs of spectral stimuli (the complementaries) when mixed produce a white sensation. Chapter 5 was devoted primarily to a particular type of mixture experiment and its use in deriving the basic chromatic response functions. In Chapters 6 and 7 these mixture results were analyzed in terms of the chromatic and achromatic response functions to account for the color appearances of spectral and broad-band stimuli.

The way lights are usually mixed in laboratory work on color problems has also been referred to several times (Chapters 5 and 6). In these situations light beams that come from separate monochromators are intermixed with the aid of lens systems, beam splitters, mirrors, prisms of various sorts, and so on. The light beams are then viewed through short-focus telescopes or eye lenses. Many kinds of stimulus fields can be arranged and several are shown in Figure 1. The apparatus shown in Figure 2 in Chapter 5 produces two overlapping circular fields, and the introduction of an additional monochromator (III) produces a surround for the mixture field. The most common arrangement is the one that presents two semicircular split fields adjoining each other. The mixture variables appear on one side of the circular field and the color to be matched on the other.

But colored stimuli can be intermixed in a variety of ways that do not require expensive optical equipment. Probably the simplest way is to place two differently colored papers at right angles to each other and interpose between them a piece of glass inclined at a 45-degree angle to each of the

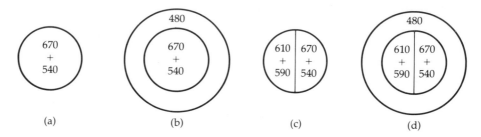

1 VARIETIES OF VISUAL FIELDS used in color-mixture experiments. (a) Two overlapping fields. (b) Two overlapping fields in a surround. (c) Bipartite field, each containing a pair of overlapping stimuli. (d) Bipartite field, each containing a pair of overlapping stimuli centered in a surround.

papers (see Figure 3 in Chapter 13). When you look down from above through the clear glass, one of the papers is seen through the glass and the other is seen by reflection from the front surface of the glass. Each colored stimulus is thus imaged on the same part of the retina and, by varying the angle of the glass, different proportions of the two stimuli can be reflected toward the eye of the viewer. The result is an ADDITIVE COLOR MIXTURE, since different stimuli are focused on the same part of the retina.

Another simple way in which stimuli can be intermixed is to use a refinement of a child's spinning top. Youngsters' tops that have differently colored segments produce a fused single color when spun rapidly because the separate stimuli succeed each other on the same retinal position at high frequencies. The uniform color that we perceive is related to the individual stimulus components and their relative time durations. This sort of color mixture is called TIME-WEIGHTED AVERAGING.

A refinement of the spinning top that finds widespread laboratory use dates back to James Clerk Maxwell of electromagnetic-theory fame, who used spinning discs in some of his experiments on color. Colored discs are slit along a radius and then interleaved as shown in Figure 2. In more modern versions of color-mixture wheels the interleaved color discs are mounted on motor shafts that are rapidly rotated. It is a simple matter to combine colored discs of various sorts (see Plate 8-1,) but more important, the proportions of the different sectors can be changed with great ease when the motor is briefly stopped. There are even differential color mixers, constructed to permit the sector disc proportions to be changed while the discs are spinning.

Projectors with colored filters (either broad-band or narrow-band) can be used to project overlapping light beams onto a surface that diffusely reflects them to be viewed with the "naked" eye (Figure 3), and instances of this sort of mixture were noted in the discussion of complementary lights in Chapter 4 (p. 49).

Color mixture is important because it is not restricted to the laboratory (although it is there that it is best analyzed) and the laws of color mixture have important implications for the mechanisms of color vision. Whenever we look at a colored light or surface that is composed of a large variety of individual wavelengths (a broad-band stimulus), additive light mixture occurs.

Consider, for example, a piece of nonselective white-appearing paper. Light rays of all wavelengths uniformly radiated from a light source are diffusely reflected from the object's surface and impinge in overlapping fashion everywhere on the retina within the image boundaries of the paper. The amounts of the different wavelengths are such that they lead to a balanced or zero chromatic neural response and we see a piece of paper as "white" because of the activity of the achromatic neural system (see Chapter 7). In this example the different wavelengths of light originate

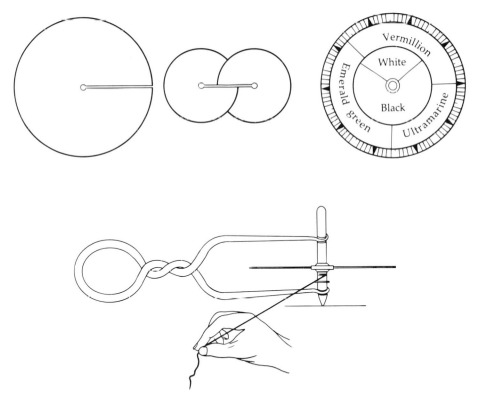

2 INTERLEAVED COLOR DISCS and the spinning arrangement used by Maxwell. By appropriate adjustment of the proportions of the inner white and black discs, and the proportions of the outer vermilion, ultramarine, and emerald green discs, upon rotation, a color match can be established between them to produce a uniform gray-appearing field. The stimulus amounts in angular degrees are read by using the fixed protractor mounted on the circumference.

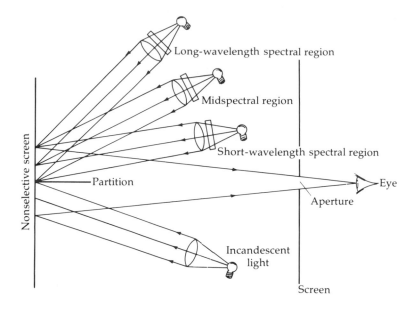

3 PROJECTORS WITH DIFFERENT COLOR FILTERS can be used to project overlapping light beams on a diffusely reflecting screen.

from the same surface before they impinge on the same retinal points. This happens with the light rebounding from the surfaces of all objects, whatever their reflective properties.

In the everyday situation, moreover, we find that additive light mixture occurs when a given object reflects not only the light of the primary source but the light that reaches it from adjacent colored stimuli as well. Thus in a situation where we have objects, papers, and books on our desks, illuminated by incandescent light, additive light mixture also occurs on the retina when the light reflected from the items on the desk mixes with the light reflected from the colored wall surfaces.

It is because of additive light mixture of the sort just described that a yellow flower picked in an open field in daylight illumination will take on an orange cast when we hold it near the red brick wall of a building. In this situation not only are mid- and long-wavelength rays reflected to the eye from the flower itself, but in addition there are long-wavelength radiations from the brick that the flower "picks up," and they are also reflected from the flower to the eye. The additive mixture gives us reddish yellow.

There are other situations in our everyday lives where we encounter additive light mixture. It is not uncommon to see ourselves reflected from a window pane in a store window display. When in a bus or train, what we see outside the window next to us is combined with reflections of objects or people from inside. We see mixtures also in viewing performers in stage productions that make use of spotlights and footlights.

Still another sort of mixture, which we might call "space-dependent," is the additive mixture that occurs when we view mosaics, pointillist paintings, and colored printed materials that are made up of very small juxtaposed spots or lines of different color. The small colored elements are too small to be resolved by the retinal grain at large distances, and taken together with small eye movements we get overlapping stimulation of the same retinal elements by the different light components (Plate 8-2).

We also encounter light mixture when viewing movies and television screens. In the latter situation the various phosphors on the cathode ray tube are excited briefly and sequentially by a scanning electron beam. These mixture situations are both space- and time-dependent.

The major point I want to make now is that *all* colors can be matched (i.e., generated) by the intermixture of *three* appropriately selected stimuli. For this discussion I shall return to the laboratory-type situation where spectral lights* are used in the mixture experiments and first discuss hue matches. Complete color matches will be covered in Chapter 9.

The hue of an intermixture of two wavelengths clearly depends both on the hues evoked by the stimuli considered individually and the relative stimulus energies of the two stimuli when they are intermixed. We discussed in Chapter 6 the use of pairs of spectral stimuli to produce unique hues.

We can mix pairs of stimuli taken arbitrarily from any spectral region. Consider, for example, a mixture of 590 nm and 570 nm. Viewed alone, 590 nm evokes a reddish-yellow hue and 570 nm evokes a greenish-yellow hue. By intermixing these two wavelengths and varying their relative energies, we can produce a variety of results. We can produce a reddish-yellow, a yellow, or a greenish-yellow mixture result. In fact, if a 580-nm stimulus is imaged in one half of a circular split field, and 590 plus 570 nm in the other half, we can vary the relative amounts of 590 nm and 570 nm to achieve a perfect hue match for the hue evoked by 580 nm alone. When this occurs it is, as we now know, because the antagonistic red and green processes evoked by 590 nm and 570 nm, respectively, are in balance. But both the 590-nm and 570-nm stimuli excite precisely the same yellow process that 580 nm excites by itself. We are dealing here again with the bucking or cancellation principle.

We can repeat this experiment with different stimulus combinations and move off to short- and long-wavelength directions with each of the

* Broad-band distributions may be used for these mixture experiments, as well as spectral lights (see Chapter 9).

individual stimuli, as noted in Chapter 6. Thus 550- and 610-nm stimuli also permit us to obtain a yellow that matches the hue of the 580-nm field; 540 and 630 nm will act in the same way, as will 540 and 670 nm. The red evoked by 670 nm can be balanced by the green evoked by 540 nm and the yellow remainder is the hue equivalent of the yellow of 580 nm.*

Note also that the hue associated with any other stimulus wavelength that lies between 540 and 670 nm can also be matched by properly adjusting the relative energies of the two mixture stimuli. If the stimulus to be matched is 650 nm rather than 580 nm and looks yellow-red rather than yellow, more of the 670 nm stimulus will have to be used in the mixture with 540 nm. If the stimulus to be matched is 560 nm rather than 580 nm, more of the 540-nm test stimulus will be needed; and so on.

If we now consider the situation for stimuli below 540 nm, we find that it is comparable in principle to the one just discussed. A wavelength of 540 nm evokes a yellowish-green hue; if we now use a 440-nm stimulus (which evokes a reddish-blue hue by itself) rather than 670 nm, we can duplicate the hues of all intermediate wavelengths from 440 nm to 540 nm by appropriate mixtures of 440 nm and 540 nm. The blue-reds of the shorter-wavelength lights are matched by using proportionately greater amounts of 440 nm and the yellow-greens by using proportionately greater amounts of the 540 nm stimulus. If the intermediate stimulus is 475 nm and blue, it is matched when the red and green systems are in balance, and the small amount of yellow that 540 nm evokes is balanced by a small amount of blue from the 440-nm stimulus.

Since it is true that any spectral stimulus beyond 650 nm can be matched in hue by 650 nm and that the hues evoked by the stimuli below 440 nm are also matchable by 440 nm, our analysis shows us why the hue of *any* spectral stimulus can be matched by the appropriate manipulation of three (and only three) mixture stimuli, say, 440, 540, and 650 nm. Three vertical lines corresponding to these wavelengths are superimposed on the chromatic response functions in Figure 4 to show their spectral loci relative to the response curves. Plate 8-3 illustrates in a gross way the perceptual outcome of such mixtures. The specific outcomes depend on the proportions in which the mixture stimuli are combined. In this schematic figure we cannot, of course, represent all possible outcomes.

In any given instance we are simply "juggling" the amounts of any one or two of the mixture stimuli to equate the perceived hue with that of a selected spectral stimulus. If the spectral stimulus is 440 nm or less, the reddish-blue 440-nm "primary" can be adjusted to match any wavelengths in this series. If the spectral stimuli lie between 440 and 540 nm

* See Chapter 16 for a discussion of the Nagel anomaloscope, an instrument that uses wavelengths close to these to diagnose various color-vision anomalies.

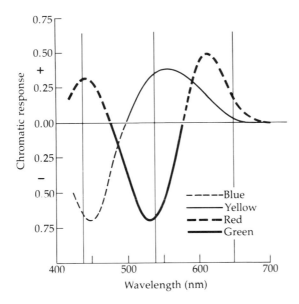

4 ALL SPECTRAL HUES can be matched with appropriate combinations of the three stimuli shown in the figure: 440, 540, and 650 nm. Other stimulus combinations that fulfill the requirements discussed in the text may also be used.

and vary from a red-blue to blue-green to green to a yellow-green, then, depending on the wavelength selected, appropriate intermixtures of the 440- and 540-nm primaries enable us to make a hue match. If the spectral stimulus lies between 540 and 650 nm and appears as a green-yellow, yellow, or red-yellow, it can be matched in hue by adjusting the two primaries 540 and 650 nm. Stimuli beyond 650 to 700 nm are yellow-reds and can be matched in hue by varying the amount of the 650-nm mixture stimulus.

We have seen that the color appearance of the spectrum ranges from the short-wavelength violets to the long-wavelength reds, which still retain traces of yellow. We have already noted that there are three spectral stimuli that are unique in hue [i.e., blue (no red or green), green (no blue or yellow, and yellow (no green or red)]. There is no spectral stimulus, however, that is uniquely red, since short-wavelength stimuli that are red are also blue and long-wavelength stimuli that are red are also yellow. If we intermix the blue-red short-wavelength 440-nm stimulus with the 650-nm yellow-red long-wavelength stimulus, we obtain a variety of hues that range from blue-reds to yellow-reds, depending on the mixture ratio. But we can carefully adjust the ratio of the two stimuli so that in this series of "extraspectral purples" we can produce a red that contains neither yellow nor blue, as we have already noted. This red has a quality that is sometimes seen in the pale reds of neon advertising signs. With appropriate amounts of the red-blue-, green-yellow-, and red-yellow-appearing stimuli, we can also produce an achromatic white-appearing field.

I have been using 440, 540, and 650 nm as the three mixture stimuli in these examples of spectral hue matching. The use of these particular stimuli is quite arbitrary. An indefinite number of stimulus triads might be used. We could use 450, 550, or 640; or 445, 550, and 630 nm; or 460, 530, and 655 nm; and so on. If we limit ourselves to three arbitrarily selected spectral stimuli for matching the hues evoked by any spectral stimuli, we must fulfill one basic condition. We must be certain that the set of mixture stimuli that we choose makes available to us all the hues when they are used separately or in combination.

Were we to select the three unique stimuli 480, 500, and 580 nm, which evoke the unique hues, blue, green, and yellow, respectively, we could get matches for spectral stimuli that are blue, blue-green, green, yellow-green, and yellow. But how could we match the stimuli from the spectral extremes? There would be no possibility with this triplex of stimuli of obtaining any blue-reds or yellow-reds. Note also that if we were working with two complementary stimuli, 580 nm (yellow) and 480 nm (blue), as primaries, we have eliminated the possibility of matching extra-spectral purples (red-blues)—assuming that one of our interests is to match, not only the hues of spectral stimuli but also hues of various broad-band distributions, among them the purples. If, on the other hand, we chose 475 nm (unique blue), 580 nm (unique yellow), and 650 nm (yellow-red) as our stimulus triad, we have no possibility of generating greens. An additional restriction on the general statement that we can choose any arbitrary three stimuli is that we should not select as one of our mixture stimuli a light that can be matched by a mixture of the other two. Such a stimulus would be redundant and would add nothing to our color-matching capabilities. In fact, it constitutes the loss of a necessary mixture stimulus. Were we to select, for example, 500 nm (green), 550 nm (yellow-green), and 600 nm (yellow-red) as the mixture stimuli, the hue evoked by 550 nm is achievable by mixtures of the 500- and 600-nm stimuli. We have gained nothing and lost the possibility of selecting a stimulus that would provide us with blue excitation.

Thus three properly selected stimuli enable us to match any spectral stimulus in *hue*. Nor are we limited to matching only *spectral hues*. We can match the hue of any colored sample regardless of its physical light distribution, since the same hue can be generated by an indefinite number of different physical distributions. What we are matching to is some common physiological state basic to the given hue experience.

In Chapter 9 we continue to discuss additive color mixture but concentrate on complete color matches, that is, matches for hue, saturation, and brightness rather than for hue alone. But first, let us look closely at the difference between subtractive and additive color mixtures, since this distinction tends to cause unnecessary difficulties.

Most of us have used paints or color pigments at some time often starting in our childhood, and have learned from our experience with colored paints that when we intermix the pigment "primaries," blue-green (cyan), blue-red (magenta), and yellow, the results are not those shown in Plate 8-3, because mixing yellow and cyan pigments or watercolors gives us green colors; yellow and blue-red (magenta), reds; and blue-red and green-blue, blues. When all three are intermixed, the yellow, magenta, and cyan pigments produce a black appearance. To get "white," the background surface is generally left unpainted (Plate 8-4).

The three pigment primaries, are, of course, the basic mixture components used in painting, printed color reproductions, and color photography (see Chapter 21). What is the meaning of this? Do these rules of SUBTRACTIVE COLOR MIXTURE for colorant materials affect in any way what we have been saying about additive color mixture? Fortunately, there is no contradiction between the results of subtractive pigment mixture and additive light mixture.

The basic fact that we need to remember is that the color experience is intimately associated with those frequencies (or wavelengths) of light that impinge on the retina. Thus if a pigment that reflects wavelengths of light that evoke a yellow is intermixed with a pigment that reflects short wavelengths that look blue and the resulting experience is green, we should ask ourselves whether there may not be something about this situation whereby only midspectral wavelengths of light are finally striking the retina. If it is true that only midspectral light impinges on the retina in such a situation, the result is as expected; the visual experience should be green. This is, in fact, the case.

Consider the filter situation shown in Plate 8-5. Sunlight is dispersed by the spectrum and we see the entire spectrum at A. By interposing a filter at this point with a short-wavelength cutoff, we see the spectrum from 490 to 700—greens, yellow-greens, yellows, orange, reds, and so on. Now let us remove the first filter and interpose a second filter at A. This has a long-wavelength cutoff and we see colors from 400 to 550 nm: blue-reds, blues, blue-greens, greens, and yellow-greens. Now let us place one behind the other: one filter at A, the other at B. The long-wavelength pass filter and short-wavelength pass filter in combination only permit wavelengths from 490 to 550 to reach the eye. Those of maximal energy are at 525 nm, say. The crosshatched area of Figure 5 shows the ultimate wavelength distribution reaching the eye. Not surprisingly, we see green. All

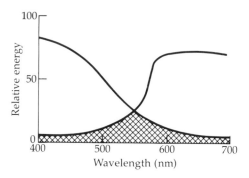

5 RELATIVE SPECTRAL LIGHT TRANSMITTANCES of appropriately selected yellow- and blue-appearing filters indicate that only the midspectral light (crosshatched area) is not selectively absorbed by the two overlapping filters.

that now remains to point out is that the pigment particles that constitute paints and dyes and other colorant materials behave essentially like filters. A yellow pigment is one that traps within its material particles all short-wavelength light rays and reflects midspectral long-wavelength light rays; therefore, we see it as yellow. A blue-appearing pigment absorbs all long wavelengths. Since the yellow pigment traps the short wavelengths and the blue pigment traps the long wavelengths, when these two pigments are intermixed, only the midspectral-band light rays can emerge to be reflected toward the observer's eye, and these midspectral rays are, as is to be expected, seen as green.

There is, in summary, no basic contradiction. What is seen depends upon the light rays impinging on the eye and retina. When we are able to work directly with light rays, their intermixture can produce a total hue gamut with a minimum of three properly selected stimuli; if we work with pigments, paints, and dyes, because of their absorptive properties and the way they reflect light rays, a complete gamut of hues can be produced from the usual set of three primaries, which are magenta, cyan, and yellow in appearance.

Background Readings

Jameson, D., and Hurvich, L. M. 1955. Some quantitative aspects of an opponent-colors theory. I. Chromatic responses and spectral saturation. *J. Opt. Soc. Amer.* 45: 546–552.

Rood, O. N. 1879. *Modern Chromatics,* Chaps. 10 and 11, pp. 124–180. D. Appleton, New York. [Reprinted 1973 with supplements, F. Birren (ed.). Van Nostrand Reinhold, New York.]

Southall, J. P. C. 1937. *Introduction to Physiological Optics,* Chap. 8. Oxford University Press, London.

Trendelenburg, W. 1961. *Der Gesichtssinn,* 2nd ed. Chap. 2, Sec. B and C, pp. 76–96. M. Monjé, I. Schmidt, and E. Schütz, (eds.). Springer-Verlag, Berlin.

9

Additive Color Mixture: Complete Matches

WITH three properly selected spectral stimuli, it is possible to match the hue of any perceived color. The three stimuli, for that matter, do not need to be spectral; three appropriately selected broad-band stimuli made up of reddish-yellow, greenish-yellow, and reddish-blue filters, used together with a light source such as daylight or incandescent light, can be intermixed—two stimuli at a time—to match any hue that we see.

So far, we have emphasized hue matching, but we can also match the brightness of any test light with the same three matching stimuli. If the combined matching stimuli appear too bright relative to the test stimulus, we can simply reduce their energies relative to that of the test stimulus. Conversely, if the test stimulus is brighter, we can raise the energy level of the matching stimuli. We can, for that matter, vary the test-stimulus energy to produce the brightness match.

Will we have achieved a complete or perfect match for the spectral test light when we have intermixed and adjusted the individual primaries, as required for a hue and brightness equation, to a given spectral light? Very likely not. How would the test and mixture fields differ in appearance? The test field with a narrow-band stimulus will in all probability look more saturated than will the mixture field produced with the variable primaries. The discussions in Chapters 5, 6, and 7 of the way single narrow-band stimuli excite the achromatic as well as chromatic mechanisms simultaneously and of why broad-band stimuli are more desaturated than are narrow-band ones have anticipated this point. We must now consider how we go about obtaining complete matches between the two half-fields.

Let us consider a specific case. Suppose that we have set out to match a test field provided by 510 nm in one half of a bipartite field with a mixture of the spectral primaries 460, 530, and 650 nm in the other half. If we examine the chromatic and achromatic response functions of Figure 15 in Chapter 5, we see that for a unit of energy, the wavelength 510 nm excites the red/green system to an amount = −0.41 red (i.e., green), the yellow/blue system to an amount = +0.10 yellow (i.e., yellow), and white to an amount = +0.50. Let us start by placing a unit amount of the 530-nm primary in the mixture side of the bipartite field. The chromatic and achromatic values associated with this stimulus are −0.66 red, +0.25 yellow, and +0.99 white. These values say that the 530-nm primary is a bit more green and considerably yellower and whiter than the 510-nm stimulus we are trying to match. To make the comparison field less green and less yellow, we can intermix with the first primary, 530 nm, some of the 460-nm primary which generates −Y (blue) activity, and +R (red) excitation and a small amount of white per unit energy. By adding blue-ness and redness, we cancel the excessive yellow and green excitations generated by the 530-nm primary. This is what we want to do, but un-fortunately the mixture of the two primaries also increases the whiteness. In fact, 530 nm by itself produces more white than does 510 nm, the test stimulus. Shall we now add the 650-nm primary to the mixture of the two primaries already intermixed in an effort to match the spectral wavelength 510 nm? This will add even more undesired redness and whiteness and obviously take us still further from our goal of a perfect match. We will only succeed in making the mixture of primaries redder, yellower, and whiter, as a reading of the response-function graph shows.

There is an alternative. What if we add the 650-nm primary to the 510-nm test stimulus instead of to the field containing the other two primaries? This gives us the necessary white excitation for the test field that we need to balance the white excitation produced by the mixture of the 460- and 530-nm primaries and it also introduces a little red to cancel the excess of green that 510 nm has (compared to the mixture of the 460-nm and 530-nm primaries). Admittedly, this procedure brings in even more yellow on the test side of the field, but we can balance this either by increasing the relative amount of the midspectral 530-nm primary or by decreasing the amount of the short-wavelength 460-nm primary.

This rough account of a single match is intended to show that a complete color equation is achieved only when we have balanced the achromatic as well as the chromatic excitations. The stimulus manipula-tions may seem complicated, but the analysis emphasizes that what we are achieving in a complete color match is a match of the hue, brightness, and saturation of the test field with the hue, brightness, and saturation of the comparison field. For complete color matching throughout the spec-trum, three primaries are necessary (and sufficient), and the hues, bright-nesses, and saturations of the matching fields are equated by adjusting the proportions of the three primaries as required. In many instances this requires that we move one of the primaries to the test-stimulus side to achieve the complete match. Given four lights, one test and three primaries, depending on the test light, a match can be achieved by a single primary, combinations of two of them, or occasionally by the addition of one primary to the test light in order to match the combination of the other two primaries.

When we analyze complete color matches in relation to the chromatic and achromatic excitations, we are not limited to approximate descriptive accounts of the sort just given. The chromatic and achromatic equivalences of the complete color-matching situation can be restated in a precise quantitative fashion in stimulus terms to tell us how much of each of the three spectral primaries is required for each match to a spectral test stimulus. The results of such an analysis are shown in Figure 1.

The curves labeled H and J are two separate sets of color-mixture curves derived by calculations based on the experimentally measured chromatic and achromatic response functions of two observers. The data for one observer (J) are shown in Figure 15 in Chapter 5. To obtain these sets of color-mixture curves from the response functions, we have selected three arbitrary primaries and calculated the ratios in which they have to

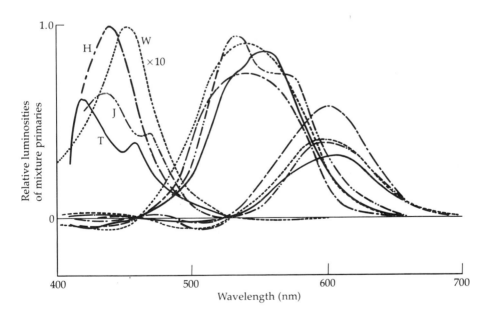

1 COLOR-MIXTURE FUNCTIONS for two observers, H and J. These color-mixture functions are computed ones based on an arithmetical transformation of the chromatic and achromatic response curve of these two individuals, assuming that the mixture primaries are 460, 530, and 640 nm. The two additional sets of curves identified by the symbols T and W are color-mixture functions determined directly with the use of these three stimulus primaries.

be mixed to match the red (or green), yellow (or blue), and white values of the visual response to any single wavelength of unit energy.

For the primaries 460, 530 and 650 nm used in this example, we know from Figure 15 in Chapter 5 how much red or green, yellow or blue, and white a unit of energy from each of these primaries provides. If the chromatic response to a given primary light is green, we remember that this green is equivalent to $-R$; if it is blue, we read it as $-Y$. We can also read from the same graph the R, Y, and Wh (or $-R$, $-Y$, and Wh) values of the test stimulus of interest. Our aim is to determine how much energy we need from the 460-, 530-, and 650-nm primaries to match the test stimulus. We can write three equations, where a, b, and c represent the unknown energies of 460, 530, and 650 nm as follows:

$$a(R_{460}) + b(R_{530}) + c(R_{650}) = R_\lambda$$
$$a(Y_{460}) + b(Y_{530}) + c(Y_{650}) = Y_\lambda$$
$$a(Wh_{460}) + b(Wh_{530}) + c(Wh_{650}) = Wh_\lambda$$

In these three equations everything is known except the energy amounts a, b, and c of the three primaries, 460, 530, and 650 nm. Solving these three simultaneous equations for the three unknowns a, b, and c gives us a color-mixture equation of the form

$$a_{460} + b_{530} + c_{650} = 1_\lambda.$$

These color-mixture curves are expressed in energy units. In the form shown in Figure 1, the curves are shown in relative light units (photometric units) which take into account the sensitivity of the eye at different wavelengths in the spectrum. (See Chapter 5 for a discussion of the whiteness or spectral luminosity function.)

Two additional sets of color-mixture functions are also shown in Figure 1. These are not indirectly derived color-mixture functions; they are not based on computations using chromatic and achromatic response functions. They are, in fact, based on actual laboratory measurements for two different individuals (T and W). To obtain these functions three spectral-light primaries, 460, 530, and 650 nm, were used to match a series of spectral-light stimuli. Since these real stimuli affect the chromatic and achromatic responses in the way shown in the computational analysis, it should come as no surprise that the experimental data for these two observers have the same general forms as those calculated for two different observers.

Color-mixture experiments of this sort are as old as the science of color. They date back to Newton's color-mixture experiments of about 300 years ago, and color matches have been redetermined with refined apparatus and with ever-increasing precision of measurement by many famous researchers. Maxwell's early apparatus is sketched in Figure 2. A much improved color-mixture apparatus was designed and used by W. D. Wright and his students to provide color-mixture data that became standard. An advanced trichromator, used to extend the standard, was designed by W. S. Stiles and is shown in Figure 3.

In Figure 4 the data obtained in a number of different investigations are shown in energy terms, and in Figure 5 some additional functions are shown expressed in relative light units. The latter are directly comparable to the data of Wright and Thomson included in Figure 1. The color-mixture data can also be presented in percentage terms and a set of such functions is shown in Figure 6.

The three primary-mixture stimuli used in the experiment that measured the color-mixture curves directly were 460, 530, and 650 nm. If we want to know in percentage terms how much of each of these primaries is needed to match a given wavelength, we need only locate the wave-

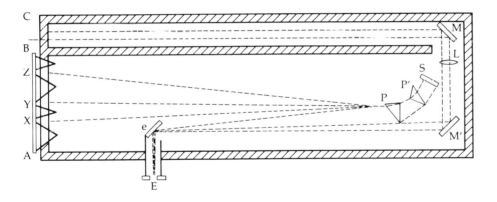

2 MAXWELL'S COLOR-MIXING APPARATUS. This apparatus, as built in 1856, was about 3½ feet long by 1 foot wide. In Maxwell's procedure all color matches were made by mixing combinations of spectral lights to match white light. The entrance slits at X, Y, and Z were adjustable both in their relative positions and widths. They were connected by hinged shutters that blocked off unwanted light. A large board covered with paper that is nonselective for wavelength was placed at the left end of the tube to reflect sunlight into the entrance slits. Two 45-degree prisms, P and P', were used and the dispersed light reflected back in a slightly displaced position through the prisms from a concave silvered mirror S. After another reflection at e, the light reaches the slit at E, where the eye is placed. The comparison white source entering between CB is reflected from mirrors M, M', and e and is seen next to the mixture colors. Maxwell used 630, 528, and 457 nm as his primaries. Matches were made to white with these three wavelengths and with a variable wavelength used in conjunction with two of the three primaries. Since the white standard was common to all matches, the spectral-color-mixture functions are derivable by simple arithmetic computations.

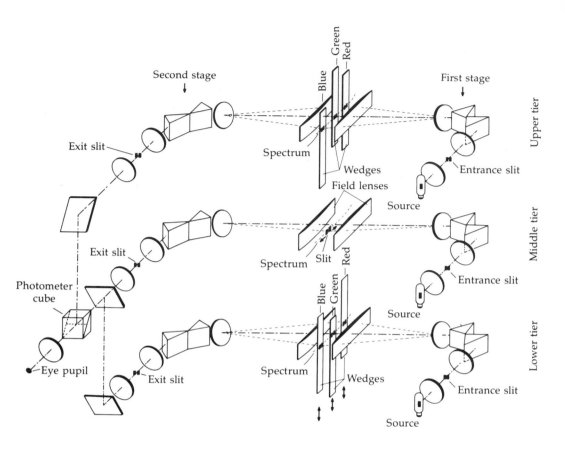

3 STILES'S COLOR-MIXING APPARATUS. This is the most recent apparatus used in color-mixture experiments. The optical system is arranged in three tiers and the entire apparatus occupies a small room. Three double monochromators are mounted vertically in the three tiers. In each case a spectrum is formed centrally. The stimuli selected from each spectrum can be recombined by the second dispersing stage to enable one to mix the selected stimuli at each exit slit as necessary. (This is a zero-dispersion system.) The central tier provides the monochromatic test light, the upper tier the three monochromatic matching stimuli, and the lower tier the desaturating stimulus that is mixed with the test stimulus. Wedges adjusted vertically control the light intensities. The beams from the top and bottom tiers are reflected into the photometer cube and the three exit slits are imaged at a common point in space. The observer sees a bipartite field, one half made up of the test field (with desaturant light as required) and the other half made up of the variable mixture stimuli.

length on the abscissa, erect a perpendicular line at that point, and read off on the ordinate the percentage of each stimulus that enters into the mixture. Thus to match 460 nm we need 100 percent of the 460-nm primary and zero amounts of the other two primaries. The same is true of the two other spectral stimuli, 530 nm and 650 nm. They, too, are matched by 100

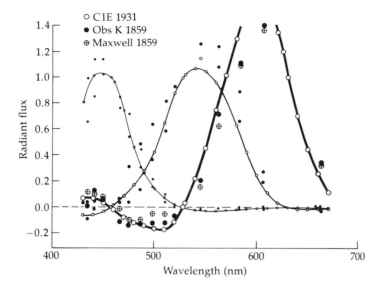

4 COLOR-MIXTURE FUNCTIONS shown in energy terms for different experiments. The three primaries are 456.9, 528.1, and 630.2 nm and show the amounts of each necessary to match a unit of energy at the various wavelengths. Observer K and Maxwell were measured in Maxwell's apparatus; the data plotted as open circles are for the 1931 CIE standard (average) observer.

percent of a single primary and zero amounts of the other two primaries. If we look now at wavelength 630 nm, for example, we see that it is matched by approximately 80 percent of the long-wavelength primary 650 nm and 20 percent of the midwave primary 530 nm. Nearly zero amount of 460 nm is needed. But now let us look at the spectral region

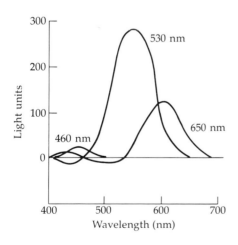

5 COLOR-MIXTURE FUNCTIONS like those in Figure 1 are plotted here in relative light (photometric) terms rather than energy. The short-wavelength function shown here is not multiplied by an arbitrary factor as in Figure 1.

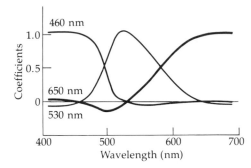

6 COLOR-MIXTURE FUNCTIONS shown in relative or percentage values.

between 500 and 530 nm—at 510 nm in particular. To match the 510-nm stimulus it appears that positive amounts of the 460- and 530-nm stimuli are mixed with what looks like a negative amount of the 650-nm stimulus. Note that negative amounts of the 530-nm primary are also evident at the short- and long-wavelength spectral extremes and negative amounts of the 460-nm stimulus are evident beyond about 530 nm.

The occurrence of a negative primary value would seem absurd if we had not already analyzed the experiment in perceptual terms. (Negative values appear in the functions in Figures 5 and 6.) What does it mean to say that a 510-nm stimulus is matched by a mixture of 97 percent of 530 nm plus 15 percent of 460 nm and a negative amount of 12 percent of the long-wavelength stimulus, 650 nm? What can we possibly mean by a negative stimulus percentage? This is not, of course, as absurd as it seems to some on first glance, nor is it as complicated as it appears at first. The meaning of negative values in color-mixture experiments can be understood either in perceptual terms or by analyzing color equations as equivalent in principle to simple algebraic equations.*

In the analysis in perceptual terms at the beginning of this chapter for a match to a 510-nm stimulus field with the three primaries, 460, 530, and 650 nm, we noted that chromatic and achromatic equivalences had to be achieved. This could be done but only by moving the 650-nm primary and mixing it with the 510-nm test field to dilute the latter and make it look "whiter." The computed color-mixture functions of Figure 1 based on the chromatic and achromatic functions express this fact in quantitative stimulus terms. The 650-nm stimulus is calculated to have a negative value at the 510-nm spectral locus.

The direct experimental measures make the same point: in order to

* Color mixture and color matches can also be analyzed mathematically in vector terms. Vectors are quantities that have both magnitude and direction. The magnitude is represented by the length of a line segment and the direction by the orientation of the line. Vectors combine according to certain rules of addition.

achieve a complete color match in certain spectral regions, one of the primaries has to be intermixed with the test light. Clearly, this additive intermixture changes the appearance of the test light that is being matched.

In color matching, however, there is no direct concern with the appearances of the spectral stimuli, either test or primaries; what is sought are the stimulus-mixture proportions of the primaries that produce an exact match to the test stimulus.

The color matches are recorded from this point of view in "shorthand" algebraic expressions such as

$$q(D) \equiv u(A) + v(B) + w(C)$$

The symbols (A), (B), (C), and (D) merely identify lights: (D) could be any spectral wavelength; (A), (B), and (C) are the arbitrarily selected primaries, and q, u, v, and w are amounts of radiation. By convention the sign $=$ is taken to mean "matches" or "is matched by." It is not a literal equality sign but can be treated as an equality sign, as in any simple algebraic equation.

We know the way simple algebraic equations behave. For example, if we have an equality between four values u, v, w, and q, such that $u + v = w + q$, we know that if we add some value z to both sides of the equation so that

$$u + v + z = w + q + z$$

the equality remains unaffected. Since $u + v = w + q$, we can remove or subtract them from both sides of the equation and the equality remains

$$z = z$$

We can multiply both sides of such a simple equation by a common factor, and the equality remains

$$2(u + v) = 2(w + q)$$

Each of these equalities remains unaffected if we subtract equals or add equals to both sides or if we multiply both sides of the initial equality by the same amount.

The same is true of color equations or matches. Regardless of the stimulus components that form the basis for the initial match, if in the laboratory we add equal amounts of the same light to both sides of the equation, we do not upset it; if we have made a match between two different sets of stimuli, we can add these matching stimuli to the original match without upsetting it; and we can double or triple the amounts of the matching lights on both sides of the light equation without upsetting it (which is equivalent to the multiplication operation).

Thus to take a simple addition example: if

$$q_1(D)_1 \equiv u_1(A) + v_1(B) + w_1(C)$$

and

$$q_2(D)_2 \equiv u_2(A) + v_2(B) + w_2(C)$$

where q_1 and q_2 are the amounts of the D_1 and D_2 stimuli to which the three primaries are matched, the resultant is

$$q_1(D)_1 + q_2(D)_2 \equiv u_3(A) + v_3(B) + w_3(C)$$

where

$$u_3 = u_1 + u_2$$
$$v_3 = v_1 + v_2$$
$$w_3 = w_1 + w_2$$

Thus, if D_1 is a yellow-red of 640 nm and is matched by appropriate amounts of three primaries, 460, 530, and 650 nm, and D_2 is a green-blue of 490 nm matched by different appropriate amounts of the same three primaries, then adding the 490-nm stimulus to the 640-nm stimulus in one half of the split field; and the second combination of the three primaries to the first combination of them, in the other half-field, will leave us with the fields matched. The match remains a match but the appearance of the matched fields will, of course, change.

The fact that lights behave this way is sometimes referred to as the RULES OF COLOR ARITHMETIC and the rules themselves are often called GRASSMANN'S LAWS OF COLOR MIXTURE, after the eminent German mathematician who systematically stated them.

We know from elementary algebra that if

$$q = u + v - w$$

then by simple transposition it is also true that

$$q + w = u + v$$

Since color equations behave like elemental algebraic equations, then if

$$q(D) \equiv u(A) + v(B) - w(C)$$

it must also be true that

$$q(D) + w(C) \equiv u(A) + v(B)$$

Thus the stimulus primary enters the additive color-mixture equation as a minus value if it has to be added to the test stimulus to effect the match. This is the meaning of a negative primary value.

Hue matches throughout the spectrum can be made, as we saw, by appropriate combinations of three arbitrarily selected primaries. Complete color matches also require three primaries, and they too can be arbitrarily selected within the limits previously noted (i.e., no two of them should be complementary, etc.). Since each spectral stimulus is specifiable by linear combinations of amounts of three others acting as primaries, it is possible to show by simple algebraic computation that any spectral stimulus can be substituted as a primary for any one of the three originally selected.

If a series of spectral lights is matched with the three primaries 460, 530, and 650 nm, we have as examples the following color equations:

$$q_1 670 \equiv u_1 460 + v_1 530 + w_1 650$$
$$q_2 610 \equiv u_2 460 + v_2 530 + w_2 650$$
$$q_3 590 \equiv u_3 460 + v_3 530 + w_3 650$$
$$q_4 550 \equiv u_4 460 + v_4 530 + w_4 650$$
$$q_5 480 \equiv u_5 460 + v_5 530 + w_5 650$$
$$q_6 410 \equiv u_6 460 + v_6 530 + w_6 650$$

If we elect to restate these equations with 460 and 530 nm as primaries and 610 nm instead of 650 nm as the third primary, since

$$q_2 610 \equiv u_2 460 + v_2 530 + w_2 650$$

it follows by simple arithmetic that

$$w_2 650 \equiv q_2 610 - u_2 460 - v_2 530$$

By simple substitution we can then write in, say, the first equation given above,

$$q_1 670 \equiv u_1 460 + v_1 530 + (q_2 610 - u_2 460 - v_2 530)$$

or

$$q_1 670 \equiv (u_1 - u_2)460 + (v_1 - v_2)530 + q_2 610$$

Matches to each spectral light can be restated in terms of 460, 530, and 610 nm. By proceeding in a similar fashion, we can substitute for 460 nm and 530 nm any other primaries we choose. Color-mixture equations using different sets of primaries are said to be LINEAR TRANSFORMATIONS of one another.

One set of transformed functions is particularly noteworthy. In order to eliminate negative values from the color-mixture functions, three "unreal" primaries are assumed for calculating them. These CIE (Commission International de l'Éclairage) functions are used by international agreement as the color-mixture curves for the "standard observer" (see Figure 7 in Chapter 20). They are in wide use in the colorimetric specification of stimuli and are discussed in Chapter 20.

Since our discussion has shown us that different stimuli that look alike imply equalities of chromatic and achromatic responses—a common physiological state—the various laws of color mixture—that equals subtracted from equals remain equal, equals added to equals remain equal, and equals multiplied by a common factor remain equal*—have a certain obviousness about them. If we have a common physiological state that correlates with a given visual experience, it makes no difference to the identity of the appearance of the color match that this physiological state is changed in exactly the same way by different stimuli or combinations of stimuli. Once an equality has been established between the response relations that underlie the comparison and test fields, modifying the response mechanisms in precisely the same way maintains the equality. To echo Gertrude Stein's statement about the rose: a match is a match is a match.

METAMERIC COLOR MATCHES, color equations between lights of different spectral distributions, are also stable or invariant with changes in chromatic adaptation at normal daylight light levels. If a color match is made between different stimuli in two halves of a split field for a neutral state of adaptation (see Chapter 15), the color match will persist regardless of the way we change the state of adaptation of the eye, provided only that the change is the same for all stimulated parts of the retina. For example, if a complete color equation is made between the stimulus wavelength 580 nm in the test field and an appropriate mixture of the two stimulus wavelengths 540 nm and 670 nm in the comparison field, this match is not upset if the observer's adaptive state becomes nonneutral.†

Thus, if an observer sets a color match in a neutral condition of adaptation and then exposes his eyes to a red-appearing adapting field, on reexamining the equation he will judge it still to be a match. This is also true if we use a green-appearing adaptation field before reexamining the initial equation. However, something does change: the *appearance* of the matched fields. After the adaptation to long-wavelength "red" light, the matched fields continue to match, but now they both look yellow-green rather than yellow. After "green" adaptation the match also persists, but both fields now look yellow-red rather than yellow.

Color equations can be expressed as equalities between stimulus quantities; they can also be expressed as equalities between neural response systems. Since photopigment absorbances link the stimulus quan-

---

* This is equivalent, as noted, to raising or lowering the energy of the matching fields by equal amounts.

† In these instances spectral lights are imaged directly on the retina. Metameric color matches are also obtainable with objects of different reflectances illuminated by the same light source (see Chapters 15, 17, and 20).

tities and the neural responses, it is not surprising that color equations can also be expressed as equalities between photopigment absorbances. For an explanation of the persistence of color matches with changes in adaptation (Chapter 15), it becomes necessary first to look at the color-matching problem as an issue of equality of photopigment absorbances. This is done in the next chapter.

Background Readings

Hurvich, L. M., and Jameson, D. 1957. An opponent-process theory of color vision. *Psychol. Rev. 64*: 384–404.

Ishak, I. G. H. 1952. Determination of the tristimulus values of the spectrum for eight Egyptian observers and one British observer. *J. Opt. Soc. Amer. 42*: 844–849.

Judd, D. B. 1966. Fundamental studies of color vision from 1860 to 1960. *Proc. Natl. Acad. Sci. USA 55*: 1313–1330.

Maxwell, J. C. 1860. On the theory of compound colours of the spectrum. *Phil. Trans. R. Soc. Lond. 150*: 57–84. *Scientific Papers,* 1890, Vol. 1, pp. 410–444. Cambridge University Press, Cambridge, England.

Stiles, W. S. 1955. 18th Thomas Young Oration: The basic data of colour-matching. *Phys. Soc. Year Book,* pp. 44–65.

Stiles, W. S., and Burch, J. M. 1959. N.P.L. colour-matching investigation: Final report (1958). *Opt. Acta 6*: 1–26.

Wright, W. D. 1927–1928. A trichromatic colorimeter with spectral primaries. *Trans. Opt. Soc. Lond. 29*: 225–241.

Wright, W. D. 1972. Colour Mixture. In D. Jameson and L. M. Hurvich (eds.), *Handbook of Sensory Physiology,* Vol. 7/4, *Visual Psychophysics,* Chap. 16, pp. 434–454. Springer-Verlag, Berlin.

Wright, W. D., and Pitt, F. H. G. 1935. The colour-vision characteristics of two trichromats. *Proc. Phys. Soc. Lond. 47*: 205–217.

Further Readings

Grassmann, H. 1853. Zur Theorie der Farbenmischung. *Poggendorff Ann. Phys. Chem. 89*: 69–84. (Translation: On the theory of compound colors. *Phil. Mag. 4,* ser. 7: 254–264.)

Hering, E. 1887. Ueber Newton's Gesetz der Farbenmischung (On Newton's law of color mixture). *Lotus, Jahrb. Naturwiss.* new ser. 7: 177–208.

Judd, D. B., and Wyszecki, G. 1975. *Color in Business, Science and Industry,* 3rd ed., Chap. 1, pp. 47–54. Wiley, New York.

Krantz, D. H. 1975. Color measurement and color theory. I. Representation theorem for Grassmann structures. *J. Math. Psychol. 12*: 283–303.

Krantz, D. H. 1975. Color measurement and color theory: Opponent-colors theory. *J. Math. Psychol.* *12*: 304–327.

Pokorny, J., Smith, V. C., and Starr, S. J. 1976. Variability of color mixture data. II. The effect of viewing field size on the unit coordinates. *Vision Res. 16*: 1095–1098.

Smith, V. C., Pokorny, J., and Starr, S. J. 1976. Variability of color mixture data. I. Interobserver variability in the unit coordinates. *Vision Res. 16*: 1087–1094.

Stiles, W. S., and Wyszecki, G. 1974. Colour-matching data and the spectral absorption curves of visual pigments. *Vision Res. 14*: 195–207.

Wyszecki, G., and Stiles, W. S. 1967. *Color Science.* Wiley, New York.

10
Color Mixture and
Cone Photopigments

A BASIC theme of this book is that there exists a correlation between experienced color and certain patterns of neural activity; changes in the neural activity are related to differences in perceived color. The pattern of neural activity may change because various internal physiological changes occur whose origins are unknown, or in response to inappropriate stimuli (see Chapter 2), or, most commonly, because light rays enter the eye and produce these neural changes.

But since light rays do not act directly on the neural tissue, we need to look at the way light first affects the eyes.

The two eyes, roughly spherical in shape, are set in the bony sockets of the head. Six muscles control the movements of each eye and enable us, even with the head fixed, to fixate, at will, over a circular area about 100 degrees in diameter. With its lens system, each eye forms images on its rear surface by focusing the light rays that enter it through the variable iris diaphragm, the pupil. For these reasons the eye is very commonly compared to the ordinary camera, but some people think a panning television camera is a better analogy since the eyes can move in the head to scan a scene. A cross section of the human eye is shown in Figure 1.

The figure shows the front, corneal surface, and the lens, which together form the main part of what is called the DIOPTRIC APPARATUS.* Variations in the thickness of the elastic lens control accommodation and make it possible, together with convergence and divergence movements of the eyes, to bring objects at various distances from the two eyes into focus on corresponding parts of their rear surfaces. The lens, incidentally, is not perfectly transparent to all wavelengths of light and an average relative transmittance curve is shown in Figure 2. As people age, their lenses become yellower in appearance and less and less of the short-wavelength light from light sources and reflecting objects is transmitted to the back of the eye.

* What it does is to bend and focus the light rays that reach it from external objects.

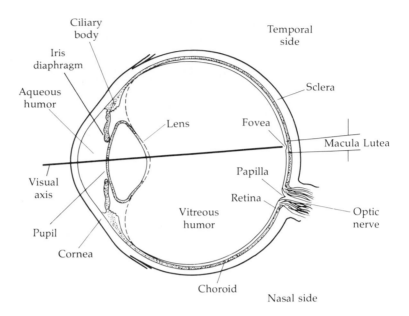

1 HUMAN EYE in horizontal cross section.

We also see in Figure 1 the iris diaphragm, which forms the pupil of the eye. This pupillary aperture is wide open at low light levels and closes down as the illumination increases. It is essentially an automatic control device that can vary the amount of light that enters the eye by a ratio of about 16:1.

At the rear surface of the eye there is a complex network of cells and neurons called the RETINA, a word that derives from the Latin word "rete," meaning "net." The retina is shown in schematic cross section in Figure 3.

There are 10 identifiable layers in this tissue, whose thickness at the equator is only 0.25 mm. There are, of course, blood vessels (not shown in Figure 3) which provide nutritional materials to the retina. They are

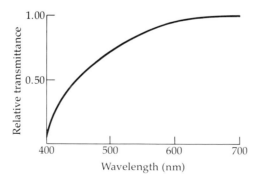

2 RELATIVE OPTICAL TRANSMITTANCE of the average human crystalline lens as a function of wavelength. Value at 700 nm arbitrarily set at unity.

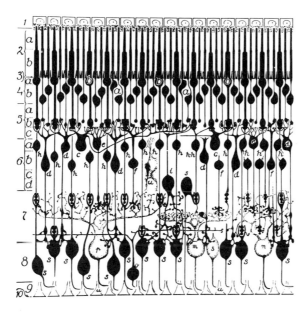

3 PRIMATE RETINA shown in cross section in a schematic diagram. There are ten layers of nerve cells.

mainly located in layers 6, 7, and 8. The light coming through the pupil reaches the receptor cells labeled a and b in layer 2, where it is absorbed only after it traverses all the other layers of transparent visual cells that lie ahead of it. In addition to the neuronal cells, another tissue that lies "ahead" of the photoreceptors in the retina should be mentioned. This is an inert yellow pigment called the MACULA PIGMENT, which diffusely covers an approximately 5-degree elliptical area of the center of the eye and, like the lens, absorbs more of the short-wavelength spectral lights than mid- and long-wavelength lights. An average spectral transmittance curve of this pigment is shown in Figure 4. The amount and distribution

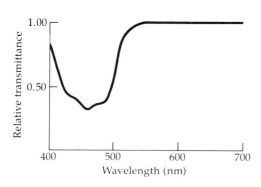

4 MACULAR PIGMENT TRANSMITTANCE as a function of wavelength. Average results. Transmittance is set at a minimum value of 31.7 percent at 457 nm.

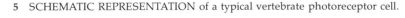

5 SCHEMATIC REPRESENTATION of a typical vertebrate photoreceptor cell.

Outer
segment

Connecting
structure
(Ellipsoid)

Inner
segment
(Myoid)

Fiber

Nucleus

Fiber

Synaptic
body

of this pigment will, of course, affect spectral color matching because it transmits relatively less short-wavelength light. Since it varies in amount from one individual to the next, it accounts for a large amount of the interobserver variability in making such matches. The presence of this built-in filter is not normally detected because we adapt to its presence, but it is seen under special circumstances (see Chapter 15).

It has long been known that there are two types of light-sensitive receptor cells, the RODS and CONES. Figure 5 shows a schematic representation of a typical vertebrate photoreceptor cell. Figure 6 shows the rods

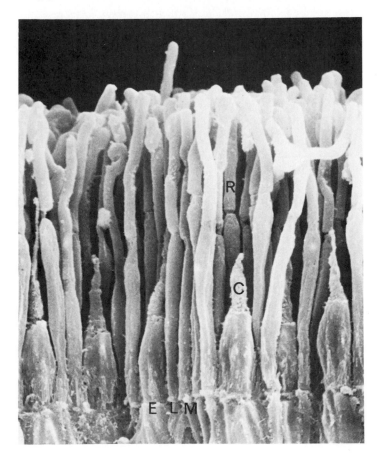

6 ROD AND CONE RECEPTOR ELEMENTS. Scanning electron micrograph of the receptor layer of a vertebrate eye (pig) with rod (R) and cone (C) elements that are very similar to human peripheral rods and cones. The cone inner segment at its widest is about five microns in diameter

and a few cones in the retina of a vertebrate (pig) eye recorded and magnified many thousands of times in a scanning electron micrograph.

The way the densely packed rods and cones—there are estimated to be something like 120 million of them—are distributed varies in different parts of the retina. Figure 7 shows this variation graphically along one meridian. The central region of the retina, called the FOVEA (see Figure 1), which is the region of sharpest vision, subtends a small angle about 1 degree in size and contains cones exclusively.* The cones are primarily concerned with vision at daylight levels of illumination (called the PHO-TOPIC LEVEL), and as we move away from the foveal region of sharpest resolution, the number of cones per unit area drops off sharply (Figure 7). There are thought to be about 6 to 7 million cones in the retina of the human eye. The rods, completely absent from the fovea, increase in number and are interspersed with the cones as we move toward the edge of the eye, the periphery. The rods are most numerous about 20 degrees from the fovea and fall off rapidly in number from this region out to the extreme periphery.

In the rod RECEPTORS, so called because of their shape, there is a photopigment called RHODOPSIN or visual purple. It is now fairly certain that when the molecules of the rhodopsin pigment absorb light quanta,

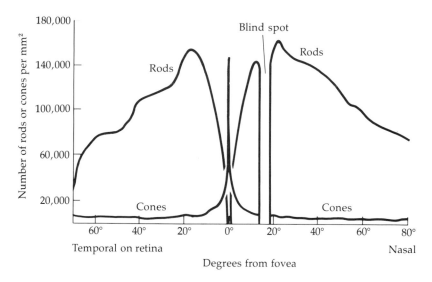

7 ROD AND CONE DISTRIBUTIONS along a horizontal meridian in the human eye.

* For most people, if one arm is held out directly in front and the thumb extended vertically, the nail portion subtends an angular image of about 2 degrees at the eye. The foveal area is thus about half this angle.

these molecules change their structure or form. These changes, in turn, trigger some kind of physicochemical change and there is an accompanying electrical change in the receptor itself. The excitation passes on down from the receptors to the various neural layers (Figure 3). The rods are thought of as most intimately connected with vision at low levels of illumination, called SCOTOPIC VISION.

The absorption spectrum of rhodopsin, the rod pigment, is shown in Figure 8. Such a curve can be described in various ways, but its meaning is that different wavelengths of light are not equally effective in producing molecular changes in rhodopsin. The pigment most effectively absorbs light of 505 nm. Other wavelengths are less effective, since more energy is required to achieve the same result. But the photopigment responds in the same way to all wavelengths: it bleaches. What appears to be a reddish material in the dark becomes pale on exposure to light. The bleaching is related to biochemical changes in the molecular structure of the rhodopsin molecule. The experiments that show this bleaching are done on extractions of the photopigment taken from the eyes of animals such as cattle or frogs.

These chemical changes have been studied with great patience and skill. Much is known about the receptor response to light and dark, but the details are beyond the scope of this book. The bleaching or molecular changes trigger in some as yet not fully understood way the nerve impulses that are necessary for light to be seen. If we measure the number of quanta of different wavelengths required to produce a just detectable flash of light in darkness, there is a very close relation between such a spectral sensitivity curve and the absorption spectrum of rhodopsin (Figure 8). The place in the spectrum where light bleaches rhodopsin with the greatest efficiency (i.e., at 505 nm) is the place where the least light is necessary in order for an individual to detect flashes in the dark. At wavelengths other than 505 nm, the amount of light energy required for vision is greater in a way that is closely related to the efficiency of the "quantum-catching" properties of rhodopsin. This close relation argues for the theory that the initial visual events are related to the photopigment absorption.

The receptors, which contain rhodopsin, seem to be linked to a neural response mechanism that signals gray or white (an achromatic signal) and regardless of which wavelength excites the rhodopsin, when this material absorbs light quanta and excites the nervous tissue "linked" to it, the experience is the same. Therefore, if we look at two different areas, one dimly illuminated with a short wavelength, 450 nm, the other illuminated by 550-nm light, they will look identical if the light level is adjusted so that the same number of quanta are absorbed by the rhodopsin molecules responding to the different wavelengths.

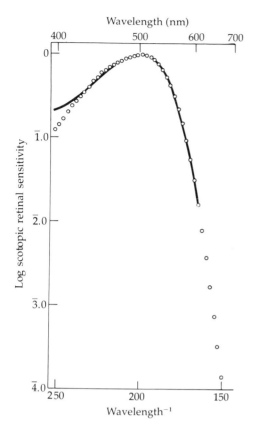

8 ABSORPTION SPECTRUM OF RHO-DOPSIN, the rod pigment, as a function of wavelength. The relative sensitivity of the human eye for the dark-adapted condition is shown by open circles.

But the rods function primarily at low illuminations and are relatively ineffective at light levels associated with color vision.* As we know, the visual receptors that are associated with the perception of light and color at ordinary daylight levels of illumination are the cones. Their name refers to the shape of these elements, even though they look more rodlike at the very center of the retina, the foveola, where they are most densely packed.

Although the rhodopsin of rods has been successfully extracted in solutions for about a hundred years, attempts by biochemists to extract photosensitive materials from the cones have failed. This is largely because in most eyes there are many more rods than cones. As a result, in extraction techniques about 1 percent of the material will come from cones and about 99 percent from rods. Nevertheless, for a long time, almost all researchers have agreed that there are three different kinds of light-sensitive pigments for color vision, and they are generally assumed to be segregated in three different types of cone receptors.

Despite the persistent failure to detect any cone-sensitive materials

---

* Many experiments are now being reported in the literature that demonstrate interactions between the rod and cone systems (see Further Readings).

with extraction techniques, let alone to detect three different kinds of such absorbing materials, why has there been almost universal agreement that three different types of photosensitive material are necessary as the first step in the mediation of color vision? The reason is based on the color-mixture data discussed in Chapter 9.

From the very first theorizing about color vision (Palmer, 1777; Young, 1802) it was recognized that we can see an indefinite number of different hues, even at one retinal location. Physiologically, this would seem to require that at each retinal locus an indefinite number of different kinds of nervous excitations can occur. This seemed to be extremely unlikely. Since all colors can be generated by appropriate mixtures of only three stimuli (three stimuli are necessary and sufficient), however, a postulate that states that only three fundamental hues need to be coded by only three different types of neural patterns or three types of cone absorptions at the initial photoreceptor state at approximately each retinal locus is in complete accord with the color-mixing facts.

This still leaves unanswered the question of the exact forms and locations of the spectral peaks of the three cone photopigment functions. Although every different set of color-mixture functions measured in stimulus terms reflects the action of the same underlying *basic* set of three cone absorption functions, each triplex set of color-mixture curves is an arbitrary one. The particular forms taken by the color-mixture functions depend on the choice of a set of three particular primaries. The big challenge to vision researchers was to make *the* appropriate transformation of their experimental color-mixture data so that it would accurately represent the "true" photopigment absorption functions. Depending upon what sorts of additional assumptions the researchers made about the color-vision mechanism, they tended to come out with different answers. Two sets of these derived data for the "candidate" cone absorption functions are shown in Figure 9.

Both sets of curves are based on color-matching data, and each set is intended to represent the forms and distributions of the three cone photopigments. There is no simple way of choosing between the two sets. In pigment absorption terms, the two sets illustrated account equally well for all the color-matching data. Two stimulus fields with different physical energy distributions match because the "quantal catches" of the three different photopigments are the same for each of the different physical distributions. This requirement is fulfilled by both "photopigment" sets illustrated. This is the equivalence of response referred to in Chapter 9, but here we are dealing with equivalent photopigment absorptions. Thus color mixture can be treated as stimulus equivalences, perceptual equivalences, or photopigment absorption equivalences.

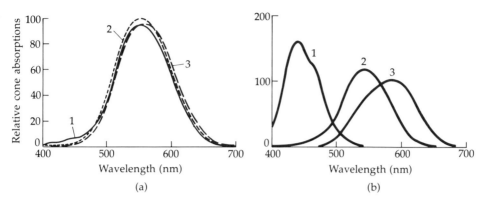

9 FUNDAMENTAL RESPONSE CURVES as derived by (a) Hecht (1934) and (b) Thomson and Wright (1953).

We are fortunately no longer dependent on indirect evidence from color-mixture results to tell us about the cone photopigments, particularly since the indirect evidence can give us such different results as those shown in Figure 9. The evidence for three types of cone photopigments located in three different types of receptors has now been fairly conclusively established using a technique called microspectrodensitometry. This evidence is strongest for cyprinid fish—goldfish and carp—a species that probably has color vision. But there are now also data for monkey and human eyes which establish the existence of three cone photopigments with absorbance peaks at three different spectral locations, approximately 450, 530, and 560 nm.* This technique uses a minute spot of light that is imaged on individual receptors taken from the eye, and the absorbance spectrum of the pigment is measured by rapidly scanning the entire spectrum. (See the discussion of the spectroradiometer in Chapter 3 for a related instrument.) Figure 10 shows the three different classes of cones, each with a different absorbance spectrum. In Figure 11 the three different photopigments are arbitrarily labeled α, β, and γ. The subscripts 450, 530, and 560 are attached to them to represent the wavelengths at which absorbance is maximal in each instance: thus the labels are α_{450}, β_{530}, γ_{560}. At any given wavelength, say 585 nm, for a unit of energy striking the retina, the three different photopigments absorb quanta in the proportions shown on the ordinate on the graph, and the forms of these functions accord with the average color-mixture data.

---

* Evidence for three types of photopigments in fish is also provided by direct electrical recording from the receptor cells, and for human beings a technique called reflection densitometry tends to support the evidence for three types of pigments. This technique is less reliable than microspectrodensitometry and gives no data for the short-wavelength pigment in the region of 450 nm.

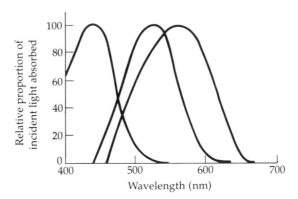

10 MICROSPECTROPHOTOMETRIC RECORDS of three classes of cones in the human retina. Peaks are located at approximately 450, 530, and 560 nm. Heights of curves are arbitrarily adjusted to the same value, unity in this case.

For any known energy we can state the number of quanta absorbed at any particular wavelength by all three photopigments, α_{450}, β_{530}, and γ_{560}. If we are using a set of three stimuli for color-matching purposes and each stimulus primary, like the test stimulus, excites the same three types of photopigments, we obtain a match when the relative energies of the mixture stimuli are adjusted so that the total α_{450}, β_{530}, γ_{560} quantal absorptions produced by the three mixture primaries are the same as those produced by the test stimulus.

This can be written in equation form. If the test stimulus is 585 nm and if q, u, v, and w represent the number of quanta, then

$$q1_{585(\alpha_{450})} = u1_{460(\alpha_{450})} + v1_{530(\alpha_{450})} + w1_{650(\alpha_{450})}$$

$$q2_{585(\beta_{530})} = u2_{460(\beta_{530})} + v2_{530(\beta_{530})} + w2_{650(\beta_{530})}$$

$$q3_{585(\gamma_{560})} = u3_{460(\gamma_{560})} + v3_{530(\gamma_{560})} + w3_{650(\gamma_{560})}$$

These equations say nothing more than that the single spectral light 585 nm has the same number of quantal absorptions in the three photo-

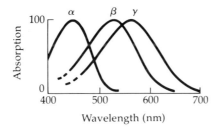

11 RECEPTOR DISTRIBUTION FUNCTIONS labeled α, β, and γ whose peaks are located at 450, 530, and 560 nm, respectively.

pigments as do the three separate lights used as primaries. This illustrative example applies to all other test wavelengths as well.

It is important to note that color equations which specify equal quantal absorptions for test and comparison lights tell us nothing at all about the *appearance* of the color-matched fields.

In and of itself knowledge of different amounts of absorbance by the three pigments means very little for color vision beyond telling us that certain mixtures of stimuli match or do not match. For a fuller understanding of the facts and phenomena of color vision, we must go beyond the receptor level and the pigments contained there to look at the various and complexly interrelated neural cells and at more central anatomical pathways.

Beyond the receptor cells in the retina there is a large variety of neuronal cells. After the photosensitive pigments are affected by the light, the electrochemical changes that take place in the receptors are communicated through these other cell layers in the retina to excite more central patterns of neural activity. The various retinal layers were shown schematically in Figure 3, and in Figure 12 an enlarged schematic representation is given of how the major cell types may be interrelated and interconnected. Excitability changes pass in general from rods and cones through bipolar cells to ganglion cells. The latter are the first elements that form the optic nerve pathway. The horizontal and amacrine cells integrate activity across large retinal areas.

The optic nerve fibers that come from the ganglion cells tend to group together and they all converge on one exit area in the back of the eye and form the optic nerve (see Figure 1). This region of the eye contains no light-sensitive elements and hence is "blind." It lies about 15 to 16 degrees away from the center of the fovea and in the direction of the nose. Therefore, objects that lie away from the center of fixation at this angle in the external field toward the temples fall on the BLIND SPOT.

The blind spot of the eye can be easily demonstrated. A simple experiment exposes its existence (Figure 13). But most people are unaware of it. How come? Objects of interest are fixated foveally and in binocular vision the seeing portion of one retina overlaps the blind spot of the other retina. But even in monocular vision there is an intriguing but little understood phenomenon that is usually labeled "filling in." A small colored field, say a yellow imaged on the blind spot, will, if surrounded by a larger field, say a blue, not be seen. Instead, we will see a uniform blue field with no gap or hole in it. Individuals with visual scotomas (blind spots) that come about because of retinal or cortical damage or disease also manifest this effect. Other instances of filling-in effects remain unexplained.

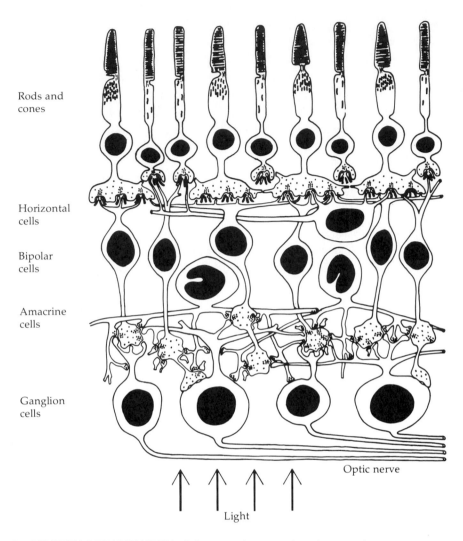

Rods and
cones

Horizontal
cells

Bipolar
cells

Amacrine
cells

Ganglion
cells

Optic nerve

Light

12 COMPLEX ORGANIZATION of the synaptic connections in a vertebrate retina.

The optic nerve fibers that are activated by events in the earlier stages of the network pass through the optic chiasma, a crossover point of a special sort, and go on to the "higher" visual centers in the occipital or visual cortex. These pathways are shown in Figure 14. It should also be noted that the neural pathways from the optic nerve tract to the brain have in recent years been shown to be much more complex than was thought earlier. The neural pathways that reach the lateral geniculate area feed signals to a number of cortical regions, but there are now known to be pathways from the optic tract that lead to areas other than the lateral geniculate area, and excitation reaches a number of cortical regions via

13 BLIND SPOT is located by shutting the right eye and fixating the upper cross with the left eye. If the book is held about a foot from the eye and its distance moved back and forth slightly, the disk on the left will disappear since it is imaged on the blind spot. If fixation with the left eye is dropped to the lower cross on the right, the gap in the lower line which falls on the blind spot will not be perceived and because of "filling-in", the black line will be seen as continuous.

these alternative pathways. These newly discovered anatomical pathways are now being intensively studied in lower organisms such as the cat.

In Chapter 11 we examine the ways in which events in the different photopigments might be related to the neural patterns or response systems that code for color.

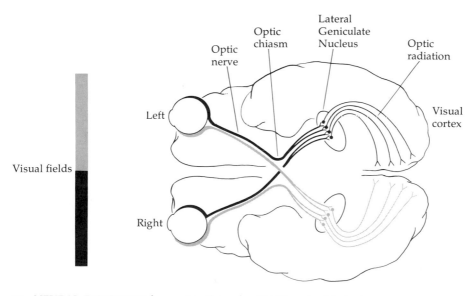

14 NEURAL PATHWAYS from retina through optic nerve tract to brain.

Background Readings

Brown, J. L. 1965. The Structure of the Visual System. In C. Graham (ed.), *Vision and Visual Perception,* Chap. 2, pp. 39–59. Wiley, New York.

Brown, P. K., and Wald, G. 1964. Visual pigments in single rods and cones of the human retina. *Science 144*: 45–52.

Dowling, J. E., and Boycott, B. B. 1966. Organization of the primate retina. Electron microscopy. *Proc. R. Soc. Lond. B 166*: 80–111.

Duke-Elder, S., and Wybar, K. C. 1961. The Anatomy of the Visual System. In S. Duke-Elder (ed.), *System of Ophthalmology,* Vol. 2. Mosby, St. Louis, Mo.

Hecht, S. 1934. Vision: II. The Nature of the Photoreceptor Process. In C. Murchison (ed.), *A Handbook of General Experimental Psychology,* Chap. 14, pp. 704–828. Clark University Press, Worcester, Mass.

Jameson, D. 1972. Theoretical Issues of Color Vision. In D. Jameson and L. M. Hurvich (eds.), *Handbook of Sensory Physiology,* Vol. 7/4, *Visual Psychophysics,* Chap. 14, pp. 381–412. Springer-Verlag, Berlin.

Kuffler, S. W., and Nicholls, J. G. 1976. *From Neuron to Brain: A Cellular Approach to the Function of the Nervous System.* Sinauer, Sunderland, Mass.

Marks, W. B. 1965. Visual pigments of single goldfish cones. *J. Physiol. Lond. 178*: 14–32.

Marks, W. B., Dobelle, W. H., and MacNichol, E. F., Jr. 1964. Visual pigments of single primate cones. *Science 143*: 1181–1183.

Miller, W. H. 1979. Ocular Optical Filtering. In H. Autrum (ed.). *Handbook of Sensory Physiology.* Vol. 7/6A, *Comparative Physiology and Evolution of Vision in Invertebrates,* Chap. 3. pp. 69–143. Springer-Verlag, Berlin.

Palmer, G. 1777. *Theory of Light.* Leacroft, London.

Polyak, S. L. 1941. *The Retina.* University of Chicago Press, Chicago.

Thomson, L. C., and Wright, W. D. 1953. The convergence of the tritanopic confusion loci and the derivation of the fundamental response functions. *J. Opt. Soc. Amer. 43*: 890–894.

Walls, G. L. 1954. The filling-in process. *Amer. J. Optom. Arch. Amer. Acad. Optom. 31*: 329–340.

Wright, W. D. 1947. *Researches on Normal and Defective Colour Vision,* Chap. 30. Mosby, St. Louis, Mo.

Wyszecki, G., and Stiles, W. S. 1967. *Color Science,* Sec. 2, pp. 202–227. Wiley, New York.

Yager, D. 1967. Behavioral measures and theoretical analysis of spectral sensitivity and spectral saturation in the goldfish, *Carassius auratus. Vision Res. 7*: 707–727.

Young, T. 1802. On the theory of light and colours. *Phil. Trans. R. Soc. Lond. 92*: 12–48.

Further Readings

Blough, D. S., and Yager, D. 1972. Visual Psychophysics in Animals. In D. Jameson and L. M. Hurvich (eds.), *Handbook of Sensory Physiology*, Vol. 7/4, *Visual Psychophysics*, Chap. 28, pp. 732–763. Springer-Verlag, Berlin.

Frumkes, T. E., and Temme, L. A. 1978. Rod-cone interaction in human scotopic vision. II. Cones influence rod increment thresholds. *Vision Res. 17*: 673–680.

Makous, W., and Boothe, R. 1974. Cones block signals from rods. *Vision Res. 14*: 285–294.

McCann, J. J. 1972. Rod-cone interactions: Different color sensations from identical stimuli. *Science 176*: 1255–1257.

Stabell, V., and Stabell, B. 1977. Wavelength discrimination of peripheral cones and its change with rod intrusion. *Vision Res. 17*: 423–426.

11
Color-Vision Models:
Receptor-Neural Linkages

THE number of independent variables necessary and sufficient to account for the various phenomena of color vision is three. Three photopigment-receptor systems as well as three opponent neural response systems are involved. The challenge is to find the simplest linkage between receptor events and neural events that will enable us to explain our color experiences and how they are related to physical stimulation.

The simplest correspondence that one might want to examine is diagrammed in Figure 1a. Biochemical activity in one receptor that has maximal absorbance in the short wavelengths would be linked to a set of nerve fibers that signals, say, a blue appearance when light absorbed by this short-wavelength photopigment excites these nerve fibers. The activity in a second type of receptor containing, say, a photopigment that absorbs maximally in the midspectral region would be linked to a set of nerve fibers that signals a green appearance when stimulated; and in such an arrangement, the long-wavelength-absorbing photopigment would be linked to a set of nerve fibers whose activity signals a red appearance when stimulated.

Simple schemas of this sort have played a prominent role in the history of color-vision research, but on close analysis such accounts do not jibe well with some obvious facts of color vision, and as they are modified to cope with difficulties, the simple schemas become excessively complex.

The simplistic "coding"* schema just outlined, which assigns each of three basic hues, blue, green, and red, to three separate photochemical-neural structures, cannot account for the appearance of the spectrum. At the short-wavelength end of the spectrum, where we see blue-reds (violets), the model leads us to expect blue hues only. As we move toward longer wavelengths, we do see blues, then blue-greens, and greens, as predicted. But what of the yellow-greens, yellows, and yellow-reds that follow? The model tells us that greens are succeeded by green-reds and then red-greens. But we know these to be nonexistent percepts.

* See Chapter 2.

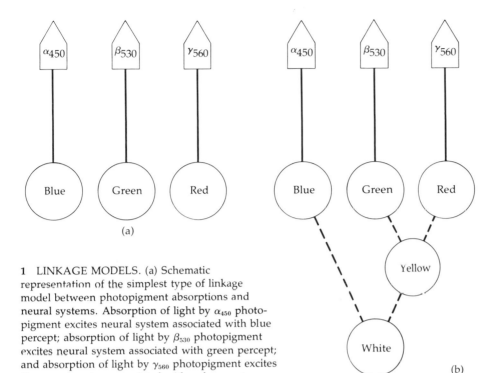

1 LINKAGE MODELS. (a) Schematic representation of the simplest type of linkage model between photopigment absorptions and neural systems. Absorption of light by α_{450} photopigment excites neural system associated with blue percept; absorption of light by β_{530} photopigment excites neural system associated with green percept; and absorption of light by γ_{560} photopigment excites the neural system associated with red percept. (b) This scheme [an ad hoc modification of (a)] shows that the neural events associated with green and red percepts are assumed to interact with each other to evoke yellow percepts. Whiteness is associated with the activation of the neural systems that underlie the occurrence of yellow and blue percepts.

As a way out of these difficulties, various interactions have been postulated to occur among the separate hue percepts. Thus red and green sensations, for example, are assumed to interact to produce a yellow sensation (Figure 1b). Such a modification abandons, of course, the simplicity of the original coding notion, but there are more serious difficulties. This sort of model, which dates back to Thomas Young* at the beginning of the nineteenth century and is associated particularly with Helmholtz, the renowned German physicist, also fails badly in trying to account for the color deficiencies (see, e.g., Chapter 17).

In recent years more complex models have been formulated that cope more adequately with the phenomena of color vision. These models also postulate interactions between events at the photoreceptor level and the neural level, and they are of a sort that are in accord with the findings of anatomy (see Chapter 10) and electrophysiology (see Chapter 12). But the interactions postulated are not interactions that occur *after* the neural events have taken on a hue coding.

* Palmer preceded Young in this view. He published in 1777.

Consider both the response functions and spectral absorbances of the photopigments in Figure 2. At the short-wavelength end of the spectrum, say at 440 nm, where light is absorbed to a greater degree by the α_{450} photopigment than it is by the other two photopigments, the color responses are blue, red, and white. Figure 3a shows this in schematic form. If the spectral stimulus is at a longer wavelength, say 540 nm, where absorbance by the β_{530} photopigment is greater than for the other two photopigments, the color-response systems that are active are green, yellow, and white. Let us diagram this in Figure 3b. Finally, suppose that

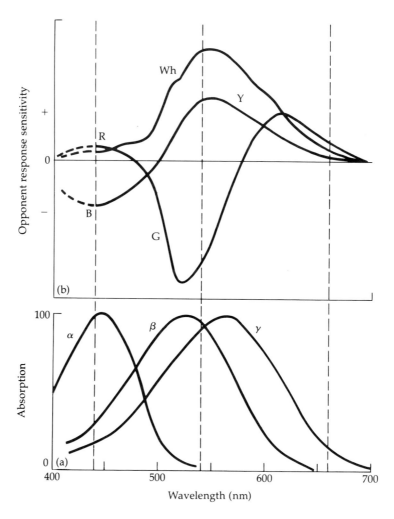

2 SPECTRAL DISTRIBUTIONS of photopigment absorptions and opponent chromatic and achromatic responses. (a) Absorptions in photopigments by 440, 540, and 660 nm stimuli are indicated by vertical dashed lines. (b) The associated responses related to these absorptions.

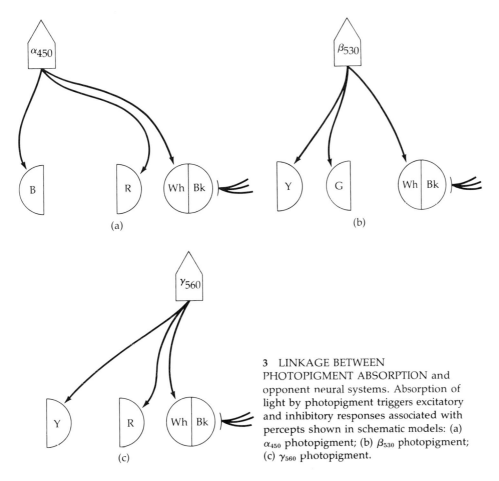

3 LINKAGE BETWEEN PHOTOPIGMENT ABSORPTION and opponent neural systems. Absorption of light by photopigment triggers excitatory and inhibitory responses associated with percepts shown in schematic models: (a) α_{450} photopigment; (b) β_{530} photopigment; (c) γ_{560} photopigment.

the spectral stimulus is 660 nm. At this wavelength the absorbance is mainly via the γ_{560} photopigment. Since the response functions show that the perceived hues are yellow, red, and white, let us diagram these relations in Figure 3c. We see that absorption by any one of the three photopigments appears to be capable of activating three kinds of neural responses:

$$\alpha_{450} \rightarrow \text{blue, red, and white}$$
$$\beta_{530} \rightarrow \text{yellow, green, and white}$$
$$\gamma_{560} \rightarrow \text{yellow, red, and white}$$

(The symbol $\rightarrow$ indicates "activates.") Thus absorptions in each of the three photopigments excite the white/(black) neural system, and in addition α_{450} and γ_{560} excite "red" in common, and β_{530} and γ_{560} excite "yellow" in common.

If we unite this set of three linkages in a single diagram and at the same time assign the plus and minus symbols that derive from Figure 2 to the three neural response systems, the overall picture is the one shown in Figure 4. (Physiologically, the plus and minus symbols represent excitation and inhibition; see Chapter 12.)

This schematic figure represents in principle the way the photopigment absorptions relate to the different modes of neural activity. It shows that the photopigment and neural linkages need not necessarily be of a simple one-to-one sort. In summary form, we can write

$$\alpha_{450} \rightarrow \text{blue}$$
$$\beta_{530} \rightarrow \text{green}$$
$$\beta_{530} + \gamma_{560} \rightarrow \text{yellow}$$
$$\alpha_{450} + \gamma_{560} \rightarrow \text{red}$$
$$\alpha_{450} + \beta_{530} + \gamma_{560} \rightarrow \text{white}$$

Keeping in mind the fact that the yellow/blue and red/green response systems are opponent and that the plus and minus signs are merely arbitrary ways of representing this antagonism, let us write these relations as follows:

$$\text{yellow/blue} = [\beta_{530} + \gamma_{560}] - \alpha_{450} \qquad (1)$$
$$\text{red/green} = [\alpha_{450} + \gamma_{560}] - \beta_{530} \qquad (2)$$
$$\text{white/(black)} = [\alpha_{450} + \beta_{530} + \gamma_{560}] \qquad (3)$$

What does a set of relations of this sort between photopigment absorptions and neural responses express? For example, consider Figure 2 and the spectral stimulus 430 nm as stimulus. All three photopigments absorb light of 430 nm. If the absorbance of photopigment α_{450} exceeds the sum of the β_{530} and γ_{560} absorbances at this wavelength, as it seems to, the algebraic total of equation (1) is a negative quantity. This indicates that the response is blue. If the absorbance values at this same wavelength

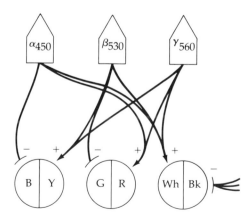

4 LINKAGE BETWEEN PHOTOPIG-MENT ABSORPTION and opponent neural systems. Composite of (a), (b), and (c) of Figure 3. Inputs from photopigments assigned + (excitatory) and − (inhibitory) coding.

(430 nm) are inserted into equation (2), the algebraic sum of $\alpha_{450} + \gamma_{560}$ exceeds the β_{530} value and the positive value indicates that the response is red. Summing all three absorbance values of α_{450}, β_{530}, and γ_{560} at this wavelength gives a positive value, indicating a white response. This rough analysis tells us that we should see reddish blue (with a whitish component).

Since we know the forms of the three absorbance (or receptor sensitivity) functions α_{450}, β_{530}, and γ_{560}, we can, for a unit of energy at any given wavelength, insert the values of these functions into the three equations given above and calculate response values as well as specify their signs. Since we are dealing with three photopigments whose maxima have been arbitrarily adjusted to the same value, it would be remarkable indeed if a calculation of this sort were to generate the chromatic and achromatic response functions of the forms we are familiar with (see Figure 2a). And, in fact, such is not the case. We can, however, determine an appropriate set of weighting factors for the three receptor sensitivities (shown in Figure 2b) that alters their relative amplitudes so that they will generate response functions with the forms and distributions that have been measured experimentally (see Chapter 5). The weighting factors for unit energy stimuli are given in the following equations:

$$\text{red}_\lambda/\text{green}_\lambda = 0.37\alpha_\lambda + 1.66\gamma_\lambda - 2.23\beta_\lambda$$
$$\text{yellow}_\lambda/\text{blue}_\lambda = 0.06\beta_\lambda + 0.34\gamma_\lambda - 0.71\alpha_\lambda$$
$$\text{white}_\lambda/(\text{black}_\lambda) = 0.01\alpha_\lambda + 0.15\beta_\lambda + 0.85\gamma_\lambda$$

Since the photopigment absorbance functions are expressable as simple linear transformations of stimulus color-mixture data (see Chapter 10) and since the achromatic and chromatic response functions are, as we see, themselves linear transformations of the photopigment functions, one might ask why we cannot bypass the photopigment functions and proceed directly from color-mixture data to the achromatic and chromatic response functions, thus specifying the latter quantitatively in terms of the former. This is a perfectly reasonable question, and equations have been written that link average achromatic and chromatic response functions with the average color-mixture data. If the color-mixture functions are used that have been designated as standard for use in applied color measurement (CIE functions, see Chapter 20), the achromatic and chromatic response functions can be calculated using the following equations, where $\bar{x}_\lambda$, $\bar{y}_\lambda$, and $\bar{z}_\lambda$ are the spectral tristimulus values (or distribution coefficients) of the CIE standard color-mixture curves:

$$Y_\lambda/B_\lambda = 0.4\bar{y}_\lambda - 0.4\bar{z}_\lambda$$
$$R_\lambda/G_\lambda = 1.0\bar{x}_\lambda - 1.0\bar{y}_\lambda$$
$$W_\lambda/(Bk_\lambda) = 1.0\bar{y}_\lambda$$

This being true, why do we concern ourselves at all with a photopigment absorbance phase that is intermediate between easily measured external stimulus mixture values and just as readily measured achromatic and chromatic response functions? The reason is that the color-mixture functions remain fixed with adaptation, whereas the response functions do not and only by concerning ourselves with the intermediate photochemical state and the way it exerts its effects upon the response system can we begin to cope with the "color-adaptation" problem and the related color-contrast problems. Furthermore, as we shall see in Chapters 16, 17, and 18, the problems of color deficiency also require an understanding of the way the photopigment absorbances are related to the response functions.

But before turning to these issues, we first discuss recent electrophysiological evidence as it relates to the postulated opponent processes red/green, yellow/blue, and white/(black). This evidence confirms the complex nature of the relation between photopigment absorptions and various types of neural responses.

Background Readings

Helmholtz, H. v. 1911. *Physiological Optics*, 3rd ed., Vol. 2. J. P. C. Southall (ed.). Optical Society of America, Rochester (1924). (Reprinted, Dover, New York, 1962.)

Hurvich, L. M., and Jameson, D. 1955. Some quantitative aspects of an opponent-colors theory. II. Brightness, saturation, and hue in normal and dichromatic vision. *J. Opt. Soc. Amer. 45*: 602–616.

Jameson, D. 1972. Theoretical Issues of Color Vision. In D. Jameson and L. M. Hurvich (eds.), *Handbook of Sensory Physiology,* Vol. 7/4, *Visual Psychophysics,* Chap. 14, pp. 381–412. Springer-Verlag, Berlin.

Jameson, D., and Hurvich, L. M. 1968. Opponent-response functions related to measured cone photopigments. *J. Opt. Soc. Amer. 58*: 429–430.

Judd, D. B. 1951. Basic Correlates of the Visual Stimulus. In S. S. Stevens (ed.), *Handbook of Experimental Psychology,* Chap. 22, pp. 811–867. Wiley, New York.

Palmer, G. 1777. *Theory of Colours and Vision.* Leacroft, London.

Wright, W. D. 1947. *Researches on Normal and Defective Colour Vision.* Mosby, St. Louis, Mo.

Young, T. 1802. On the theory of light and colours. *Phil. Trans. R. Soc. Lond. 92*: 12–48.

Further Readings

De Valois, R. L., and De Valois, K. K. 1975. Neural Coding of Color. In
E. C. Carterette and M. P. Friedman (eds.), *Handbook of Perception,*
Vol. 5, *Seeing,* Chap. 5, pp. 117–166. Academic Press, New York.

Guth, S. L. 1971. A new color model. *Proc. Helmholtz Mem. Symp. Color
Metrics, Driebergen,* pp. 82–98.

Walraven, P. L. 1973. Theoretical Models of the Colour Vision Network.
In *Colour 73.* The Second Congress of the International Colour Association, pp. 11–20. Hilger, London.

12
Opponent Processes and Electrophysiology

I F physical-chemical changes in neural cells are correlated with the phe-nomena of color vision, these phenomena must provide us with a direct readout of the net effect of specialized nervous activity of some as yet unknown sorts. A variety of visual phenomena, such as contrast effects, after images, colors seen in peripheral vision, color-deficient vision, and the way our color experiences are most efficiently systematized and or-dered, have all been cited to argue that the "coding" of color experience at the neural level is organized in a three-variable opponent-process fash-ion; there are three independent systems of neural opponent processes: red/green, yellow/blue, and white/black.

But an analysis of this sort is inferential. However sensible the pro-cedure is, given the basic premise, it provides us with no *direct* information on the nature of the physical-chemical events that may occur, let alone provide us with any clues as to where in the anatomical pathways leading from eye to brain the significant neural events may be occurring. To get at these processes more directly, it has long been the practice to monitor the electrical activity of the nervous system and measure the electrical currents (ionic changes) that are generated in various cells when the eye is stimulated.

Appropriate electrodes, amplifiers, oscilloscopes, and cameras have long been used to analyze receptors, nerve fibers, muscle fibers, synaptic events, neuromuscular junctions, and so on. Computer technology is now widely used in this kind of experimentation to control the stimulation and to do more sophisticated analyses of the results. Our major concern here is with neural events related to visual excitation, and the currents recorded are those set off by stimulating either visual receptor cells with light or other relevant neural cells with electrical stimuli.

It is known that the electrical potentials recorded from cellular tissue depend upon the concentrations of a variety of ions, such as potassium, sodium, and chloride, the differences between the concentrations on the inside and outside walls of the cell membrane and the changes in selective permeability of this membrane for the different ions that occur when a stimulus excites the cell. The details of these mechanisms are available in textbooks. The electrical potentials are called ACTION POTENTIALS and carry signals rapidly over large distances in the nervous system. Although action potentials vary in size from one neural element to the next, each neuron obeys what is called the ALL-OR-NONE LAW. It fires or does not fire, and when it does the spike size is uniform; only firing *rate* (spiking rate) may change with changes in applied energy.

The evidence is now overwhelming that nervous tissue is capable of a "biphasic" opponent response. When unstimulated, most neural cells are in a "resting" state, and in this "resting" state show a "spontaneous" relatively slow rate of firing. When stimulated, such cells may respond in either one of two ways. Depending upon the conditions of stimulation and measured from the level of spontaneous activity, they can increase or decrease their firing rates.

Using the excised eye of the frog, Hartline reported in 1938 that all nerve fibers did not react in the same way to light onset and light offset. What he found was that there were at least three different classes or types of nerve fiber leading from the ganglion cells (Figure 1). There are ON-CELLS, which fire with a sustained burst of impulses when the light is turned on and subsequently gradually become quiet. There are ON-OFF CELLS which show short transient bursts of spiking both when the light is turned on as well as when it is turned off. Between the periods of spiking are quiet periods. A third class of cell, which ceases any spontaneous activity when first stimulated but responds with a burst of electrical impulses when the stimulus light is turned off, is also found.

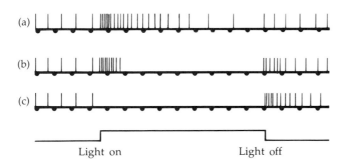

1 THREE TYPES OF RESPONSE in retinal fibers in the frog. (a) On-cell, fiber that responds with a sustained burst of activity. (b) On-off cell, fiber that responds to onset and cessation of light. (c) Off-cell, fiber that responds only to cessation of light. In each record the signal that marks the duration of the stimulus fills the white line above the time marker. Time is in fifths of a second.

Granit (1947), in particular, established the fact that the on- and off-responses in the frog and cat optic nerves were manifestations of true physiological antagonism in the neural processes. When experiments were so arranged as to cause both on- and off-discharges to impinge simultaneously on the same ganglion cell, they canceled each other. The on- and off-discharge phases were thus shown to be mutually antagonistic.

The first discovery of wavelength-specific neurophysiological responses in individual cells of the retina was made by Svaetichin working on the eyes of shallow-water fish. The electrical signals that Svaetichin recorded in this particular work were not action potentials but localized potentials. The LOCALIZED POTENTIALS, as their name implies, act only over short distances, in contrast to the action potentials. Also in contrast to the latter, the local potentials are graded potentials and not fixed in size. The voltage change recorded intracellularly with fine electrodes implanted in the cell body varies with the electrical voltage that may be applied to the cell, or with the energy, say, of a light stimulus, or with the nature of the light stimulus itself.

Svaetichin showed that the potentials that he recorded varied in size as he changed the light stimulus impinging on the eye of the fish from one wavelength to the next. Not only were the responses differently graded for the different wavelengths of the same energy, but what was even more startling was his discovery that some cells showed a reversal of electrical sign at different spectral regions. There was little reason to anticipate that the electrical sign of a single cell's response would shift from "positive going" (hyperpolarization) to "negative going" (depolarization) as the spectrum was traversed from, say, short to long wavelengths of light. The sort of result obtained by Svaetichin for a series of different spectral wavelengths is shown in Figure 2. In connection with this finding of spectrally opponent-type responses in a single cell, it is important to know that many shallow-water fish have been tested in well-controlled behavioral experiments and have been shown to have good color discrimination.

Svaetichin reported two major types of cells, those that he labeled "C" type, which showed reversal of polarity of the electrical-graded potential as the wavelength changed, and another type, which he labeled "L" type. The latter did not show a polarity reversal, as the spectrum was traversed; he associated cells of this type with the "whiteness" or brightness response. All of these graded potentials are now called "S" potentials, in recognition of Svaetichin's discovery of them. Among those that reverse their polarity with wavelength change, Svaetichin reported several variations, and some of these are shown in Figure 3. These records are, of

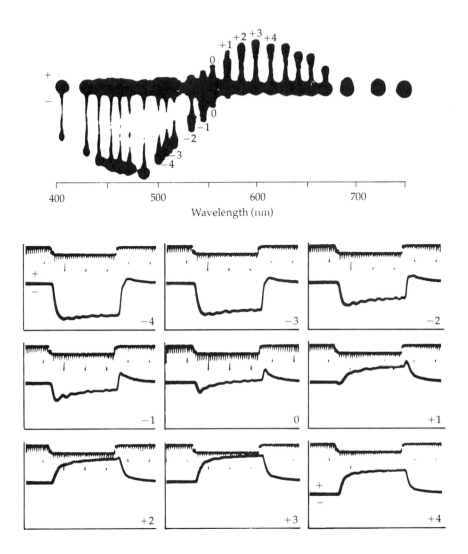

2 HYPERPOLARIZATION AND DEPOLARIZATION RESPONSES in a single cell as a function of wavelength. These microelectrode records of graded localized potentials (called "S" potentials in honor of their discoverer, Gunnar Svaetichin) were obtained from the retina of a fish. Response amplitude as well as polarity varies with wavelength. The records in the single frames are made with an expanded time base.

course, reminiscent of the opponent-response curves measured in the human and the labels B-y, b-Y, and r_2-G-r_1 are intended to represent the blue/yellow and red/green responses. Although we can establish the sorts of wavelength discriminations fish can make using the techniques of animal psychophysics and make various inferences about fish color vision,

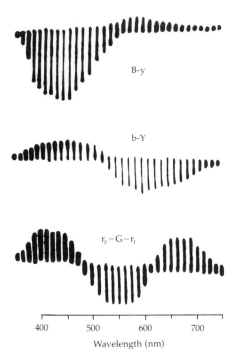

B-y

b-Y

$r_2 - G - r_1$

400   500   600   700

Wavelength (nm)

3 REVERSAL OF POLARITY of electrical graded localized potentials as a function of wavelength.

there is, of course, no way of knowing whether the terms "red," "green," "blue," and so on, have any direct counterparts in the fish visual experience.

Svaetichin's experimental results have now been confirmed in the retinas of many vertebrate species and by different investigators in different laboratories. Their source in the retina is now accepted as being mainly in the horizontal cells (see Figure 12 in Chapter 10).

I have already said that both Hartline and Granit were concerned with recording on and off types of spike discharge. The former worked with frogs and the latter primarily with mammals such as the cat and the guinea pig, and the recordings were being made at a "higher" neural level than the horizontal cells of the retina. They were working at the level of the ganglion cells and their axons that form the optic nerve fibers. But it was only after Svaetichin's work was published that the electrophysiologists were alerted to the way the spike discharges were related and correlated with the graded potential events. The result was a large body of evidence that shows the existence of spectrally opponent cells in a variety of organisms and at different levels beyond the horizontal cells in the neural chain from retina to cortex.*

* Antagonistic responses that show reciprocal spatial interactions are discussed in Chapter 13.

One example of this work is shown in Figure 4, which shows the response with a change in wavelength of a single ganglion cell of the goldfish retina. In a way that is similar to the graded potential responses that reverse their polarity with a change in wavelength, this cell reacts differently to short-wavelength lights from the way it does in the longer-wavelength region. When short-wavelength light stimulates the retina, spiking is recorded from the cell at the onset of stimulation and suppression of spiking at stimulus offset; at the longer wavelengths there is suppression of spike discharge at stimulus onset followed by a burst of spikes at stimulus offset. Sometimes the on-responses occur with long-wavelength light stimulation and the off-responses with the short-wavelength light. As Figure 4b shows, a small wavelength change, about 10 nm, can flip the cell's response from on to off. These are antagonistic or

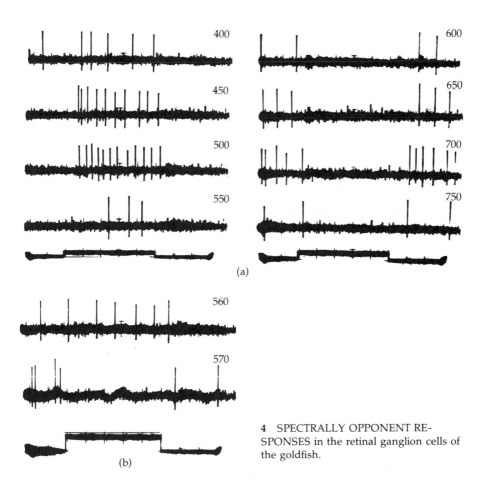

4 SPECTRALLY OPPONENT RE-SPONSES in the retinal ganglion cells of the goldfish.

opponent cellular reactions that could be related to the perceptual antagonisms discussed earlier.

Spectrally opponent ganglion cells and optic nerve fibers are also reported in the carp, macaque monkey, spider monkey, and ground squirrel, and there are similarly behaving cells in a somewhat higher anatomical layer in the goldfish, the "optic tectum." Furthermore, similar results have been obtained in the cells of the lateral geniculate nucleus (LGN), where the optic nerve fibers terminate for the macaque and for the squirrel monkey. They are also found in some areas of the visual cortex of the monkey. Figure 5 shows a series of records for a spectrally opponent cell in the macaque LGN, an animal about which we shall have more to say below. If we look, for example, at wavelengths 586 nm and 603 nm, we see that a change occurs from spiking upon stimulation at the 586-nm wavelength to suppression of spontaneous discharge during stimulation and an after-discharge of spiking at the 603-nm wavelength.

In the face of all this evidence, we need no longer have any doubt

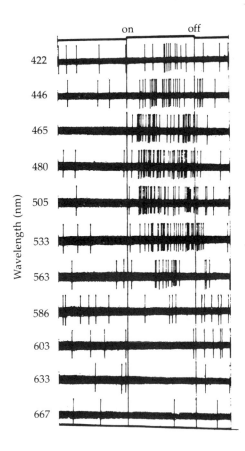

5 SPECTRALLY OPPONENT RESPONSES in the lateral geniculate nucleus of the macaque monkey. Responses are shown in each record for a 1-second period before, during, and after light stimulation by light of specified wavelengths.

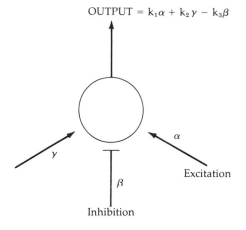

$$\text{OUTPUT} = k_1\alpha + k_2\gamma - k_3\beta$$

γ

α

Excitation

β

Inhibition

6 CELL OUTPUT is dependent on both excitatory and inhibitory inputs to it. The α and γ inputs are shown as excitatory, the β input as inhibitory. Output = $k_1\alpha + k_2\gamma - k_3\beta$, where the k's are weighting factors.

that cells of the nervous system are capable of opponent-type responses to different wavelengths. The evidence now mustered has convinced the most skeptical, and neurophysiologists have accepted the fact that cells act under the influence of two types of input, usually called EXCITATION and INHIBITION. The two different inputs act by means of different transmitter substances released or secreted across junctions between the different receptor-neural (or neural-neural) elements to activate a common postsynaptic neuron. The output of this cell, say, a ganglion cell, depends upon the difference between the two separate types of inputs (Figure 6). Since the ganglion cell has a steady-state spontaneous level of excitation (background rate of firing), the two antagonistic modes of response are associated with firing rates greater than this background level and less than this background level. The inputs on individual cells are, of course, multiple ones coming from many excitatory and inhibitory inputs, not simply two, as diagrammed for simplicity.

Figure 4 in Chapter 11 shows the relation between three different photopigment absorptions, on the one hand, and the opponent neural events, on the other. We have incorporated the essence of the kind of interplay schematized in Figure 6 as operating on a single cell. If the inhibitory input from, say, α, exceeds the excitatory input arriving from β and γ photochemical inputs, the minus quantity signifies "blueness." If the sum of the β and γ excitatory inputs exceeds the inhibitory input, we have a "yellow" signal; and so on. The neural elements, labeled as, say, B/Y, will respond *either* with the B or Y aspect, never with both simultaneously.

The electrophysiological data that have aroused the greatest interest in connection with opponent-process-type color theories come from the laboratories of De Valois and his co-workers.

Figure 7 shows the results obtained in a single LGN cell in the monkey in response to a series of different spectral lights. On top we see the number of spikes produced in this single cell as the spectrum is traversed from, say, short to long wavelengths of light. In the bottom portion of the figure, the number of spikes produced in each 10-nm section of the spectrum is plotted. Note that the cell is inhibited by short-wavelength light stimulation and excited by long-wavelength light stimulation. This firing pattern is taken to be evidence of a spectrally opponent cell and it has been arbitrarily called a +R, −G (+red, −green) cell. We shall return shortly to the naming of these cells.

If a large number of LGN cells are sampled, the results that are obtained are summarized in Figure 8. Basically, there are opponent red/green cells, opponent yellow/blue cells, and one nonopponent cell type that presumably codes a white/black signal. The two opponent and one nonopponent type are shown on the left side of the figure. They are called the *red-excitatory, green-inhibitory* (+R −G) cells; *yellow-excitatory, blue-inhibitory* (+Y −B) cells; and *white-excitatory, black-inhibitory* (+Wh −Bk) cells.

On the right-hand side of the figure, we have what are essentially mirror images of the firing patterns on the left. Here we have +G −R, +B −Y, and +Bk −Wh cells. For the "chromatic" cells excitation occurs in the spectral region that evokes inhibition in the first set of cells, and vice versa. The +Bk −Wh cell shows an inhibitory pattern of response throughout the spectrum.

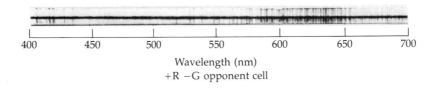

Wavelength (nm)

+R −G opponent cell

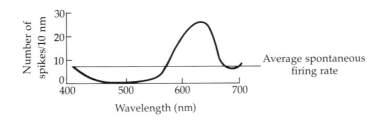

7 RESPONSES OF AN OPPONENT CELL in macaque LGN to different spectral lights. Upper graph shows the result of a wavelength sweep with a monochromator. Bottom record is a plot of number of spikes found in each 10-nm section of the spectrum. Cell is excited by long wavelengths of light and inhibited by shorter wavelengths of light.

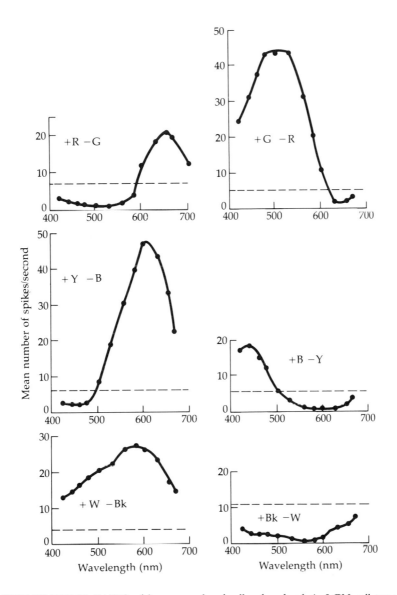

8 AVERAGE FIRING RATES of large sample of cells of each of six LGN cell types as a function of wavelength. Top four cells are spectrally opponent ones and bottom two are spectrally nonopponent cells. The cells on the left are, in principle, "mirror images" of those on the right.

These results are found using rather large diffusely illuminated test fields, and similar results are reported by others. They provide the best evidence that the neural color-processing system of the higher primates is organized in a manner that closely resembles the opponents schematization presented in earlier chapters.

The fact that electrophysiological recordings from the LGN of the monkey resemble in a general way the chromatic and achromatic response functions of human beings does not mean that we know how the nervous system is organized to provide color information. Strong support for the view that we are on the right track comes from the color discrimination performance of the monkeys from whom the electrophysiological data are obtained since their discriminations are very nearly like that of human beings. Behavioral measures of spectral sensitivity, color matching, and color discrimination (saturation and wavelength discrimination; Chapter 15) all indicate that both the monkey and human color systems have very similar properties. It makes sense, therefore, to use the electrophysiological data from the animals in order to compare them with human color experience and discrimination.

We must, however, be careful not to go overboard in the belief that the electrophysiological data in hand necessarily provide the whole story. There is still the important problem of how the information from the two-opponent and one-nonopponent system is integrated physiologically. Since the paired opponent processes are assumed to occur in separate cells, we must know what the pattern of activity is across different cell types if we are to be able to specify the color experience. Where and how are the excitations of independent cells (or are they?) compared or combined?

Other questions still need answering. The data obtained on human beings in cancellation-type experiments are unequivocal in establishing two pairs of opponent systems: red/green and yellow/blue. Is the existence of two separate opponent response systems established with equal rigor for the electrophysiological data? The answer is not certain. Records from individual cells show considerable variability from one to the next. However, by adopting an arbitrary criterion to create separate classes, statistical tests have been made of the various distributions of peak responses as well as the crossover points in the spectrum from excitation to inhibition and these suggest just two spectrally opponent types (four, if the mirror images are included). We have to remember that the different physiological types, red/green and yellow/blue, have been so named because of the way the test stimuli that produce certain impulse frequencies look to the experimenter. Spikes are spikes and they carry no color names. Without the human psychophysical data and the perceptual data it is certain that sorting different LGN cells into appropriate bins would be a more difficult task.

We should remember, moreover, that the LGN is usually thought of only as a way station for the flow of visual information toward the visual cortex, and further processing of the information is to be anticipated beyond the LGN. We know that the cortex is very complexly organized, but the information we have about the physiological basis of color at this level is rather meagre. Suffice it to say that there is some evidence of color-specific striate cortex cells, multiple-color striate cells, and color-specific cells in an area of the cortex labeled V 4.

For the sake of completeness we should also mention that electrical responses can be recorded from the visual system in the intact organism without discomfort or injury to the observer. The visual evoked cortical potential (VECP), which is a gross electrical response, is recorded by placing electrodes on the scalp over the occipital cortex.* With its use, differential responses among various wavelengths of light can be demonstrated. There are also experimental data obtained with cortical recordings in intact human beings that provide evidence for opponent-color responses for some individuals.

The organization of the visual cortex for the processing of a variety of information other than color (e.g., form, shape, and pattern) has been explored in great detail by many investigators. There is considerable information available about the way the various levels of the eye/brain system are interrelated, how the two eyes are coordinated in their visual activities, what the developmental stages are, and how the visual cortex is organized in columnar structures from an anatomical point of view. But these topics are outside the scope of this book; interested readers should check the Readings for more on this topic.

I have presented an account of some of the basic physiological properties of the visual system, noting only once (and in a footnote) that there is not only a spectrally opponent physiological system but that there is a spatially opponent one as well. Furthermore, the complex spatially opponent system may be spectrally opponent at the same time. Chapter 13 will treat spatial contrast effects and show that there is a neurological basis for these types of antagonisms.

Background Readings

Abramov, I. 1972. Retinal Mechanisms of Colour Vision. In M. G. F. Fuortes (ed.), *Handbook of Sensory Physiology.* Vol. 7/2, *Physiology of Photoreceptor Organs*, Chap. 15, pp. 567–607. Springer-Verlag, Berlin.
De Valois, R. L., and De Valois, K. K. 1975. Neural Coding of Color. In E. C. Carterette and M. P. Friedman (eds.), *Handbook of Perception,*

---

* Electrical records can also be made by placing electrodes on the cornea of the intact organisms. Although results have been obtained for the photopic light-adapted condition, the electroretinogram is a gross response whose properties primarily reflect the activities of rods.

Vol. 5, *Seeing*, Chap. 5, pp. 117–166. Academic Press, New York.

De Valois, R. L., Abramov, I., and Jacobs, G. H. 1966. Analysis of response patterns of LGN cells. *J. Opt. Soc. Amer. 56*: 966–977.

Gouras, P. 1972. S-Potentials. In M. G. F. Fuortes (ed.), *Handbook of Sensory Physiology*, Vol. 7/2, *Physiology of Photoreceptor Organs*, Chap. 13, pp. 513–529. Springer-Verlag, Berlin.

Granit, R. 1947. *Sensory Mechanisms of the Retina*. Oxford University Press, London.

Hartline, H. K. 1938. The response of single optic nerve fibers of the vertebrate eye to illumination of the retina. *Amer. J. Physiol. 121*: 400–415.

Kuffler, S. W., and Nicholls, J. G. 1976. *From Neuron to Brain: A Cellular Approach to the Function of the Nervous System*. Sinauer, Sunderland, Mass.

MacNichol, E. F., Jr., and Svaetichin, G. 1958. Electric responses from the isolated retinas of fishes. *Amer. J. Ophthalmol. 46*: 26–40.

MacNichol, E. F., Jr., Feinberg, R., and Harosi, F. I. 1973. Colour Discrimination Processes in the Retina. In *Colour 73*, pp. 191–251. The Second Congress of the International Colour Association. Hilger, London.

Ripps, H. 1978. Electrophysiology of the visual system. *Invest. Ophthalmol. 17*: (Suppl.) 46–54.

Stevens, C. F. 1966. *Neurophysiology: A Primer*. Wiley, New York.

Svaetichin, G. 1956. Spectral response curves from single cones. *Acta Physiol. Scand. 39*: Suppl. 134, 17–47.

Svaetichin, G., and MacNichol, E. F., Jr., 1958. Retinal mechanisms for chromatic and achromatic vision. *Ann. N.Y. Acad. Sci. 74*: 385–404.

Svaetichin, G., Fatehchand, R., Drujan, B. D., Laufer, M., Witkovsky, P., Negishi, K., and De Testa, A. S. 1963. Interacción glia-neuronal: Su dependencia metabólica. Una nueva teoría acerca del funccionamiento del sistema nervioso. *Acta Cient. Venez.* Suppl. 1, 135–153.

Yager, D., and Thorpe, S. 1970. Investigations of Goldfish Color Vision. In W. Stebbins (ed.), *Animal Psychophysics*, Chap. 12, pp. 259–275. Appleton-Century-Crofts, New York.

Yamanaka, T., Sobagaki, H., and Nayatani, Y. 1973. Opponent-colors responses in the visually evoked potential in man. *Vision Res. 13*: 1319–1333.

Further Readings

Brown, K. T. 1968. The electroretinogram: Its components and their origins. *Vision Res. 8*: 633–677.

De Valois, R. L., Morgan, H. C., Polson, M. C., Mead, W. R., and Hull,

E. M. 1974. Psychophysical studies of monkey vision. I. Macaque luminosity and color vision tests. *Vision Res. 14*: 53–67.

Gouras, P. 1974. Opponent-colour cells in different layers of foveal striate cortex. *J. Physiol. (London.) 238*: 583–602.

Hubel, D. H., and Wiesel, T. N. 1968. Receptive fields and functional architecture of monkey striate cortex. *J. Physiol. (Lond.) 195*: 215–243.

Hubel, D. H., and Wiesel, T. N. 1972. Laminar and culumnar distribution of geniculocortical fibers in the macaque monkey. *J. Comp. Neurol. 146*: 421–450.

Jacobs, G. H. 1977. Visual capacities of the owl monkey (*Aotus trivirgatus*). I. Spectral sensitivity and color vision. *Vision Res. 17*: 811–820.

Zeki, S. M. 1973. Colour coding in rhesus monkey prestriate cortex. *Brain Res. 53*: 422–427.

13
Spatial Contrast and Assimilation Effects

CHAPTER 1 discussed the way in which a small stimulus field of fixed energy and light distribution changed from white to darkish gray as the illumination on the field surrounding it was changed. In Figure 1a the two small circular fields reflect the same amount of light, yet the one on the left in the lighter background looks darker or blacker than the one on the right. If, in a piece of paper of uniform reflectance, we cut two round holes of the same size and separation as the two small gray fields and place this "mask" over the figure so that the two small circular fields are seen in a uniform background, the two fields look equal in brightness: the two grays are the same. If the two surrounds are less different from each other than they are in Figure 1a, the difference in appearance between the two physically equal test fields is less noticeable.

This phenomenon is known as SPATIAL CONTRAST (and also as simultaneous contrast, simultaneous brightness contrast, and brightness induction). Since percepts mirror neural events, it shows that neural activity set up in one retinal region affects the ongoing neural activity in other retinal regions. The neural organization of the visual mechanisms makes it extremely likely that there would be considerable interdependence among neural activities in neighboring regions of the retina and its associated neural pathways.

The appearances of the smaller test stimuli depend upon the whiteness or blackness of adjacent objects or surrounds and usually the change in appearance of a test stimulus is in a direction opposite to the different surrounding or inducing areas. As the surround becomes increasingly white, the center test field becomes increasingly dark or black, and as the surround becomes increasingly black the test field becomes progressively light or white. The effect is summarized in Figure 1b for a single small field equal in size and energy but shown in a series of backgrounds ranging from white to black. Most people speak of the stars as "coming out" at night. They know, of course, that the stars are always there and it is only their contrast with the dark sky that "comes out" at night.

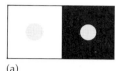

(a)

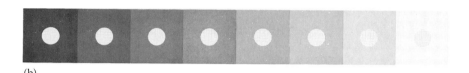

(b)

1 SIMULTANEOUS CONTRAST EFFECT. (a) Central gray areas are of the same reflectance and hence the same light level. Surrounds are of different light levels. (b) Central gray areas are of the same reflectance and hence the same light level in each of the eight rectangular surrounds. Surround illumination varies in steps from high to low light level.

Unless special care is taken to keep the eyes fixed when viewing these various figures, successive contrast (see Chapter 14) also enters as a factor. But controlled brief exposures of fractions of a second make it clear that these effects can be purely spatial contrast ones.

Spatial contrast effects are, of course, not limited to the whiteness/blackness or achromatic dimension. We have already seen an illustration of contrast effects that involve the opponent-hue pairs in Plate 2-2. In that demonstration of simultaneous color contrast, we saw that a narrow strip looks yellowish when surrounded by a blue background and grayish red when surrounded by a green background. Needless to say, the physical radiation reaching the eyes from the narrow strips is fixed and invariant. The fact that a grayish area is used in the narrower field to produce a good visual effect should not mislead us into thinking that the contrast effects are present only under these conditions. Any stimulus located in the center of a surrounding field is subject to the contrast action. Thus a yellow test field on a green background appears somewhat more reddish than it does on a gray background; a blue test field on a red background, more greenish. In fact, a yellow test field on a blue background, in accordance with the opponent principles, will become more yellow (more saturated) than on a gray background and a yellow test field on a yellow background will become less yellow (it will become desaturated). The effect of two differently colored backgrounds on an identical set of four colors is illustrated in Plate 13-1.

These phenomena have been known since time immemorial, particularly to artists. The effects can be very vivid and it is sometimes difficult to convince an individual that a certain color appearance is the result of contrast action. Chevreul, the famous French chemist, who among his many other careers was from 1824 to 1883 the director of dyes at the Gobelin tapestry works, wrote a treatise on contrast effects in which he analyzed the practical visual problems that arose in the execution of complicated woven colored patterns. For example, buyers who contracted for calicos with red and black patterns would complain that the black dyes were of inferior quality and had a greenish cast rather than the black stipulated in their orders. Having established that the black dyes were stable, Chevreul had to resort to masking techniques (appropriately designed cutouts in papers of uniform reflectance—see the discussion of Figure 1) to convince buyers that, in fact, the dyers and weavers had done their job properly and that the green aspect of the pattern was purely visual, the result of a contrast effect. By appropriately manipulating the dyes, the unwanted color appearances could be eliminated.

Contrast effects are operative at all times in our visual field, as the simple masking procedures that eliminate them reveal. But scientists who are interested in the effects per se and the neural mechanisms related to them have had reason to try to develop ways of accentuating the effects.

The simple "background" type of contrast effect I have been discussing and for which one uses achromatic and colored papers can be accentuated simply by placing a piece of tissue paper or translucent white paper over the entire stimulus pattern. This acts both to blur the edges between the fields and to desaturate the hues. By using Maxwell discs of the sort discussed in Chapter 8, one can vary the proportions of achromatic and chromatic stimulation in both test and surround areas (Figure 2) to study the effects quantitatively. By appropriately adjusting the disc proportions of the annular test area in which the contrast colors are induced by the

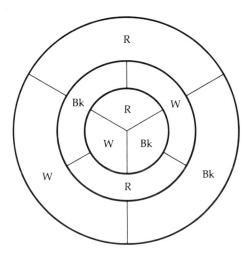

2 ROTATING DISC ARRANGEMENT for measuring simultaneous contrast effects. The inner and outer fields are the inducing fields and the annular area is the test area. The contrast effects produced by the inducing fields can be offset by appropriately adjusting the test field color. For example, if the inducing fields are red and induce some green in the annular field, the induced color can be offset by the introduction of a small amount of red color in the annulus.

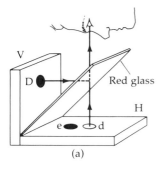

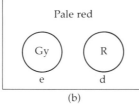

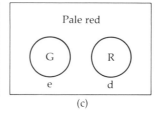

(a) (b) (c)

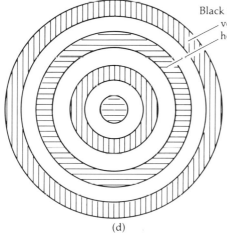

Black rings mounted on
vertical surface
horizontal surface

(d)

3 DEMONSTRATION OF SIMULTANE-
OUS COLOR CONTRAST. (a) Mirror
method devised by Ragona Scina. The
glass is a colored one, say, red, and the
two surfaces V and H at right angles to
each other are nonselective reflecting surfaces. To an eye looking down at the
glass from above, the light from V is
mainly "white" in ordinary room illumination, since it is reflected from the upper
surface of the inclined colored glass. The
light that passes through the colored glass
plate is seen as red. Thus the mixture
reaching the observer's eye is a pale red.
If a small black disc is placed at point D, no "white" light reaches the eye from this area and
its image is seen at d; it looks red (and redder than the background) since the light from
position d passes through the red glass. The second black disc, e, on the horizontal surface,
which would ordinarily be seen as black, looks grayish because "white" light is reflected
from the inclined surface at that location. The stimuli as described perceptually would be
expected to look as sketched in (b). In actuality, they look as sketched in (c). A series of
black rings of increasing diameters placed in alternating fashion on the vertical and horizontal
surfaces create even more striking contrast effects (d).

inner or outer surrounds, one can cancel the contrast color produced by
the surround discs.

More than a century ago, Ragona Scina, an Italian astronomer, devised a mirror experiment that requires only a transparent color glass, two
pieces of white cardboard placed at right angles to each other, and two
small pieces of black paper to produce contrast effects that are quite vivid
(Figure 3). But without question the most extraordinary colored contrast
effects are produced with the use of two different light sources that are
arranged to cast a double shadow of an opaque object. The essence of the

4 DOUBLE SHADOW EFFECT to illustrate simultaneous contrast. Two incandescent light sources, A and B, are set up in a darkened room and illuminate an opaque object, for example, a rod. What we see on a screen set up at an appropriate distance behind the rod are two neighboring dark shadows of the rod at A′ and B′. If we place a colored filter in the beam of source A, a colored filter that looks red, for example, the area in shadow at B′ that is illuminated by the radiation from light B is seen as green. However, area A′, which receives no yellowish-appearing light, since the rod blocks it, but receives only light from source A, is seen as red. If source A is switched off, B′ looks yellowish white. If projector A is switched on, B′ instantly becomes greenish. If the relative light energies of sources A and B are properly adjusted (this is most easily done by varying the relative distances of A and B from the screen), it is impossible to tell which of the two shadows is colored by contrast with the background.

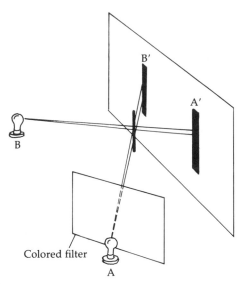

procedure is shown in Figure 4. Figure 5 clarifies the stimulus situation for the double-shadow contrast effects.

The colored-shadow contrast effect, whereby the shadowed "white" portion of the screen takes on a hue that is opposite in color to the color of the surround, can be extended to create a progressively more complex pattern of multiple shadows simply by interposing many rods as shadow casters and by varying the depth of the shadows by manipulating the positions of the opaque rods relative to the two light sources. The shadow casters need not be opaque ones. They can be graded in opacity and have different degrees of transparency. With a progressive buildup of a complex shadow picture, with multiple shadows of different darknesses distributed irregularly over the screen, different amounts of contrast are produced in different areas. Starting from the simplest case of a double shadow we can generate a varicolored image pattern. It is not too difficult to imagine a shadow picture of this sort that contains a multiplicity of reds and greens of different saturations as well as various grays, even though only two light sources, say, a red and white one, are used, just as in the simple double-shadow demonstration.

A conventional technique of color photography, preparing black-and-white separation negatives by photographing a scene through three different colored filters, can be used to create striking color-contrast effects based on the colored-shadow principle (Figure 6). This technique, which uses a "white" and a colored light source was demonstrated in conjunction

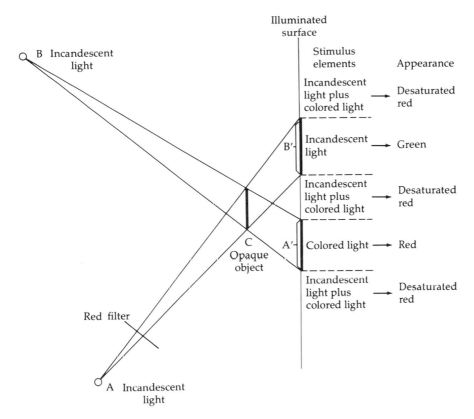

5 LIGHT DISTRIBUTION in double shadow effect. One shadowed area is illuminated only by the broad-band illuminant, incandescent "white," and the other only by the colored light, red. Both shadowed areas are surrounded by a mixture of the two illuminations. The contrast effect occurs in the shadowed area that is illuminated only by the yellowish-white light but which is an area bordered on both sides by the desaturated red stimulus. The contrast colors induced depend on the colors of the light sources, and contrast effects are obtained even when illuminants A and B differ only slightly from each other.

with two appropriate transparent black-and-white photographs (shadow casters) with great effectiveness by Ralph Evans of Eastman Kodak Company. Later, Edwin Land of Polaroid generated similar complex shadow pictures that rather stunningly illustrated simultaneous induction or contrast, and his demonstrations mystified many physicists and others who had thought of color hues as being directly tied to particular wavelengths of light.

Many aspects of simultaneous contrast have been studied, particularly the way variations in stimulus parameters affect the phenomenon. Usually, the parametric variations are concerned with changes in small central fields that are seen in the presence of larger surround fields and most of

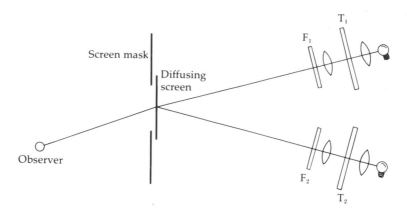

6 MULTIPLE-SHADOW-CASTING ARRANGEMENT. Two black-and-white positive transparencies are prepared by using conventional color photography technique. One scene is photographed twice, each time through a different color filter: one, say, a yellow-red, the other a yellow-green. These transparencies (T_1 and T_2) are then projected so that they overlap on a common diffusing screen. The projection filters are yellow-red (F_1) and neutral (F_2). Because of simultaneous contrast effects, the colors seen are not limited to a variety of yellow-reds of different saturations. Blues, yellows, blue-greens, and grays are also seen.

our discussion has dealt with contrast effects induced in the smaller field by the large one. But it is important to note that the contrast interaction between spatially adjacent fields is not one-way.

That simultaneous color contrast is a reciprocal contrast interaction between different parts of the visual field can be made very obvious if we examine experimentally the contrast effects that two targets of the same size, placed side by side, exert on each other. A simple way of determining how colored simultaneous contrast acts is first to place a small colored stimulus, say, a yellow-red, within a black or dark surround. If we call this small colored square the "focal" area, we can, by using a series of standardized Munsell sample chips that are available for specifying colors (see Chapter 20), select the Munsell chip that most closely matches or resembles this focal stimulus. We can now place a second, different-colored stimulus next to the first (yellow-red) one, say a green one, and cover the first one with the same black material that is used for the background. The second stimulus—the green one—is also matched by choosing the Munsell sample chip that most closely resembles it. We have in this way specified or "measured" the two stimuli seen independently.

Suppose now that we expose both stimuli simultaneously and side by side in the dark surround. The situation is as shown in Figure 7a. The observer is asked to look at the left square, the yellowish-red one, arbitrarily designated the focal area, F_1, and to match it in the presence of the green area to its right, now arbitrarily labeled the inducing area, I_1. The matching procedure is the same as in the first step in the preceding example: a Munsell sample is selected that most closely matches the focal test stimulus on the left. This matching procedure is now reversed: the green stimulus is regarded as the focal stimulus (F_2), and the observer fixates it in the presence of the adjacent yellow-red stimulus (I_2) and selects a matching Munsell sample by alternating his or her gaze between the series of standard Munsell samples available and the focal test stimulus. (Successive contrast is, of course, involved to some extent, but let us disregard this for the time being; see Chapter 14.)

If we analyze the match made to the focal area (F_1) in the presence of the inducing area (I_1), we find that the observer selects a slightly redder-appearing Munsell chip in this situation than when F_1 was seen in isolation. We find also that F_2 (F_2 = green area as focal) is matched with a slightly greener- and slightly bluer-appearing Munsell chip when I_2 (yellow-red) is present than when F_2 is matched in isolation. If we record the differences between matching Munsell samples for individual stimuli presented in the isolated condition (dark surround) and in the presence of the inducing stimuli, these differences provide us with a measure of the amount of contrast produced. The contrast effect is shown to be a reciprocal "two-way" one when this experiment is carried out.

We do not, of course, have to limit ourselves to two test areas that directly abut each other as in Figure 7a in order to study reciprocal contrast effects. Nor for that matter do the targets have to be uniform in size. In fact, Dorothea Jameson and I studied contrast interactions where the total pattern was like the one shown in Figure 7b. Here we were interested in the appearance of each of the six differently shaped areas when they were seen in the context of the entire configuration as compared with their appearances when seen in isolation. Each area was shown to be affected

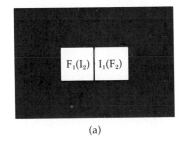

(a)

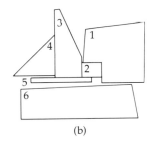

(b)

7 EXPERIMENTAL ARRANGEMENTS to measure color contrast effects. (a) Focal and inducing fields. (b) Complex test-stimulus pattern made up of six elements of various shapes and sizes.

by the total stimulus pattern and, not surprisingly, different areas were affected in somewhat different ways.

For a more systematic study of the complex mutual contrast interactions we used the more regular pattern of Figure 8a made up of five different small squares on a large background. We could then determine not only the way a focal pattern was affected by an adjacent stimulus that abutted it but also the way it was changed if the focal and inducing areas touched only at a corner or if the focal and inducing stimulus were not directly contiguous but separated by a dark area. It is also clear from inspecting Figure 8b that other combinations of focal and inducing areas can be used.

A systematic series of experiments was first carried out for the two-element spatial configurations shown in Figure 8b. Rather than give all the details of the original research, it suffices here to say that we can convert the Munsell sample chip specifications that were selected for the matches to the X, Y, Z tristimulus values of the CIE system of colorimetric specification (see Chapter 20). Since CIE X, Y, Z standardized color-mixture values, like any other color-mixture measures can, in turn, be transformed to the quantified chromatic response values of the opponent-color scheme (see Chapter 9), the contrast effects can be analyzed in perceptual terms. Thus if we have determined the redness or greenness, and the yellowness or blueness, of a given area in isolation (i.e., in the absence of induction

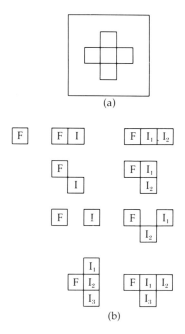

(a)

(b)

8 COMPLEX TEST-STIMULUS PATTERN. (a) Five similar elements on a square background used to measure color-contrast effects. (b) Focal and inducing area combinations derived from the stimulus pattern of (a).

areas), and the measured redness or greenness, and yellowness or blueness, in the presence of other inducing areas, the differences in measured hue qualities for the two conditions express the way the area has changed in perceived hue. This change can be expressed in relation to the chromatic responses of the inducing areas since they too have been evaluated independently using dark surrounds as masking fields.

Our measurements indicated that when two squares abutted, the contrast effect was twice as effective as when they touched only at a corner, and this in turn was twice as effective as when they were separated by a square "space." If we take this into account and "weight" the relative effectiveness of the spatial interaction in the ratios 4:2:1 for the three different contiguity conditions, we find that the way redness or greenness and yellowness or blueness are related to the strength of the chromatic response of the inducing stimuli is as shown in Figures 9 and 10.

The $+\Delta R'$ values are the increments in the redness direction and the $-\Delta R'$ values are the greenness increments. That is, a greater $-\Delta R'$ value indicates a larger increase in greenness. The values on the abscissa, the $+R'$ values, are the redness values of the inducing fields. Plus and minus Y' values and $\pm\Delta Y'$ values have similar meanings but related to the yellow/blue dimension. From both figures we can conclude that as redness of the inducing area increases, the focal area becomes increasingly green or less red; and as the yellowness of the inducing area becomes greater, the focal area becomes increasingly blue or less yellow. Needless to say, the different chromatic changes represented separately in the figures could

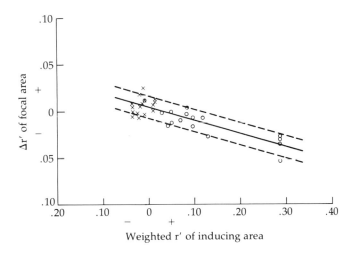

9 CHANGE IN REDNESS OR GREENNESS of the focal area as related to the redness or greenness of a single inducing area. Results are appropriately weighted for separations of focal and inducing areas.

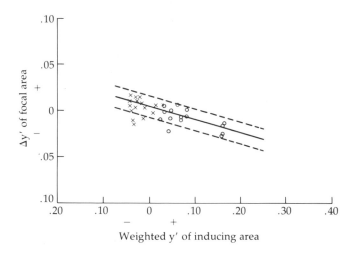

10 CHANGE IN YELLOWNESS OR BLUENESS of the focal area as related to the yellowness or blueness of a single inducing area. Results are appropriately weighted for different separations of focal and inducing areas.

and did occur at the same time (i.e., with a yellow-red inducing field present, the induced color was a bluish green; etc.).

For these particular conditions the chromatic response activity induced, $(R\text{-}G)_i$, $(Y\text{-}B)_i$, in a focal area, by a neighboring inducing stimulus is, for any given contiguity of the two stimulus fields, opposite but proportional in magnitude to the chromatic response activity aroused by the surrounding, inducing stimulus, $(R\text{-}G)_s$, $(Y\text{-}B)_s$. We can thus write

$$(R\text{-}G)_i = -k_1(R\text{-}G)_s$$
$$(Y\text{-}B)_i = -k_2(Y\text{-}B)_s$$

The values k_1 and k_2 are induction coefficients and appear to have the same value for both the red/green and yellow/blue response systems. And they seem to be related systematically to the contiguity of the two areas. Thus for focal and inducing areas separated by their own width, $k = -0.14$; for areas tangent at a single point, $k = -0.28$; and for areas having a common side, $k = -0.56$. This reflects the 4:2:1 ratio noted above.

Our discussion has dealt with pairs of small areas that are side by side, diagonal to each other, or separated by the distance of one square. What of the more complex stimulus situations?

When more than a single inducing area is present in the stimulus configuration, we have to take into account not only the induced color effects "suffered" by the focal area, but we also have to deal with the mutual contrast interactions among the various areas of the complexly composed inducing field itself. Consider, for example, three distinct points, P_1, P_2, and P_3, in the retinal image plane. When P_1 (the focal area) is illuminated alone, a certain visual reaction occurs. When P_2 is illuminated together with P_1, the response to P_1 is altered by the simultaneous P_2 stimulation (and vice versa). If P_3 illumination is added, the effect at P_2 is altered (by induction from P_3) and hence the inducing effect on P_1 exerted by the altered P_2 response also undergoes a change. Since the inductions are mutual and opponent, it seems obvious that the introduction of additional inducing (surround) areas will *not* show a simple summative effect with respect to the changes brought about in an arbitrarily selected focal area. Rather, if the pattern of surround stimuli is variegated, the mutual interactions among added elements would tend to counterbalance the effect of increasing the total area of surround stimulation.

Our analysis of complex fields therefore rests on the working assumption that the mutual interaction among all the various areas of the complex inducing field results in an averaging, rather than a summation, of the individually effective surround stimuli. Our quantitative data for complex surrounds analyzed in this way give essentially the same results as those we found for the contrast effects produced by single, homogeneous inducing areas (Figure 11). The induction effects result from mutual interactions among all the excited elements of the visual field.

It would be an error to assume that the mutual reciprocal interactions

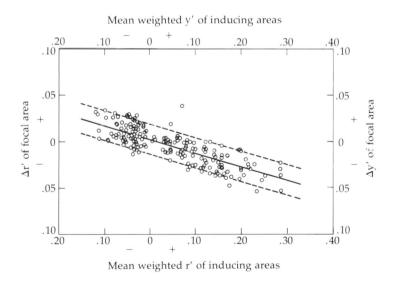

11 CHANGES IN REDNESS OR GREENNESS and yellowness or blueness of focal area and the average redness or greenness and yellowness or blueness of inducing areas. Results are appropriately weighted for different separations of focal and inducing areas.

among stimulus fields are limited to situations where the focal and inducing fields are of different energies and colors. Even when every element in a stimulus field has the same energy, there is a mutual interaction among the elements. Thus an isolated stimulus object of fixed reflectance will change in appearance if we vary its spatial dimensions even in a uniformly dark surround. Changes in size will produce changes in hue, saturation, and brightness. For example, a colored stimulus usually increases in saturation as its visual angle is increased up to about 20 degrees, but beyond this size it seems to decrease in saturation. There are also systematic hue changes that accompany changes in size. Objects that look green-blue tend to look much less blue or simply greenish when their retinal images are very tiny. And objects that look yellow-red lose their yellow hue when very small. The smaller the size of a colored object, the less likely it is that we will be able to see whether it is yellowish or bluish, even when we can still report with certainty whether it is red or green. This size effect is called "small-field tritanopia," which relates it to a rare form of congenitally deficient color vision known as tritanopia (Chapter 17).* Of course, if the retinal image is made sufficiently tiny, and the object did not look very bright to begin with, its brightness will be diminished to the point of disappearance in the dark surround. This is why we use telescopes to magnify the very distant stars.

On the other hand, because of the mutual and opposite interactions, a large field of uniform illumination can look less bright than an isolated piece of the field. (Any large field can obviously be considered as being constituted of a large number of individual components of the same unit size.) To see this, we need only compare the appearance of, say, a uniform cloud as it looks in free viewing with one eye with the way it looks when seen through a rather small hole punctured in a large piece of black cardboard or paper. Similarly, a large dark surface looks less dark than any small part of it seen alone and isolated in a light field. The mutual interactions among all the elements of the larger fields reduce the brightness of the larger fields, or their darkness, as the case may be.

Contrast effects of the sort that we have been describing seem to be uniform over the entire surface area over which the contrast is induced, and these effects have been named SURFACE CONTRAST. The general definition of perceived color must take these contrast effects into account, and in opponent-colors formulation we write

$$C = f[(r\text{-}g)_f + (r\text{-}g)_i, (y\text{-}b)_f + (y\text{-}b)_i, (w\text{-}bk)_f + (w\text{-}bk)_i]$$

where the induced chromaticity responses in the focal areas are, as we

* Note the parallel between size changes and light-level changes (see p. 72).

saw earlier, related in opponent fashion to the chromatic responses in the surround.

The same is true of the achromatic response, and we can relate the magnitude of the responses in both focal area and surround to the light level. The response in any area is composed of its own primary responses to light plus the response induced in it by neural activities in neighboring regions. Thus

$$R_f = cL_f{}^n + I_f$$

where $L_f{}^n$ is the light level in the focal area raised to a power, I_f the induced activity in the focal area, and R_f the response in the focal area (c is a constant). The same generalized relation holds for the surrounding area designated by the letter s. Thus

$$R_s = cL_s{}^n + I_s$$

Since the induced activities I_f and I_s are in each instance proportional to, but opposite to, the response activity in neighboring areas, we can write

$$I_f = -k_1R_s$$

and

$$I_s = -k_2R_f$$

Now by simple substitution we have, for the achromatic response, two equations that represent the responses to light stimulation in a focal and a surround area*:

$$R_f = c_1(L)_f{}^{1/3} - k_1R_s$$

and

$$R_s = c_2(L)_f{}^{1/3} - k_2R_f$$

Ernst Mach first called attention to the strong, unanticipated and rather dramatic contrast effects at the edge between two fields of different relative energies. If two uniformly illuminated fields of different energies are placed abutting each other, the surfaces are obviously of different brightnesses. If we then examine the interface or edge between the two fields carefully with rigorous fixation on the edge, we may see that the brighter field has a sharp line of exaggerated brightness at the interface and the darker field an exaggerated darkness at the interface. This effect becomes more evident if we use a step table of white-gray-black as in Figure 12. There is enhanced contrast at each edge despite the uniform distribution of light energy within each step.

* The exponent $1/3$ is an experimentally determined vaiue applied to L, a psychophysical measure of light level.

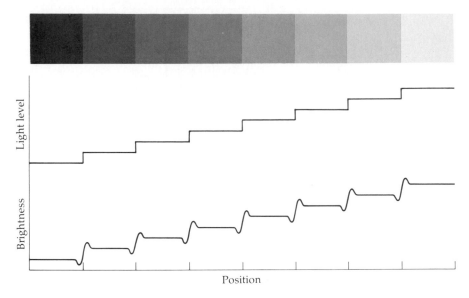

12 EDGE CONTRAST EFFECT. Step table of white-gray-black in which each step is of uniform intensity, yet at each edge there is a relative enhancement and darkening on the two sides of the edge.

The heightened contrast effect seen where two areas of different relative energies and hence different brightnesses abut is called BORDER CONTRAST or EDGE CONTRAST, for obvious reasons. In recent years it has also come to be referred to as the "Mach band effect" or "Mach contrast." These effects are particularly strong when the light energy changes gradually between the two fields, rather than sharply. If the shadow of the edge of a sunlit opaque screen is cast on a homogeneous white surface, the light distribution is that shown in Figure 13a. What we see (Figure 13b) is a relatively brighter band located at p and a relatively darker one at q. For the stimulus distribution shown in Figure 13a, we can sketch the way in which brightness varies (Figure 13c).

Stimulus-energy gradients of different slopes are most easily generated by using appropriately designed black-and-white discs that can be rotated on color wheels. The visual effect is shown in Figure 14; Figure 13a is a graph of the light-intensity distribution from the center of the rotating disc to the periphery. When the disc is spinning, the light level is high and uniform from the center out to point p. As the amount of black sector increases, there is a progressive decrease in the light level until point q is reached. Thereafter, the light level is uniformly low. Normally, we would anticipate that the inner central area of white would be seen as being surrounded by a ring gradually increasing in darkness, and that the outer area would be seen as black. These percepts would relate directly to the way the physically measured light distribution in the star pattern changes. What we do see, however, is a ring located at a point corresponding to point p, which is even brighter than the adjoining central white area, and at the point on the figure that corresponds to q we see a dark ring that is even darker than the black at the edge of the disc. The bright and dark lines occur where there are inflection points in the light energy distribution, and these are points or areas where the light energy is either above or below the average of the light energy in the adjacent regions (i.e., on both sides of the inflection point).

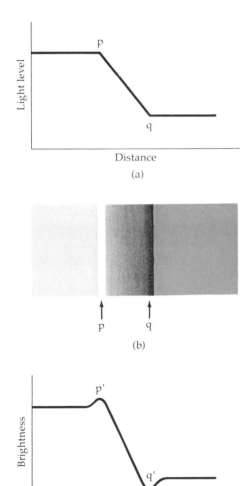

(a)

(b)

(c)

13 LIGHT DISTRIBUTION AND VISUAL EFFECTS. (a) Schematic of the light distribution when a shadow is cast on a homogeneous white surface by the edge of an opaque screen in sunlight. (b) A simulation of the Mach band effect produced by the light distribution in (a). (c) Representation of the variation in brightness when Mach bands are seen.

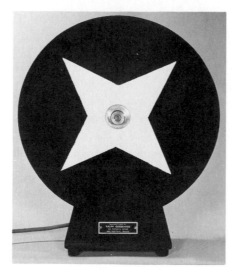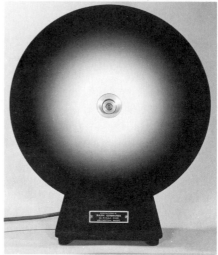

14 STAR PATTERN to produce Mach band effects. The light-intensity distribution and schematic representation of brightness distribution seen are given in Figure 13.

There has been disagreement about whether border contrast effects or Mach rings are seen if the adjacent areas vary in color only and there are no associated light level differences. Does a yellow area next to a blue one, for example, enhance their respective edges? We would expect border contrasts of this type to occur, because we often see hue contrast with surfaces that are equally bright. These edge effects, however, have not been easy to demonstrate, although in recent years a number of investigators have reported that colored Mach band effects are seen by many of their observers.

Everything we have discussed regarding spatial contrast effects—both brightness and color-contrast effects—supports the statement made at the beginning of the chapter: There appears to be an almost complete interdependence among the neural activities in the retina and its associated pathways. The phenomena of simultaneous contrast arise from these neural interactions. We have seen in our discussion of the anatomy of the visual system that in the retinal structures alone, there is a complex of interrelated nerve cell tissue organized in a way that would permit stimulation at any one retinal locus to reach a number of disparate loci further along in the chain of neural interconnections. A diagrammatic representation of the various retinal structures and their synaptic interrelations in the vertebrate retina is shown in Figure 15a. We see that the receptor cells form synaptic contacts with both bipolar and horizontal cells, and bipolars are synaptically related to both horizontal and amacrine cells as well as serving in the "transmission line" between receptors and retinal ganglion cells. It is easy to see that discharges in ganglion cell G_1 can be affected by light absorption that occurs in both receptors R_1 and R_2. The same is true for ganglion cell G_2. Figure 15b schematizes the essence of this situation.

This simple conceptualization applies, of course, to a retinal surface made up of millions of receptor cells that are linked to many hundreds of thousands of ganglion cells via the intermediate neural structures mentioned. That is, activities set up by one stimulus imaged on the retinal surface stimulate retinal receptors, which, in turn, excite the ganglion cells connected to them. If a different stimulus is imaged on an adjacent retinal region, the converging neural pathways leading from the second set of receptor cells will serve to increase the activity in the already excited

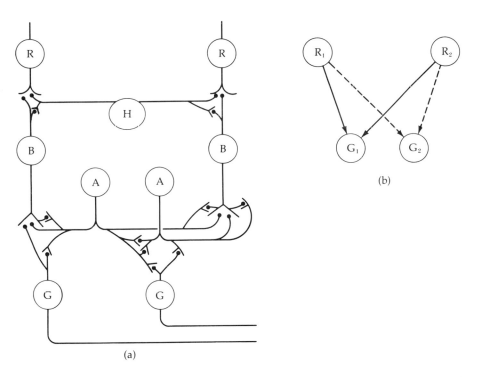

(a)

(b)

15 RETINAL STRUCTURES and their synaptic interrelations. (a) Sketch based on the work of Dowling and Werblin (1969) on the vertebrate retina. Receptors R drive both bipolar B and horizontal H cells, horizontals synapse laterally on adjacent bipolars, bipolar terminals to both ganglion G and amacrine A cells. Amacrines make feedback synapses on bipolar terminals, feed-forward synapses on ganglion cells, and feed-forward and lateral serial synapses on other amacrine cell processes. (b) Interrelations between two receptor cells and two ganglion cells, schematized for simplicity.

ganglion cells. But contrast effects are opponent in nature. If we are to conceptualize the spatial interaction among the neural elements in a meaningful way, we must look for neural interactions that are antagonistic or opponent ones. This requires a scheme whereby the receptor elements that feed into a common neural system do so in both an excitatory and an inhibitory fashion.

The basis for such a scheme has already been given. Figure 4 in Chapter 11 shows the relations between cone absorptions and opponent response functions. The neural elements blue/yellow, green/red, and white/black are linked in both excitatory and inhibitory fashion to the cone elements as indicated. This simple diagram can be taken as being representative of the linkage between a trio of receptor cells and their associated neural cells at one retinal location. The figure presents what might be called the "vertical" relations between the receptor units and the opponent neural response pairs. To provide a mechanism that will encompass the various kinds of contrast effects—both simultaneous and successive—the conceptual opponent process model has to be extended and modified.

In extending the model to deal with spatial contrast effects, we assume that specific lateral interconnections exist such that activities aroused in a given paired system, whether in a blue/yellow, green/red, or white/black system, both influence and are reciprocally influenced by ongoing activities in adjacent and surrounding neural systems of corresponding types (Figure 16). This influence is assumed in the model to be both mutual and opponent, that is, if, say, blueness-coded activity is ongoing in one functional unit of the opponent blue/yellow system, opposite-coded activity is induced in adjacent functional units of the same coding. The mechanisms operate in the same way, according to the model, in the opponent red/green system, where redness activity induces greenness activity in neighboring units, and vice versa, and in the opponent white/black system as well. The achromatic white/black system differs from the hue-coded opponent pairs only with respect to symmetry of arousal. There is no external stimulus to excite blackness directly (see Chapter 5).

In terms of what we called the vertical interrelations, all three types of cone activities arouse activities of common sign in the achromatic system and the code is "whiteness." The oppositely signed blackness response comes about only indirectly as an aftereffect of the direct focal stimulation of the retina, or through the system of laterally induced opponent activities. It is the lateral, opponent, induced activities that are, we believe, responsible for the phenomena of simultaneous contrast. Since the conceptual model has been developed in a quantitative way that also expresses these lateral opponent effects in equation form, we can derive quantitative psychophysical functions to express the amount of hue and brightness contrast effect produced for a variety of stimulus parameters.

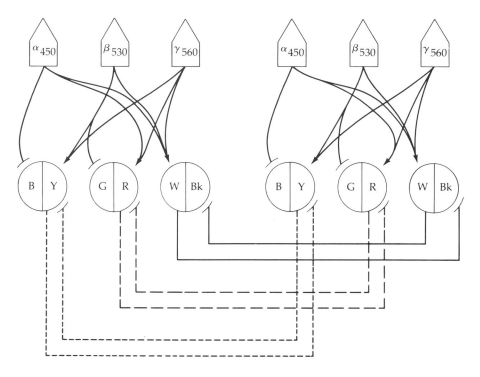

16 RELATIONS BETWEEN CONE ABSORPTIONS and opponent response processes expanded and schematized to represent the reciprocal lateral influences at the opponent process level.

Conceptualizations of this sort to explain surface contrast effects date back to the nineteenth century. Ernst Mach, more than a hundred years ago, concluded that the border contrast effects he observed were indicative of reciprocal interactions among adjacent retinal neural regions. The brilliant insights of both Hering and Mach, who argued the physiological case on the basis of the perceptual phenomena, have now been universally accepted because the reciprocal physiological antagonisms that they postulated have been found to occur in physiological preparations of a variety of organisms. What are some of these findings?

Some of the first systematic studies of the opponent spatial organization of the visual system were carried out on the individual nerve cells of the retina of the cat. If a very small electrode is used to record from a single ganglion cell and light stimuli are imaged on the retinal surface, any one ganglion cell responds not simply to a small punctiform stimulus located within a very tiny region of this surface but also to such a stimulus imaged anywhere within a relatively large retinal region. This region of responsiveness is known as the RECEPTIVE FIELD of the cell and one such

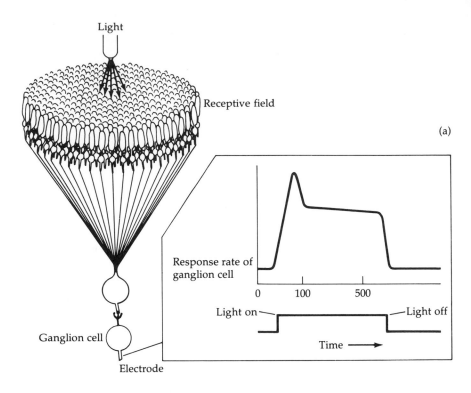

Light

Receptive field

(a)

Response rate of
ganglion cell

0   100   500

Light on   Light off

Time

Ganglion cell

Electrode

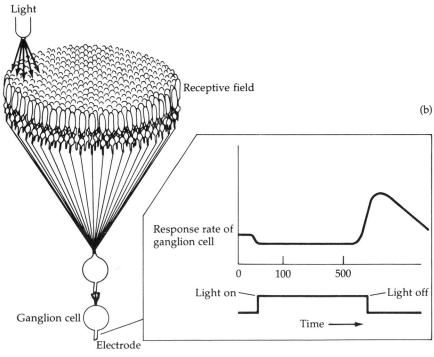

Light

Receptive field

(b)

Response rate of
ganglion cell

0   100   500

Light on   Light off

Time

Ganglion cell

Electrode

17 RECEPTIVE FIELD with electrode in ganglion cell. Light stimulus in center of field in (a) and at edge of receptive field in (b). Response of ganglion cell to light onset and offset is shown in the inset in each figure. With central stimulation there is an on-response; with peripheral stimulation there is an off-response.

receptive field is shown in perspective view in Figure 17. But the responses evoked by a small light stimulus differ in different regions of the receptive field. Figure 18 shows a receptive field map of a ganglion cell in top view. Light focused on the center (0.1 to 1.0 mm) of the field evokes, say, on-responses; that is, the cell fires when the light is turned on. But when the light is imaged on the periphery or surround area of receptivity, the cell responds in an opposite way. In this case, cell firing is inhibited during stimulation with subsequent off-responses when the light is extinguished. (In other cells, the surround area is excitatory, the center region inhibitory.)

A good deal of electrophysiological work on the retinas of a variety of species other than the cat, such as fish, ground squirrel, rat, rabbit, and monkey, has established that the receptive fields are typically organized into a roughly circular center with an antagonistic annular surround.

Figure 19 shows in diagrammatic form the essence of the opponent spatial organization that emerges from assuming specific relations between groups of retinal receptor units, on the one hand, and single neural cells on the other. The representation of Figure 19, which is a vertical cut through the perspective view of Figure 17, shows a cell with a spatially

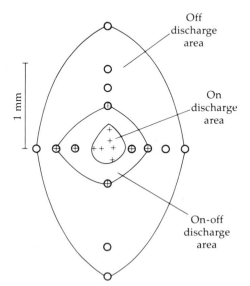

Off discharge area

On discharge area

1 mm

On-off discharge area

18 RECEPTIVE FIELD MAP of ganglion cell in cat retina. Crosses represent on-discharges (central region), circles represent off-discharges (peripheral region). Both on- and off-discharges occur in intermediate region.

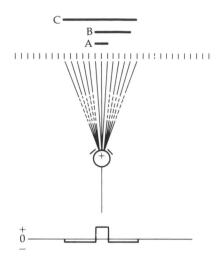

19 SPATIALLY OPPONENT RECEPTIVE FIELD ORGANIZATION shown diagramatically in cross section. Central stimulation is excitatory, peripheral stimulation is inhibitory. The bottom part of the figure diagrams the response profile, called the neural unit. The central receptor cell stimulation gives a plus response, the receptor elements in the periphery produce a negative response. A unit-magnitude stimulus A (shown centered over the three middle elements) triggers a plus excitatory response of magnitude shown in the response profile. Stimulus B triggers both excitatory (plus) and inhibitory (minus) responses; the net response is the difference between the plus and minus magnitudes. Stimulus C triggers more inhibitory responses and the net outcome is less positive than for either A or B.

opponent receptive field organization (but no wavelength specificity) with respect to type of response. What we see is that the neural (say, ganglion) cell is being influenced by activities engendered when light is incident upon and absorbed by a relatively large number of receptors on the retina. The inputs from the receptors in the center of the receptive field of this cell are associated with one mode of response (positive) and the inputs from the other receptors in the periphery of the cell's receptive field are associated with the opposite mode of response in the same cell (negative). If the cell produces excitatory bursts when the center is stimulated, stimulation of the periphery leads to inhibitory responses, and vice versa.

The response profile of such an arrangement is shown in the lower part of the figure. It has been called a NEURAL UNIT. With stimuli of appropriate dimensions, such an organization is ideally suited to heighten contrast; thus a weak light falling on the receptors in the center of the receptive field would cause some firing in such a cell, but a stronger light falling on the receptors in the surround of the receptive field would inhibit the firing rate of the cell. The net responses of the cell would then be equivalent to or even less than what it might be were there no light at all impinging on the receptors centered in the receptive field. So because of this arrangement, a gray spot centered in a light surround would, in terms of the physiological coding, appear darker or blacker than it would if the response depended on the light level of the gray spot alone.

There are, of course, many thousand cells whose receptive fields on the retinal surface overlap, and if we analyze the situation mathematically for a multiplicity of receptor cells, the outcome is the same with respect to the heightened contrast just described for the single cell under the influence of an organized field of receptor inputs.

A particularly dramatic example of heightened contrast is seen in Plate 13-2. In this geometrical design of Vasarely's there are no light-energy counterparts to the bright diagonals (Figure 20a). If we used a photocell to measure the light energy in each quadrant, we would record a decrease in light level in step fashion from the center to the figure's edge. If we measure the light energy along any perimetric strip, we would record no

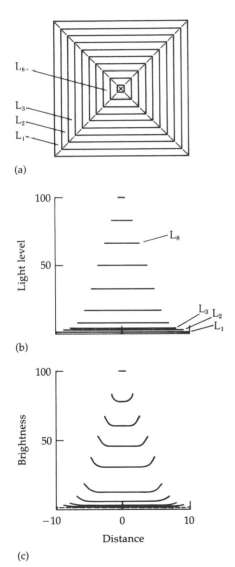

(a)

(b)

(c)

20 LIGHT DISTRIBUTION IN THE VA-SARELY COMPOSITION. (a) One of the four quadrants of the Vasarely composition. L_1 is the lowest light level, L_2 is greater than L_1 and less than L_3, and so on. (b) Measured light levels in step fashion from the center to the perimeter. (c) Brightness predictions made using a model that postulates a 5-min. receptive field center. Note that there is a brightness increase at each corner. If we visualize the brightness distributions for the three other quadrants placed next to one another, we see that there is a direct correlation with the perceived "glowing" diagonals of Plate 13-2.

variation in light level (Figure 20b). However, a model based on sets of overlapping neural units with spatially opponent receptive fields enables us to calculate the way the brightness along any perimetric strip is predicted to vary. With specific assumptions about the excitatory inputs, their sizes, the relative proportions of excitatory center diameters of the receptive fields and the width of their inhibitory flanks, and their relative scaling factors, Dorothea Jameson has determined the net outputs for specific types of light-level distributions in the retinal image. These results for one set of asssumptions (receptive fields, sizes, etc.) are shown in Figure 20c.

Similar mathematical analyses can be made for the Mach band type of contour or edge effect. But the way effects come about can be understood qualitatively without mathematical computation. The brightness variations plotted in Figure 13 are dependent upon the relative degrees of excitation and inhibition that occur at any given retinal locus. The inflection points p and q in Figure 13a show loci of increased and decreased brightness relative to their surrounding areas. The neural response at the p locus is "inhibited" to a lesser degree by the areas to its right, which are at a lower light level than are the loci to the left of p, which are all at the same high light level. The reverse is true at the q locus. Here the light levels on the retinal areas adjacent to q progressively increase going to the left of q and those to the right of it are relatively low and remain fixed. The neural response at the q locus suffers a greater inhibitory effect than do the loci to its right, which are all equally illuminated. It therefore looks darker relative to the areas adjacent to it.

I have been discussing the concept of spectral opponent action throughout this book. In Chapter 12 we reviewed some of the electrophysiological evidence that supports the notion. How can the spectral-opponents notion be coordinated with the spatial-opponents notion in receptive field terms? The spatial organization would remain as it has been described here, but it would be necessary for spectral opponency that the center portion of the field also be wavelength-specific and manifest excitation or inhibition to light from different spectral regions. Furthermore, the periphery of such a receptive field would also need to be wavelength-specific but with a reversal of the excitation/inhibition organization so that it is opposite to that of the center of the field. Cells of this type would have the properties shown in Figure 21. In sensitivity terms it would have the mirror-image form shown in Figure 21. Such a "double opponent" cell would relate meaningfully to hue and its wavelength length dependencies and to the phenomena of simultaneous hue contrast. But only a few cells of precisely this type have been reported, although approximations to this kind of organization are not uncommon.

The discussion of electrophysiological evidence for spatial and spectral

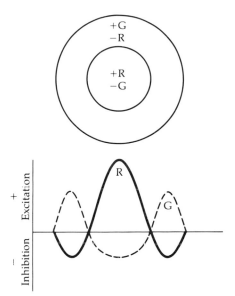

21 RECEPTIVE FIELD of a spectrally and spatially opponent cell. R and G are presumed hue coding of responses to long and midspectral wavelengths in the cell.

opponency can be extended to discuss experiments on mechanisms more central than the retina and its ganglion cells. But the way in which spectral and spatial specialization are coordinated at the cellular level gets less clear as we look more centrally in the visual nervous system and as higher-level primates are studied. Some double-opponency cells are reported in the primary visual cortex of the monkey, for example, but the cortical cells show a preponderance of other sorts of receptive field organizations and, unfortunately, the same types of cellular specialization are not found to be duplicated at different neural levels in a given species (i.e., LGN and cortex). The broad outlines are clear, nevertheless. Specifics await further experimentation.

Whatever the shortcomings of the direct physiological evidence at the moment, the "fine-grain" receptive field theoretical model with which we can account for a variety of contrast effects—whether of the surface contrast or border contrast type—has an additional advantage: we can use it to suggest a possible physiological basis for the long known but little understood visual effect which is the opposite of the contrast effects. This is the BEZOLD SPREADING EFFECT or "assimilation phenomenon" (Plate 13-3).

The effect is best seen in repetitive patterns of certain dimensions where there is a pulling together or blending of the adjacent colors rather than an accentuation of their differences, as in color contrast. The colors that we perceive in this effect are not the result of optical mixture of the conventional pointillist sort. The individual elements of the pattern are seen as discrete elements (stripes or curves) despite the color blending.

There is in the assimilation situation a blending of the adjacent hues and/or brightnesses that form a pattern of, say, alternating stripes. The grating pattern remains quite distinct when the assimilation or blending occurs. What we have is not simply an averaging process but a process in which averaging and differencing occur simultaneously.

Dorothea Jameson and I believe that the physiological basis of this effect is the spatial nonuniformity of the retina and its cellular organization, and we have consequently incorporated some known facts of receptive field organization into our model. Receptive field sizes vary from periphery to fovea and they also show considerable variation in any given retinal region (Figure 22). Thus when a grating pattern is imaged on the retina, some visual cells that have broad receptive fields will, in effect, pool the light from adjacent stripes and respond as if the light were actually mixed on the retina, while other cells that collect light over a smaller region of the retina respond as "contrast" cells and in this way maintain the spatial resolution of the linear pattern of physiological responses. The net result of calculations for physiological systems with receptive fields of different sizes agrees with this interpretation: there is a blending of hues and brightnesses (assimilation) but a maintenance of spatial pattern resolution.

The spatial contrast problem is currently being analyzed by many investigators by the use of sine-wave grating stimuli of different spatial frequencies. Such stimuli permit mathematical analysis in Fourier waveform terms, and any description of these studies requires understanding the appropriate mathematics. Analysis of the underlying physiological mechanisms, however, leads to considerations of neural receptive field properties much like those described in the preceding discussion.

The mechanisms of simultaneous contrast that I have been discussing serve very useful functions. Like all optical devices, even the most costly, the optical system of the eye is not a perfect one. A point in outer space is not imaged on the retina as a true point, but rather as a somewhat more diffuse area usually called a BLUR CIRCLE. In any optical system, the size of the blur circle depends on a variety of factors, and is influenced by the amounts of the various aberrations inherent in the system. The most common of these are chromatic aberrations, which lead to colored fringes around the edges of images formed by white light, and spherical aberrations, which produce distortions in the shape of the image from the center to its outer edges. In the human eye, these aberrations are actually quite large. Moreover, as light penetrates the eye, a good deal of it is dispersed in more-or-less random fashion as it passes through the various media and undergoes multiple reflections from the various surface boundaries. This optical process distributes a diffuse overlay of "stray" light over the

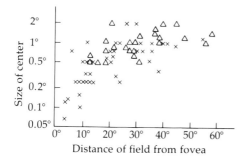

22 SIZES OF RECEPTIVE FIELDS. The diameters of receptive field centers are plotted here in degrees (in a logarithmic scale) against the distance in degrees of each field from the fovea. The receptive fields become larger in general as the distance from the fovea increases, and at any given retinal locus there is considerable variation in receptive field size. (×, on-center units; Δ, off-center units.)

entire image plane. The net effect of all these imperfections in the optical system of the eye is that the images formed on the retina are not, in fact, of very good quality. They are not extremely sharp, as is, for example, the shadow cast by an object in direct sunlight, but more like the relatively blurred shadow of the same object when the source of illumination is diffuse skylight and not the direct sun. Nevertheless, we do not see the outlines of well-delineated objects as indistinct or somewhat blurred in the way the optical system of our eye actually images them on the retina, but rather we see good sharp edges. These sharp edges or contours come about by the action of simultaneous contrast. This physiological "device" compensates for the blurred edges of objects that might otherwise be seen.

Simultaneous contrast effects, moreover, aid in offsetting the effects of stray light and irradiation. If we have a strongly illuminated object imaged on the retina, it tends to scatter light into adjacent areas of the eye because of the eye's imperfect optical imagery. This would lead to creating blurred edges and the brightness of the object would be seen as tapering off into the surround. But as we have seen, bright lights induce strong darkening effects in the neighboring regions, and the effect of this is to make the stray light dispersed into the adjacent regions visually ineffective or at least dampened in its action. Hence the outline of the strongly illuminated object is sharper. The same analysis applies to the hue mechanisms, and, although the spatial dimensions may differ somewhat, the color-contrast mechanisms also serve to make colored focal objects more sharply differentiated from neighboring objects.

Background Readings

Abramov, I. 1972. Retinal Mechanisms of Colour Vision. In M. G. F. Fuortes (ed.), *Handbook of Sensory Physiology*, Vol. 7/2, *Physiology of Photoreceptor Organs*, Chap. 15, pp. 567–607. Springer-Verlag, Berlin.

Burnham, R. W. 1952. Comparative effects of area and luminance on color. *Amer. J. Psychol. 65*: 27–38.

Chevreul, M. E. 1839. *The Principles of Harmony and Contrast of Colors.* (Reprinted 1967, Van Nostrand Reinhold, New York.)

Dowling, J. E., and Werblin, F. S. 1969. Organization of the retina of the mudpuppy, *Necturus maculosus*—I. Synaptic structure. *J. Neurophysiol. 32*: 315–338.

Evans, R. M. 1943. Visual processes and color photography. *J. Opt. Soc. Amer. 33*: 579–614.

Farnsworth, D. 1955. Tritanomalous vision as a threshold function. *Die Farbe 4*: 185–197.

Fiorentini, A. 1972. Mach Band Phenomena. In D. Jameson and L. M. Hurvich (eds.), *Handbook of Sensory Physiology,* Vol. 7/4, *Visual Psychophysics*, Chap. 8, pp. 188–201. Springer-Verlag, Berlin.

Helson, H., and Rohles, F. H., Jr. 1959. A quantitative study of reversal of classical lightness-contrast. *Amer. J. Psychol. 72*: 530–538.

Hering, E. 1878. *Zur Lehre vom Lichtsinne.* Carl Gerold's Sohn, Vienna.

Hering, E. 1920. *Grundzüge der Lehre vom Lichtsinn.* Springer-Verlag, Berlin. (Outlines of a Theory of the Light Sense, Chap. 10. Translated by L. M. Hurvich and D. Jameson. Harvard University Press, Cambridge, Mass., 1964.)

Hubel, D. H., and Wiesel, T. N. 1960. Receptive fields of optic nerve fibers in the spider monkey. *J. Physiol. Lond. 154*: 572–580.

Hurvich, L. M., and Jameson, D. 1960. Perceived color, induction effects, and opponent-response mechanisms. *J. Gen. Physiol. 43*(6): (Suppl.), 63–80.

Hurvich, L. M., and Jameson, D. 1969. Human color perception. An essay review. *Amer. Sci. 57*: 143–166.

Hurvich, L. M., and Jameson, D. 1974. Opponent processes as a model of neural organization. *Amer. Psychol. 29*: 88–102.

Jameson, D. 1972. Theoretical Issues of Color Vision. In D. Jameson and L. M. Hurvich (eds.), *Handbook of Sensory Physiology,* Vol. 7/4, *Visual Psychophysics*, Chap. 14, pp. 381–412. Springer-Verlag, Berlin.

Jameson, D. 1975. Color vision: Mechanisms, models and perception. John F. Shepard 1975 Memorial Lecture, University of Michigan.

Jameson, D., and Hurvich, L. M. 1959. Perceived color and its dependence on focal, surround, and preceding stimulus variables. *J. Opt. Soc. Amer. 49*: 890–898.

Jameson, D., and Hurvich, L. M. 1961. Opponent chromatic induction: Experimental evaluation and theoretical account. *J. Opt. Soc. Amer. 51*: 46–53.

Jameson, D., and Hurvich, L. M. 1964. Theory of brightness and color contrast in human vision. *Vision Res. 4*: 135–154.

Jameson, D., and Hurvich, L. M. 1975. From contrast to assimilation: In art and in the eye. *Leonardo 8*: 125–131.

Judd, D. B. 1960. Appraisal of Land's work in two-primary color projections. *J. Opt. Soc. Amer. 50*: 254–268.

Kuffler, S. W. 1953. Discharge patterns and functional organization of mammalian retina. *J. Neurophysiol. 16*: 37–68.

Linksz, A. 1952. *Physiology of the Eye,* Vol. 2, *Vision.* Grune & Stratton, New York.

Musatti, C. L. 1957. *Problèmes de la Couleur,* Chap. 5. Service d'Edition et de Vente des Publications de l'Education Nationale, Paris.

Thompson, B. 1794. An account of some experiments on coloured shadows. *Phil. Trans R. Soc. Lond.* Pt I, 107–118.

Tschermak, A. 1903. Über Kontrast und Irradiation. *Ergeb. Physiol.* II, 2: 726–798.

Vasarely, V. 1970. *Vasarely II.* Translated by H. Chevalier. Éditions du Griffon, Neuchâtel.

Further Readings

Green, D. G. 1968. The contrast sensitivity of the colour mechanisms of the human eye. *J. Physiol. Lond. 196*, 415–429.

Mach, E. 1914. *The Analysis of Sensations.* Open Court, La Salle, Ill.

Marsden, A. M. 1969. An elemental theory of induction. *Vision Res. 9*: 653–663.

Michael, C. R. 1978. Color vision mechanisms in monkey striate cortex: Dual-opponent cells with concentric receptive fields. *J. Neurophysiol. 41*: 572–588.

Plateau, J. 1878. Bibliographie analytique des principaux phénomènes subjectifs de la vision. Cinquième section. Phénomènes ordinaires de contraste. Sixième section. Ombres colorées. *Mém. Acad. R. Belg. 42*(5): 1–35; (6): 1–36.

Ratliff, F. 1965. *Mach Bands: Quantitative Studies on Neural Networks in the Retina.* Holden-Day, San Francisco.

14
Temporal Contrast Effects: Afterimages

WE saw in Chapter 13 that when the stimulus properties (constant energy, wavelength, and time of stimulation) are fixed, changes in stimulus size produce resultant changes in appearance. This is also true of stimulus duration if energy, wavelength, and size are fixed.

To see this for yourself, place a white piece of paper to the right of the × in Plate 14-1 to cover the yellow region that lies to the right of it. Stare at the fixation cross for 30 seconds or so. Then quickly remove the white mask while continuing to stare at the fixation ×. Note the relative saturations of the left and right halves of the yellow rectangle. The yellow half-field that has been stimulating the eye continuously for 30 seconds looks pale compared to the yellow half-field that excites the eye freshly.

Suppose, to take another example, that you are sitting in an unilluminated dark room whose walls are painted white. A single electric bulb is turned on behind your head and the room instantly brightens. The light energy is known to rise rapidly and reach a maximum, where it remains as long as the illumination stays on (Figure 1a). But if we observe closely the way the brightness of the white walls changes with time after the light is turned on, we would obtain a result like the one shown in Figure 1b. Following the light onset, the brightness rises quickly, reaches a maximum, and then slowly decays to an intermediate, relatively stable level at which it remains as long as the light stays on. These effects are subtle ones and require careful observation.

The way the light appearance changes over time can be analyzed in terms of an interaction that occurs between two opposed reactions: a "whiteness response" and a "blackness response". In the absence of external light, while we sit in the dark, the entire visual system is assumed to be in a balanced equilibrium state and the whiteness/blackness system is also assumed to be in balance. (This equilibrium state corresponds to the spontaneous level of neural discharge [see Chapter 12]). The stimulus onset is shown in Figure 2a. As shown in Figure 2b, the whiteness process

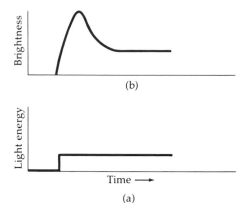

1 LIGHT-ENERGY OUTPUT (a) of an electric light bulb rises very rapidly, reaches a maximum, and stays fixed when the light is turned on. (b) Brightness changes seen do not directly parallel those of the stimulus but in time follow the course shown by the curve.

is activated by light stimulation and rises rapidly at first to reach a level plateau at some time after stimulus onset. The stimulus energy level continues unchanged. The "action" or whiteness process, in turn, sets off a "reaction" or blackness process. The blackness reaction is somewhat delayed in its onset because it is a response initiated by the whiteness process stimulated by the light. This reaction is represented as a drop

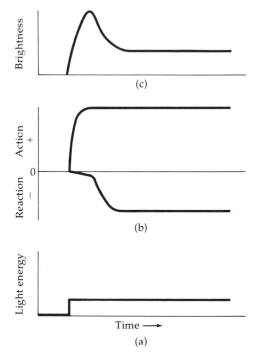

2 BRIGHTNESS CHANGES that occur are the outcome of a dual process. (a) Stimulus onset and continued fixed light output. (b) Activation of "action" or whiteness process. Rapid rise to a maximum and leveling off. "Reaction" or blackness process initiated by whiteness process. (c) Resultant of opposed action/reaction processes.

from the baseline in the negative direction opposite the positive whiteness action. The blackness response, which is of smaller magnitude than the whiteness response, also shortly reaches a steady level. The resultant of the opposed action/reaction process is shown in Figure 2c. The net outcome is the difference between the action and reaction, or whiteness and blackness, magnitudes at any moment. As we saw in Figure 1, brightness rises steeply initially and then falls back to a more intermediate level. The effects we have been discussing take place within a few seconds. If we fixate the light bulb there is an initial burst of light that is often glaring and uncomfortable. It is best described as an "overshoot" and it is followed by a settling down to a steady level of brightness.

The time course of brightness variations can be measured by using light flashes of different durations. The brightness of these flashes is matched by varying the light energy of a continuously exposed light source. Among the first experiments of this sort were those carried out by two French scientists, Broca and Sulzer. The stimulating times they used were very short ones, varying from about 0.025 to 0.125 second. They tested lights of different spectral composition and at various energy levels. A typical result is shown in Figure 3 for light levels arbitrarily labeled L_1, L_2, and L_3. Notice that stimulus L_3 looks brighter if exposed, for, say, only 0.03 second than if it is exposed for a longer time, say, 0.10 or 0.20 second. This is an initial brightness "overshoot" and then a brightness decrease, just as in the longer stimulations I have been discussing. Furthermore, note in Figure 3 that a stronger stimulus (L_3) reaches its brightness peak earlier and its visual effectiveness drops more rapidly than it does when a less intense stimulus (L_2) is used. We are simply dealing with different

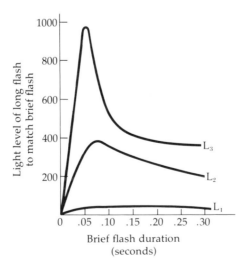

3 BRIGHTNESS VARIATIONS of briefly exposed stimuli of different light intensities. These variations are measured by adjusting the light energy of a continuously exposed stimulus to match the effects produced by the brief flashes.

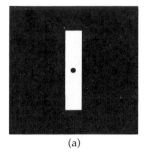
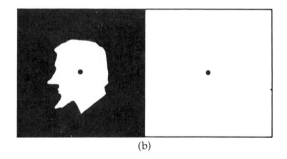

(a)   (b)

4 AFTERIMAGES perceived after extinguishing or cutting off stimulation. (a) The small white stripe on the figure is viewed with rigorous fixation for about 20 to 30 seconds; when the eyes are shut the white stripe takes on a dark appearance. The background, on the other hand, lightens. (b) If a white figure is projected on a neighboring white area after fixation, the brightness relations are again reversed. In this case the brief bright flash that may be seen when the eyes are closed does not occur.

rates of rise and different time courses of the dual action/reaction process, and these factors are responsible for the different results.

Antagonistic events are intrinsic to all sorts of equilibrium systems: physical, chemical, or biological ones. In discussing physiological systems most investigators prefer, instead of action/reaction, to use the term excitation/inhibition to describe the antagonistic physiological events.* These terms were used in Chapter 13 in discussing simultaneous contrast effects.

The situations we have been describing up to now are concerned mainly with the way the perceived brightness of either briefly exposed or long-duration stimuli vary in time following stimulus onset. Let us now concentrate on the light extinction phase. What happens when a light is turned off? Even the most casual observing reveals that we often "see" colors even after the physical light stimulation is cut off. These phenomena, as discussed and illustrated in Chapter 2, are called AFTERIMAGES, and many types have been described and catalogued in the visual literature.

Another illustration of afterimages is obtained with the aid of Figure 4a. If we look at the small white stripe on the black surface for about 20 to 30 seconds and then shut our eyes, the white stripe takes on a dark

* Flicker and flicker fusion (visual persistence effects), which use repetitive brief alternating light and dark stimulus pulses, are very closely related to neural events of this sort. Flicker research, which is primarily concerned with the temporal resolution properties of the eye, is now being worked on experimentally mainly with sine-wave-modulated light stimulation in conjunction with Fourier waveform types of analyses (Figure 3 in Chapter 3 illustrates the sine-wave form). It would take us too far afield to go into the various phenomena and theoretical issues raised by flicker and flicker-fusion studies, but see page 188 for a brief statement about flicker effects in connection with the discussion of "subjective colors."

appearance, and simultaneously or a few seconds later the background is seen to lighten. We ignore here the brief whiteness flash that may be seen on first closing the eyes. There are many afterimage phases that depend on the light energy, state of the visual system, and so on. In addition, brief persistent stimulus effects like the whiteness flash may also be reported. If, instead of closing our eyes, we "project" the afterimage on an illuminated white surface, for example, the bright phase is not seen (Figure 4b). The central area darkens immediately while the surround brightens.

When we look at Figure 5 we see that for a stimulus duration that is finite, the separate opponent white and black processes return to the baseline when the white light is cut off. If the two "recovery" processes occur at different rates, as we might expect, since these "rates of recovery" will be dependent on the relative magnitudes of the action and reaction processes at the moment the light goes off, the net outcome will be as indicated in the figure. A fairly sharp increase in darkness ("negative" afterimage) occurs just as the light stimulus is turned off, and the net response then returns to the baseline equilibrium state.

But I have also called attention to the fact that the surround, which

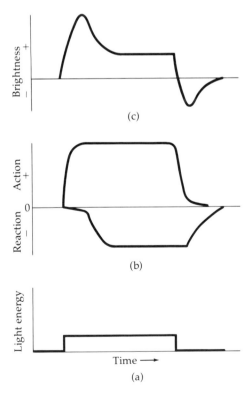

5 OCCURRENCE OF NEGATIVE AF-TERIMAGE analyzed in terms of action/reaction processes following stimulus offset. (a) Stimulus onset followed by offset. (b) Action and reaction processes at onset, during, and at offset of stimulation. (c) Resultant of opposed action/reaction processes. Reversal to darkness response shown as negative in (c) is the net outcome of different rates of decay of whiteness/blackness responses.

was initially dark, brightens. Here, too, we have a simple reversal: darkness turns to lightness in the afterimage. The antagonism between the two processes can in a sense be observed directly if in Figure 4a we observe the way the initial brightness of the white stripe darkens as we continue to stare at the fixation point. If we attend carefully to the neighboring black regions while still fixating rigorously, we can also see the way these areas start to lighten. Slight eye movements which reveal both brighter and darker edge effects emphasize that reciprocal antagonistic processes are in play.

To understand the phenomena of afterimages we must also recall that neural events that occur in any delineated area of the visual system are linked with neural events in neighboring regions, as we have seen in discussing the phenomena of simultaneous contrast. What this implies for successive contrast or afterimage phenomena is that the changes over time are also affected by spatial interactions and as in the simultaneous contrast situation, they do so in opponent fashion. Thus there is not only an opponent interaction over time in the nervous system at the place corresponding to the white stripe, where the white excitatory process entrains (essentially simultaneously) an opposite blackness reaction, but in accordance with the model shown in Figure 16 in Chapter 13, which emphasizes lateral interactions, the blackness process in the fixated region itself entrains an antagonistic whiteness process in the adjacent neural areas that correspond to the dark surround.

One can also place a small dark test field on a white background and examine the successive contrast effects by fixating the dark focal area rigorously for a short while before transferring one's gaze to either large black or white secondary fields. In all cases, the effects are those to be anticipated from an opponent process analysis that postulates antagonistic responses to occur in any one area over time and reciprocal antagonism to be in play between the neural events in, say, the focal and surround areas.

The antagonistic or opponent reactions that occur with chromatic stimuli were referred to in Chapter 2. Each of the linked neural pairs yellow/blue and red/green are assumed to act in an associated action/reaction way. Like the examples discussed there, Plate 13-1 can be used to demonstrate complementary afterimage effects in a single viewing. Fixate the center of one side of this figure for 30 seconds and look over to a piece of white paper. The afterimage hues are complementary to those seen initially.

The antagonistic response of red is green and of yellow, is blue, and vice versa. For example, if a single small red chromatic stimulus lying on a white ground is inspected for 30 seconds, the focal afterimage is vivid green and careful observation will reveal that the background, especially in the region closest to the focal stimulus, is pale red. The focally stimulated red-appearing region entrains a green opponent response, which in turn entrains an antagonistic redness response in the surround areas (Plate 14-2). On shifting fixation to the white ground, a green afterimage is seen in a pink surround.

If instead of inspecting a small red test field on a white ground we do the reverse and center a small white field in a red background (Plate 14-3), on transferring our gaze to a large white secondary field we see a red focal area where white was initially seen. However, it is also clear that the surround afterimage is a green one. Precisely the same principles are operative in the two situations. During fixation, some darkening occurs in the central white area, as expected, while the red surround area entrains an opponent green response, and this surround activity in turn acts to entrain redness events in the focal area. These hue changes can actually be seen while still inspecting the white test figure, but they become even more pronounced when the gaze is turned to a uniform white field.

Needless to say, excitation by chromatic focal fields on white surrounds which are then projected on chromatic backgrounds leads to predictable results. For example, since the opponent reaction to a red stimulus is a green aftereffect, it is seen as more saturated when projected on a green background than on a white or red one. Other hue combinations also behave as we might anticipate.

Afterimages have been studied and analyzed for several centuries now and there is a staggering amount of data on the topic. When we reflect that the primary or focal stimulus may vary in energy, duration, size, in its spectral distribution, and in its patterning; that the region of the eye stimulated may differ if we vary our fixation; that the overall adaptation of the eye may vary as well (Chapter 15); and that the secondary stimulation (i.e., the field on which the afterimage is projected) can also be varied in many ways, it is not surprising that the variety of effects reported is almost countless.

Yet there is a lawfulness that underlies their occurrence: afterimages express the fact that there are antagonistic neural processes underlying the perceived events. With careful manipulation of the stimulation, one can reduce the many complexities reported in the literature to a meaningful statement about reciprocal interaction (both spatial and temporal) between the two members of each of three pairs of opponent processes.

The evidence regarding varieties of on-off cellular responses discussed in Chapter 12 can be regarded in a most general way as indicating that the neural organization of the retina provides a physiological mechanism of antagonistic responses of the type that correlates with the afterimage phenomena. If for a given type of chromatic cell, for example, we regard the on- or off-discharges of nerve impulses as signaling one hue, and the silent phase—the nonspiking phase—as correlated with the antagonistic opponent hue, we can simply interpret the spiking as signifying, say, a red hue and the nonspiking as signifying say, its complement, a green hue.

We have examined briefly situations where the afterimage occurs in the dark, or is projected on achromatic or chromatic backgrounds after some primary excitation. If the primary excitation in a small foveal field in an otherwise dark surround is produced by, say, 500 nm, it looks green while the stimulus is on. If we turn the stimulus off and look at a small, not-too-bright achromatic surface, we see a red afterimage. If the afterimage is superimposed on a small red field, we perceive a SUPERSATURATED red ("supersaturated" means more saturated than the saturation of a narrow-band spectral stimulus of the same hue). A direct parallel to this perceptual effect has been reported for a spectrally opponent, presumably red-green-coded, cell of the macaque monkey (Figure 6). When the cell is stimulated directly by 650-nm light, it fires and we can interpret the spikes as coding "redness." The silent nonspiking period may be regarded as signifying green and when the 500-nm stimulus is cut off it produces a neural rebound, "redness." Now as we switch from a 500 nm to a 650-nm stimulus, an increase in firing rate occurs. Supersaturation?

Afterimages are usually not noticed as such but AFTEREFFECTS of the sort we have been describing have their real importance for vision in

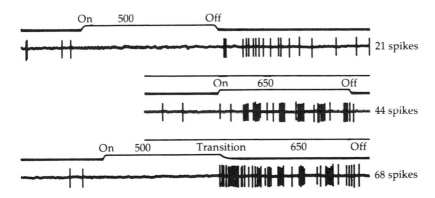

6 SPECTRALLY OPPONENT CELL of macaque monkey. The silent nonfiring period may be interpreted as signifying "greenness," and spike firing may be interpreted as signaling "redness." Stimulation by 650-nm light fires the cell and cutting off 500-nm stimulation likewise produces firing. If 500-nm stimulation is succeeded by 650-nm stimulation, there is an increase in firing rate. Both the neural rebound from 500-nm stimulation and direct 650-nm stimulation produce a redness signal.

successive contrast. Just as in the case of simultaneous contrast, where the sharpening occurs to offset the optical defects of the imaging system, successive contrast sharpens and accentuates differences if we fixate successively one part of a visual scene after another. Since the eye moves about continually in the visual field, a bright object, for example, is repetitively imaged on areas where the sensitivity for whiteness is high. The area first stimulated reacts with a "whiteness" response, and when the eye is moved elsewhere the area where the whiteness excitation first occurred reacts with a "blackness" response. If the gaze shifts back to the same area, it now encounters a more excitable region, which can be reactivated afresh.

Earlier in the chapter, when discussing the eye's capacity for temporal resolution, we noted that an examination of flicker phenomena is beyond the scope of this book. However, a brief descriptive statement about flicker is necessary at this point in order to discuss a variety of visual effects that depend on stimulus alternation but that are not usually classified as afterimages. Flicker effects are generated by alternating brief bright and dark light pulses. Should the rate of alternation be sufficiently high (e.g., 60 Hz), fusion occurs and we do not perceive flicker effects. This is true of our conventional home and office lights, for example, which are usually driven by alternating electrical currents at a rate of 60 Hz. For average illumination levels and lower frequency rates we may begin to see coarse flicker and finally a clear separation between the bright and dark pulses.

As noted in the discussion of color mixture (Chapter 8), we can also use Maxwell discs to produce an alternation of different chromatic stimuli. At sufficiently high rates of alternation we get fusion and color mixture. At lower alternation rates we begin to separate out the alternating stimulus components.

It is in this context that I want to call attention to SUBJECTIVE COLORS, a visual effect long known and frequently reported on in the visual literature. Something more than simple flicker occurs with slow pulsations of achromatic stimuli.

The essence of subjective colors also called FECHNER'S COLORS or "Fechner-Prevost colors," is that varied chromatic sensations are seen when variously patterned achromatic stimuli are presented to the eye at slow frequency rates far below fusion rates. Figure 7 shows a number of discs with different black/white patterns which when mounted on color wheels and spun slowly (5 to 15 revolutions/sec) generate subjective colors of varied hues. Similar phenomena are also seen if the eyes are moved over certain kinds of regular patterns that remain stationary. Figure 8, for example, is a stationary target conducive to producing a variety of desaturated hues when the eyes scan it back and forth slowly. Subjective color

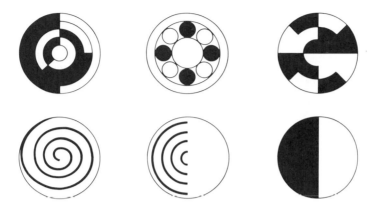

7 DISCS OF VARIED BLACK/WHITE PATTERNS. When spun slowly (5 to 15 Hz/sec) "subjective colors" of various hues are seen.

8 STATIONARY BLACK-AND-WHITE PATTERN in which pastel-like hues are seen as the eyes move slowly over the pattern.

effects have also been produced in recent years with the use of pulsing stimuli on cathode ray oscilloscope tubes or on television screens. In fact, subjective colors are perpetually being "rediscovered." Since achromatic stimuli of the sort shown in Figures 7 and 8 reflect a wide range of wavelengths a basic prerequisite for evoking chromatic effects is present in all these stimuli. The stimulus situation is, however, a complex one and not until recently has it been sensibly analyzed. It has been said that the laws of falling bodies would never have been discovered by Galileo had he set a cartwheel bounding down a hilly road and pursued its every gyration and eccentric path to the bottom of the hill, while timing its descent. The history of the subjective color situation bears a strong resemblance to this description. Many have been pursuing bounding cartwheels, stopwatch in hand.

BENHAM'S DISC is shown in Figure 9. It, too, generates subjective colors and is probably the best known pattern used to produce these phenomena. Furthermore, the pattern lends itself to fairly simple stimulus analysis. If rotated at a speed of 5 to 10 revolutions/sec, colored rings are seen. When rotated in a clockwise direction, for example, the outermost set of lines look bluish, the center ones greenish, and the innermost ones reddish. If the direction of rotation is reversed, the color sequence reverses from center to periphery (i.e., the innermost ones are bluish, etc.). The analysis of the stimulus pattern emphasizes the importance of the areas adjacent to the black radial lines and makes it clear that it is the temporal sequencing and spatial relations among stimulus elements that is impor-

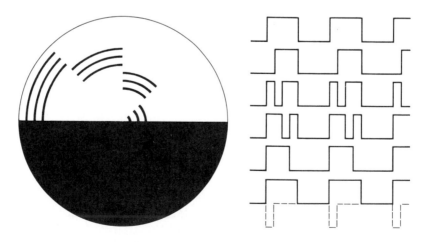

9 BENHAM'S DISC. The light-intensity distribution as a function of time is represented to the right of the disc for each different black/white sequence in the disc.

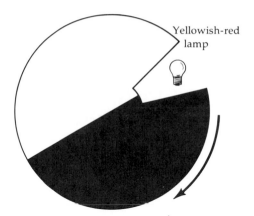

Yellowish-red
lamp

10 BIDWELL'S DISC. In this situation,
with the 650-nm stimulus alternately exposed behind a white/black rotating disc,
the observer never sees a yellowish-red,
only a bluish-green, afterimage.

tant. But, in fact, a rotating disc is not at all essential to produce the
effects, as we have seen.

In the usual afterimage situation, the primary stimulus is first seen
and it is then followed by, say, an afterimage. Thus stimulation by a long-
wavelength red-appearing stimulus leads to a complementary green afterimage, as we have seen. The BIDWELL PULSATIVE AFTERIMAGE is then of
particular interest because the stimulus arrangement is such that, unlike
the situation just described, a complementary afterimage is continually
seen, whereas the primary stimulus that generates it is never seen. The
stimulus setup is shown in Figure 10. If the sector disc is rotated so that,
say, a red 650-nm stimulus is exposed through the cutout 30-degree sector
for about 0.05 second, followed by the white portion of the disc (which is
illuminated with a broad-band achromatic source) and then the black
portion, only a green afterimage is seen. If the observer is kept in ignorance
of the nature of the primary stimulus, he could well think the light source
itself was a midspectral green one, with a wavelength peak of, say,
530 nm.

A different class of aftereffects is generated when there is a very slow
alternation (10 seconds, 10 seconds, . . .) of patterned fields. A horizontal
grating made up of green and black stripes is alternately exposed in the
center of a screen with a vertical grating that is made up of red and black
lines. The observer scans each grating exposed by itself for 10 seconds or
so, and the alternation continues for, say, 5 to 10 minutes. At the end of
this time, a black-and-white target made up of both horizontal and vertical
stripes is then presented for the observer to look at (Figure 11). What the
observer sees are greenish vertical lines (and black ones) and pinkish
horizontal lines (and black ones). If the head is tilted 90 degrees so that

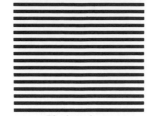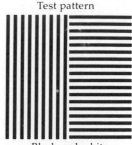

Black and red   Black and green   Black and white

11 PATTERN OF VERTICAL RED and horizontal green bars is looked at for 5 to 10 minutes with alternating 10-second fixations on each. At the end of this period, a test pattern made up of horizontal and vertical black and white bars is viewed. Pale greens are usually reported where the vertical bars are seen and pale reds where the horizontal bars are seen. This color contingent aftereffect is called the McCollough effect.

the two eyes are now one above the other rather than side by side, the physically vertical lines are now seen as pinkish and black and the physically horizontal ones are seen as green and black. This color aftereffect, called the McCOLLOUGH EFFECT after its discoverer, is contingent on the line orientations used in the inspection figure and the phenomena differ in certain surprising ways from conventional afterimages.

One important difference is that it is absolutely necessary to maintain rigorous fixation for some interval of time in order to generate an ordinary afterimage. This is not necessary in the McCollough effect. The eyes can wander over the inspection figures with no loss in effect. Another important difference is in the persistence of the McCollough effect. Conventional afterimages can be very strong, but they fade rather rapidly. The contingent color aftereffects are known to persist for hours, days, and even several months! They are, however, very weak.

Many varieties of CONTINGENT AFTEREFFECTS have been studied and we know many variables that influence their appearance and duration. Among these are effects contingent upon the direction of motion that is paired with hue in moving striped patterns. For example, upward-moving red and black stripes are viewed in alternation with downward-moving green and black stripes. After a short inspection period of this alternating sequence, a black-and-white striped field is presented. When it is moved in the upward direction, green aftereffects are seen, and when it moves in the downward direction pinkish ones are seen. Some investigators think of these long-lasting contingent aftereffects as the result of desensitization or fatigue of systems of highly specialized cells in the visual cortex. Others think of them as akin to conditioned responses not unlike the salivation responses of Pavlov's dogs. We shall have to learn more than we now know about the visual system before being able to account for these intriguing effects in a more certain and satisfactory way.

Background Readings

Benham, C. E. 1894. Notes. *Nature (Lond.)* *51*: 113–114. Letters to the Editor, 1895. *Nature (Lond.)* *51*: 321.

Bidwell, S. 1901. On negative after-images and their relation to certain other visual phenomena. *Proc. Soc. Lond. B 68*: 262–285.

Broca, A., and Sulzer, D. 1902. La sensation lumineuse en fonction du temps. *C. R. Acad. Sci. 134*: 831–834; 1903, *137*: 944–946; 1046–1049.

Campenhausen, C. v. 1968. Über die Farben der Benhamschen Scheibe. *Z. Vergl. Physiol. 60*: 351–374.

Cohen, J., and Gordon, D. A. 1949. The Prevost-Fechner-Benham subjective colors. *Psychol. Bull. 46*: 97–136.

De Valois, R. L. 1973. Central Mechanisms of Color Vision In R. Jung (ed.), *Handbook of Sensory Physiology,* Vol. 7/3, *Central Visual Information A,* Chap. 3, pp. 209–253. Springer-Verlag, Berlin.

Eichengreen, J. M. 1971. Time-dependent chromatic adaptation. Ph.D. thesis, University of Pennsylvania.

Hering, E. 1878. *Zur Lehre vom Lichtsinne,* Part 3. Carl Gerold's Sohn, Vienna.

McCollough, C. 1965. Color adaptation of edge-detectors in the human visual system. *Science 149*: 1115–1116.

Mansfield, R. J. W. 1973. Brightness function: Effect of area and duration. *J. Opt. Soc. Amer. 63*: 913–920.

Parsons, J. H. P. 1924. *An Introduction to the Study of Colour Vision,* 2nd ed. Sec. V, Temporal Effects. Cambridge University Press, Cambridge, England.

Plateau, J. 1878. Bibliographie analytique des principaux phénomènes subjectifs de la vision. Première section. Persistance des impressions sur la rètine. Deuxième section. Couleurs accidentelles ordinaires de succession. *Acad. R. Belg. 42*: 1–59.

Further Readings

Brown, J. L. 1965. Flicker and Intermittent Stimulation. In C. H. Graham (ed.), *Vision and Visual Perception,* pp. 251–320. Wiley, New York.

Franklin, B. 1769. *Experiments and Observations on Electricity Made in Philadelphia in America,* p. 469. David Henry, London.

Kelly, D. H. 1972. Flicker. In D. Jameson and L. M. Hurvich (eds.), *Handbook of Sensory Physiology, 7/4, Visual Psychophysics,* Chap. 11, pp. 273–302. Springer-Verlag, Berlin.

Stromeyer, C. F. 1978. Form-Color Aftereffects in Human Vision. In R. Held, H. W. Leibowitz, and H-L. Teuber (eds.), *Handbook of Sensory Physiology,* Vol. 7, *Perception,* Chap 4, pp. 97–142. Springer-Verlag, Berlin.

Wade, N. J. 1977. A note on the discovery of subjective colors. *Vision Res. 17:* 671–672.

15
Color Adaptation

THE previous two chapters contain many examples of the way the appearance of lights or objects of fixed spectral-energy distributions change as a result of simultaneous or successive contrast. In a sense, most of these perceived changes are artificial. We must carefully and deliberately arrange the stimulus situation to provide clear demonstrations of the existence of these usually little noticed contrast phenomena. But in the usual run of events, our world of colored objects changes very little with considerable changes in illumination. What of this seeming paradox? We will find before we are through that there is no paradox and that the objects in our visual world remain relatively stable despite large variations in external illumination partly because contrast effects contribute to producing this stability.

The visual system has the remarkable property that it can function efficiently over a very wide range of illuminations. It functions well at very low levels of illumination as well as at high ones. The eye sees dimly illuminated objects because the visual system adapts. When light is imaged on the retina, the pupillary aperture through which it passes widens at low light levels and allows more light to enter the eye, but the major increase in sensitivity comes about mainly because the rods are more active at low illuminations and they contain the sensitive rhodopsin photopigment, which is increasingly reconstituted the longer the rods are protected from bleaching light levels (see Chapter 10). The eye not only dark-adapts to increase its sensitivity, it also light-adapts to enable it to function more efficiently at moderate light levels and to protect itself from overstimulation by extremely bright lights. The cone system is operative at the higher illumination levels. The eye's sensitivity to light can thus decrease or increase depending on illumination conditions.

The visual system not only adapts to different light levels, it also adapts to color. COLOR ADAPTATION refers to changes in the eye's sensitivity when it is exposed to chromatic light stimulation. Here the changes in sensitivity tend to compensate for the spectral quality of the light rather than for changes in its overall level.

We have already encountered instances of the way chromatic light stimulation modifies the eye's sensitivity in discussing successive color contrast and afterimages. If we view a surface that reflects light nonselectively and that is judged to be "white" under what we may call an equilibrium condition, the same surface will look bluish green if the eye is preexposed for a short while to a long-wavelength stimulus that looks reddish yellow. By exposing the eye to the reddish-yellow stimulus we have altered the balance of the opponent color systems and sensitized green and blue responsiveness at the expense of red and yellow.

If we keep away from all light stimulation for a long time—one-half hour or so—by staying in a dark room with our eyes closed, what we see is usually described as shifting clouds of "retinal light." All we see are intrinsic retinal light swirls, sometimes called "light dust," "intrinsic gray," or "intrinsic brightness or darkness." Recently, the term retinal noise has become a favorite descriptive term for what is seen in the balanced equilibrium dark-adapted state. Note that this visual experience is *not* one of blackness. As we have already seen, only when there is room illumination or "white" light surrounding an object do we experience deep blacks as well as whites. The visual experience of the rested eye is a basic gray experience.

Under conditions of rest there is a neutral balance of sensitivities. However, sensitivity increases greatly during the long dark-adaptation period. A neutral balance of sensitivities, or NEUTRAL STATE OF ADAPTATION, as it is called, can also be achieved in an equilibrium system even without an extremely long period of dark adaptation. The cone system largely dominates in this state of rest and balance. This condition can be achieved by remaining in a darkened room for 10 minutes or so. (A neutral state of adaptation can also be reached in the presence of appropriately selected broad-band "white" stimuli that stimulate the component mechanisms equivalently [see below]).

Figure 1a illustrates a selected set of α, β and γ component sensitivities for a neutral balance of sensitivities. If we convert or transform these functions to determine the form and spectral distributions of the achromatic and chromatic functions, the result is as shown in Figure 1b. An analysis of the red/green and yellow/blue functions will show each to be in balance; hence they represent a situation with zero chromatic response. The achromatic system alone produces a signal, which is, of course, neutral or white.

If a visual system that initially has a neutral balance of sensitivities of this sort is then exposed to, say, north-sky daylight (color temperature = 10,000°K; see Chapter 3) which is rather heavily weighted with short-wavelength radiation, it looks bluish. This is because there is a prepon-

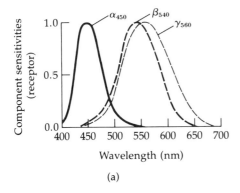

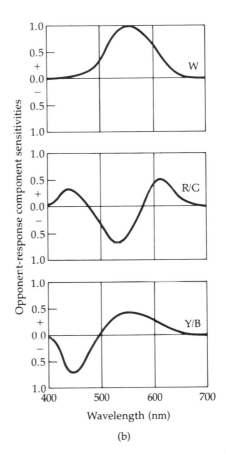

1 NEUTRAL BALANCE of component sensitivities (a) at the receptor level for equal energy at the cornea of the eye and (b) at the opponent-process level. (These curves are not adjusted for ocular transmission or quantal absorption.)

derance of α absorption, which, as we know, triggers blue (and red) chromatic events. If we continue to look at a relatively large nonselective surface illuminated by this source, it soon loses the blue appearance and becomes white or neutral. If instead of outdoor daylight illumination, we use incandescent indoor lights (2800°K) which are relatively weighted with long-wavelength radiation, the surface now appears yellowish or orange to a neutrally balanced system. In this case there is a preponderance of β and γ absorption, which triggers yellow and red chromatic responses. With continued exposure this yellowish-red-appearing illumination also appears white or neutral. How can we explain these appearance shifts or chromatic adaptation effects?

The German physiologist von Kries developed a principle now called the VON KRIES COEFFICIENT LAW which addresses this question directly. What he did was to specify quantitatively the way the photopigment absorption functions would be expected to change with chromatic adaptation. If α_λ, β_λ, and γ_λ, represent the spectral distributions of the three cone-receptor types for one state of adaptation (say, a neutral one), the *forms* of these distributions do not change with exposure to chromatic illumination, but their relative amplitudes do. Thus, if α'_λ, β'_λ, and γ'_λ represent the changed sensitivities of these elements brought about by exposure to chromatic illumination, they are related to the original α_λ, β_λ, and γ_λ by simple multiplicative coefficients:

$$\alpha'_\lambda = k_1\alpha_\lambda$$
$$\beta'_\lambda = k_2\beta_\lambda$$
$$\gamma'_\lambda = k_3\gamma_\lambda$$

The magnitudes of k_1, k_2, and k_3 are interpreted as being inversely related to the relative strengths of activation of α, β, and γ by the particular energy distribution of the chromatic light in question.

Thus in the specific instance where we are continuously exposed to outdoor illumination, such as north-sky light, the sensitivity of the α cone receptor, the one that is excited most strongly by the short-wavelength radiation, is depressed to a greater extent than are the sensitivities of the other two receptor types, β_λ and γ_λ, since they are less strongly excited. But the sensitivity of β_λ is depressed relatively more than that of γ_λ since it is initially excited to a greater degree than is γ_λ. Since the relative decrements in sensitivity are proportional to the degree of stimulus excitation, as the chromatic stimulation continues, in time the outputs of each cone receptor type become equivalent. The products of the altered receptor sensitivity × stimulus energy are equalized for the three receptor types. With equal excitation of the three selective mechanisms, we are once again back to a neutral response. The chromatic responses of each opponent system are nulled and the visual appearance is neutral white. Precisely the same logic applies to the 2800°K stimulus, which initially appears yellow-red (or orange). In time, the sensitivities of the various cone receptors are reduced in proportion to the degree to which they have been excited (the γ cone receptor most, the β one less, and the α one least) and the outputs of the three cone receptor systems are again balanced. The surface that initially appeared yellowish now also appears neutral gray or white in the incandescent light. In short, in these examples, the receptor visual sensitivities are adjusted to the degree of excitation in such a way that the balanced output always remains the same (i.e., a neutral one). The same analysis applies to any broad-band illuminant, whatever its spectral distribution.

An account such as the one I have given explains why the "white" paper of this book does not change its color from yellow to blue as we take it along with us from the yellow illumination of our rooms to peruse it under bluish daylight illumination while sitting on a park bench. Similarly, "white" shirts and blouses do not vary from yellow to blue with these shifts in illumination. Despite the change from incandescent to daylight illumination, the object continues to have approximately the same neutral white appearance. We have here an example of what is called APPROXIMATE COLOR CONSTANCY.

What is true for the spectrally nonselective objects (e.g., paper, shirts, or blouses) applies equally well to colored objects. Colored objects, whatever their colors, might be expected to look different as the light falling on them changes. But as our everyday experiences teach us, this does not happen to any great extent. The clothes we wear, and the objects and books we carry from indoors to outdoors, continue to look more or less the same as we go from indoors to outdoors and vice versa.

There are limits here, however, and hence the phrase "approximate color constancy." It is because of these limits that objects purchased in stores and shops under one form of illumination sometimes do take on different appearances when seen in the home under a different illumination from that in the shop or store where the purchase was made. (This is particularly true if the store illuminants are fluorescent ones and those in the home are incandescent, or vice versa.) Thus an object may look a little bluer in daylight than in incandescent illumination. The degree to which a shift in illuminant will produce changes, however slight, in the perceived color of the object will also depend to some extent on the reflectance of the object being viewed. If it is a high-reflectance object, it is likely to take on a bit of the illuminant quality when examined closely. Thus a white might be a cold white (bluish) in outdoor illumination and a warmer white (yellowish) in indoor illumination. On the other hand, if the object is of low reflectance, it may have a tendency to look more bluish in yellow incandescent light than it does in daylight illumination, when it might be seen as more yellowish.

The von Kries balance of sensitivities notion permits us to state precisely what receptoral changes take place with changes in adaptation. Since these changes are in turn reflected in changes in both the achromatic and chromatic response functions at the neural level, the forms of the latter can also be specified precisely for any given adaptation change.

If the eye is subjected to continued stimulation by a spectral light of 650 nm at a moderate light level, the von Kries coefficient law tells us that compared to a neutral balance of sensitivities, the new balance of sensitivities is as represented in Figure 2a. Since the 650-nm light has a tenfold greater effectiveness for the γ_{560} component than for the β_{540} one, its continued action is assumed to have a tenfold greater desensitizing effect on the γ_{560} component than on the β_{540} one.

The postreceptoral antagonistic neural responses controlled by these receptoral events are shown in Figure 2b. These are obtained by a linear set of transformation functions of the type discussed in Chapter 11. Al-

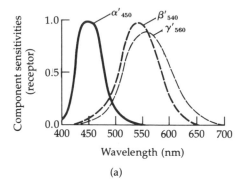

(a)

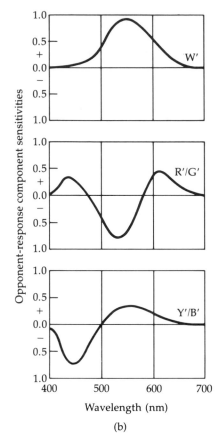

2 ALTERED BALANCE of component sensitivities (a) at the receptor level on exposure to a 650-nm spectral light and (b) at the opponent-process level following exposure to a 650-nm spectral light.

(b)

though it is small, note that the main effect of adaptation to the 650-nm light is on red/green distribution function. After adaptation the long-wavelength red amplitude is decreased, the midspectral green amplitude is increased, and the red/green transition wavelength at which unique yellow is predicted to occur is shifted by about 6 nm toward longer wavelengths.

Figure 3 illustrates the way the chromatic response functions may be expected to look after the cone system has adapted to a unique green stimulus, say, 500 nm.* Notice the change in the relative sizes of the red and green limbs of the red/green chromatic response function. (Figure 4 shows the chromatic response functions for the neutral state for comparative purposes.)

Another illustration of the way the chromatic functions may be expected to change both in form and magnitude following exposure of the eye to, say, a unique blue stimulus (475 nm) is given in Figure 5.* The

* These are theoretical functions. No account is taken of induction factors (discussed in Chapter 13 and later in this chapter), which will also alter these curves in predictable ways.

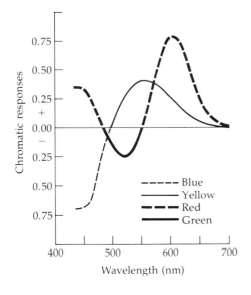

3 CHROMATIC RESPONSE FUNC-
TIONS following adaptation to a 500-nm
stimulus (green). These are theoretical
curves that do not take induction or contrast effects into account.

yellow/blue function is now the one mainly affected by changed amplitudes of the cone-receptor sensitivities. What we see is that there is in
each of these instances a relative sensitization of one member of the
opponent hue pairs and a desensitization of the other member. Thus with
green adaptation the red limb is magnified relative to the green one, which
constricts, and with blue adaptation the blue one constricts relative to the
yellow one, which expands over a wider spectral region.

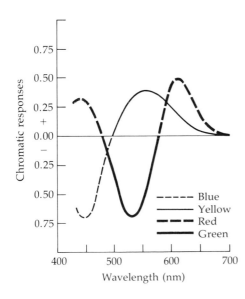

4 CHROMATIC RESPONSE FUNC-
TIONS for a neutral state of adaptation.

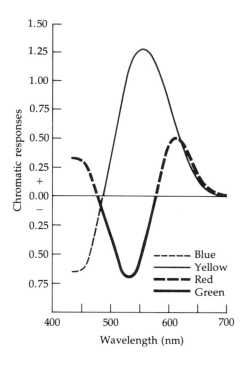

5 CHROMATIC RESPONSE FUNC-
TIONS following adaptation to a 475-nm
stimulus (blue).

The changes illustrated in Figures 3 and 5 are relatively large ones compared to those seen in Figure 2b. It should be noted, therefore, that the precise way these functions change and the degree of change depend on a large number of variables, particularly the energy, duration, and size of the adapting chromatic lights.

That changes in the chromatic response functions consequent upon adaptation can be rather large ones is related to the fact that the simple equations that relate the linkages between cone absorptions and chromatic responses are DIFFERENCE EQUATIONS. For example,

$$R - G = \alpha + \gamma - \beta$$

For neutral adaptation, at the unique spectral locus 580 nm, the sum of $\alpha + \gamma - \beta = 0$ and there is neither a red nor a green response. With adaptation to a long-wavelength stimulus, a very slight decrease in γ absorption relative to the β change will send the equation in a negative direction and the response outcome will be green. On the other hand, a slightly greater depression of β relative to γ will occur if the adapting stimulus moves in a short-wavelength direction, and in this case the summed $\alpha + \gamma$ value will increase and the outcome will be redness ($+R$).

Electrophysiological findings in single cells of the lateral geniculate nucleus (LGN) of the monkey, for example, exhibit direct parallels with the human psychophysical data on adaptation. A given cell that manifests excitatory responses (positive) to a given wavelength, say, 590 nm, will after the monkey's eye is exposed to long-wavelength light respond in an inhibitory fashion (negative). Similarly, if the adaptation is to midspectral light the excitatory response to the 590-nm stimulus will be greater and. the crossover spectral locus from excitation to inhibition will occur at shorter wavelengths.

We can, using the chromatic and achromatic response functions that are specified for different states of adaptation, calculate both hue coefficients and saturation coefficients in the way we specified them for a neutral adaptation condition (see Chapters 6 and 7).

Figure 6 shows an example of the hue coefficient function for partial chromatic adaptation to a unique yellow stimulus. The hue coefficient function for this state of adaptation may be summarized by noting that compared with the neutral-state situation (Figure 2 in Chapter 6), the proportion of the adapting hue (yellow) is reduced wherever it occurs in the spectrum. Relative decreases in the adapting hues must, of course, result in a relative increase in the associated disparate hue pair at any wavelength location. Thus if yellow adaptation produces a general decrease in the yellow coefficient, both the green and red coefficient functions will increase correspondingly at the wavelengths in question (see Figure 6). Note that the adapting stimulus represents a wavelength that evokes a pure or unique yellow hue sensation. Thus the hue of the adapting stimulus is itself unaffected. The wavelength locus of the opponent, or complementary, unique blue hue is also unaffected.* What about the third unique locus?

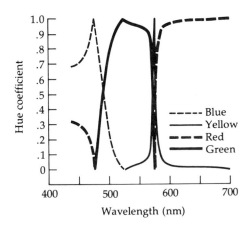

6 HUE COEFFICIENT FUNCTION for spectral lights following partial chromatic adaptation to a 580-nm stimulus (yellow).

---

*This statement does not accord with some recent experiments in which very short exposure times were used. This is probably the result of different reaction rates at the photoreceptors and neural levels, which take on increasing importance as the stimulus duration shortens.

Table 1 Hue Shifts in Chromatic Adaptation

ADAPTING STIMULI

	Neutral	Blue	Green	Yellow	Red
Blue	Blue	Blue	Reddish blue	Blue	Greenish blue
Green	Green	Yellowish green	Green	Bluish green	Green
Yellow	Yellow	Yellow	Reddish yellow	Yellow	Greenish yellow
Red	Red	Yellowish red	Red	Bluish red	Red

TEST STIMULI

Table I summarizes generally the hue shifts that occur with various types of chromatic adaptation. Saturation coefficient functions, like hue coefficient functions, will vary for different adaptations. The saturation coefficients, as we saw in Chapter 7, are the ratios of the chromatic responses to the sum of the achromatic plus chromatic responses and represent the percentage of chromatic component in the total sensation.

The data for computing these saturation values are derived from the equations relating chromatic and achromatic responses to photopigment absorptions for the various adaptations. Figure 7 illustrates such saturation coefficients for white, blue, green, yellow, and red adaptations. These functions differ markedly in form for the different chromatic states. In general, a specific adaptation tends to minimize saturation in the wavelength regions corresponding to the hue of the adapting stimulus and to increase saturation in the wavelength regions that normally evoke the opponent hue. Thus, as compared with the function for the neutral (white) state, blue adaptation, for example, brings about a decrease in saturation in the 470-nm region and greatly increases saturation in the 570-nm region.

Hue and saturation coefficients can, of course, be calculated not only for individual spectral lights but for reflectance samples or filters which reflect or transmit light throughout the entire visible spectrum, as we saw in Chapter 7.

I have referred to the neutral state of adaptation as an equilibrium balanced condition achievable by remaining in the dark a short time. We have also noted that a neutral condition of adaptation is achievable in the presence of light stimulation and have referred to a neutral state of adaptation produced by "white" light. But as we have seen, many broadband stimuli (10,000 to 2800°K) which initially look bluish or yellowish quickly take on a white appearance as we continue to look at them. They look white because the visual system is, in fact, no longer in a neutral state. It is the deviation from the neutral state that is related to their white appearance.

We now have a clue to help us seek out broad-band stimuli that appear white and that do not at the same time unbalance the visual system away from neutrality. The chromatic response functions obtained under adaptations to chromatic stimuli make it clear that there are large shifts in locations of specific unique hues. The affected loci depend, of course, on the adaptation stimuli used. If we experimentally test and find among a variety of broad-band stimuli those lights that appear neutral and that *also* do not shift the unique hue spectral loci away from their neutral positions (measured when all light is excluded), we may conclude that they are lights that maintain the system in a balanced state.

When such experiments are performed, the same results are obtained for a 5500°K broad-band stimulus as are obtained in a situation where there is no external adapting light. The distribution curve of the color temperature of a mixture of sunlight and skylight at high noon, 5500°K, can be mimicked in the laboratory with appropriately selected light sources and filters. Its use can be assumed to guarantee a neutral, bright-adapted balanced equilibrium condition of adaptation for most observers (see Figure 7 in Chapter 3).

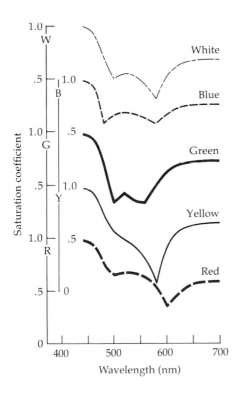

7 SATURATION COEFFICIENTS based on theoretical calculations for white, blue, green, yellow, and red adaptations.

In Chapter 9 we discussed the fact that metameric color matches (i.e., color matches between lights of different spectral distributions) are invariant with changes in chromatic adaptation. A color match made for a neutral state of adaptation persists regardless of the way the state of adaptation of the eye is changed. Since matching stimuli produce identical photopigment absorbances and generate identical neural responses, the persistence of metameric color matches accords perfectly with the von Kries conceptualization. The relative sensitivity of each receptor mechanism changes uniformly with adaptation. There is no change in the *form* of the spectral distribution of each separate cone sensitivity function; there is only an alteration in the *amplitudes* of the functions. These *amplitude* changes alter the balance among the various types of photoreceptors. The following numerical example illustrates this. For simplicity the analysis is made for the two receptor types, β and γ, whose absorbances are mainly involved in the specific color match used in the illustration.

Let a, b, and c represent the energies of three spectral lights at 580, 540, and 670 nm, respectively, where a_{580} matches the combination of b_{540} and c_{670}. We write

$$a_{580} \equiv b_{540} + c_{670}$$

Assume that a_{580} produces 1000 quantal absorptions in the β cone and an identical number in the γ cone:

$$a_{580} \rightarrow 1000\beta + 1000\gamma$$

The β cone absorbs relatively more quanta at 540 nm than at 670 nm, and the reverse is true for the γ cone. Thus we can assume that

$$b_{540} \rightarrow 900\beta + 100\gamma$$

and

$$c_{670} \rightarrow 100\beta + 900\gamma$$

Now, for

$$a_{580} \equiv b_{540} + c_{670}$$

we can write

$$1000\beta + 1000\gamma = (900\beta + 100\gamma) + (100\beta + 900\gamma)$$

or

$$1000\beta + 1000\gamma = 1000\beta + 1000\gamma$$

The summed $\beta + \gamma$ values are equivalent for the 580-nm stimulus and the combination of 540- and 670-nm stimuli. If we decrease the magnitude of any photopigment's response by some fixed percentage of its original value, the same percentage reduction will be effected for all stimuli entering into the match and the equality remains the same. A 10 percent reduction in γ absorbance and a 5 percent reduction in β absorbance applies equally to all stimuli entering into the match, and now

$$a_{580} \rightarrow 950\beta + 900\gamma$$
$$b_{540} \rightarrow 855\beta + 90\gamma$$
$$c_{670} \rightarrow 95\beta + 810\gamma$$

Thus for

$$a_{580} \equiv b_{540} + c_{670}$$

we can write

$$950\beta + 900\gamma = (855\beta + 90\gamma) + (95\beta + 810\gamma)$$

or

$$950\beta + 900\gamma = 950\beta + 900\gamma$$

Note that the match is preserved. Note also that by referring to the altered achromatic and chromatic response functions of Figure 2b, the *appearance* of the matched fields has to change with a change in adaptation.

Metameric color matches are also obtainable with objects of different reflectances illuminated by the same light source. Figure 8 shows the spectral reflectance curves of two different surfaces. When both are illuminated by a daylight source, if they are equally bright they appear as identical greens to the average observer. In the case of these reflectance samples, however, if the illumination is changed to incandescent tungsten (and with it the adaptation of the eye) the two samples, even if equally bright, will no longer match. The surface labeled A now looks brown; B continues to look green. The reason for this is that with a shift in illuminant we actually change the stimulus energies reflected from the two surfaces. In the first instance, where the illumination is daylight, the summed cross products of the light distribution × reflectance × response curves throughout the visible spectrum is the same for the two samples; in the second instance, with a shift to a tungsten illuminant, there is no longer an

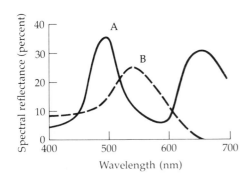

8 SPECTRAL REFLECTANCE CURVES of two colored samples that match in daylight but not in tungsten illuminations.

equality between the two summed cross products of light distribution $\times$ reflectance $\times$ responses.

The von Kries concept, which treats the adaptation effects as a change in the balance of sensitivities, adequately handles many of the phenomena of color adaptation. It does not, however, provide us with a complete account. We turn next to a situation where it fails to account for the observed phenomena. We alluded to the difficulty earlier when we said that a high-reflectance object may take on the color of the illuminant, whereas a low-reflectance object may tend to take on the opponent hue, for example look bluish in a yellowish illumination.

Suppose that we take a nonselective reflecting sample and place it on a larger nonselective reflecting background. Now let us illuminate both with the same chromatic light source. If the reflectance of the smaller test stimulus is approximately the same as that of the background, the sample will tend to appear neutral in color as soon as we have adapted. However, if the reflectance of the sample is considerably higher than that of the background, the test sample takes on the color of the illuminant. With a reddish illuminant the test area therefore looks slightly reddish or pink. On the other hand, if the test sample is of relatively low reflectance, it will in this instance look slightly greenish. If exposure to chromatic illumination merely changes the balance of sensitivities of the three cone types while leaving the forms of their sensitivity functions unchanged, there is no reason to expect a sample that is nonselective for wavelength to take on different hues, which range from the hue of the illuminant to its complementary. As the amount of light reflected from the test object changes, we expect that the product of the stimulus distribution and the three sensitivity distributions will increase or decrease. But the three products for the three sensitivity distributions would continue to bear the same relations to one another at all levels of test stimulation. Therefore, the von Kries analysis gives us no reason to anticipate the hue changes that are seen.

The changes I have described can be accounted for very simply as soon as we recognize that in addition to any sensitivity changes that may be present, there are also contrast effects. As we already know from earlier discussions, the physiological "redness" activity produced by the long-wavelength illuminant in, say, the surround, induces an opposite "greenness" response in the neural tissue associated with the test area. In the situation where the test and surround field are of equal reflectance with the reciprocal interactions between test and surround, we tend to see a uniform neutral or gray area with continued viewing. When the test area is of higher reflectance, the greenness induction produced in the test area by the red surround is insufficient in magnitude to offset the redness evoked by the illuminant directly. When the test reflectance is low, the greenness induced in this area by the surround becomes perceptible. Only by taking incremental opponent induction effects into consideration can we gain a clear comprehension of perceived effects of the sort described.

A system that operates in the way we have described it—a system that provides for "approximate color constancy"—has advantages over one that would give us perfect color constancy. Because the system is to a large extent compensatory, it enables us to continue to recognize objects despite illumination changes. Experience also enters importantly. Psychologists have long recognized the importance of what they call MEMORY COLOR; the color in which we most consistently see an object is impressed indelibly on our memory. This is what people tend to call the real color of an object. And, of course, a system that is partially compensatory for illumination changes is required if we are to build up stable memory colors.

But because the system is not perfectly compensatory it permits us at the same time to recognize pretty well both the level and quality of the illumination. We are not unaware of changes in illumination. We know whether we are close to high noon or that sunset is approaching. If we are observant, we detect subtle changes in the colors of objects and shadows, and in the sharpness of apparent contrast between objects and their surroundings, and we can make these judgments because both receptor sensitivity changes and neural interaction effects take place.

We have seen in the examples in this chapter that the appearances of various chromatic stimuli depend on the state of adaptation of the visual system. It is not surprising, therefore, that differences between chromatic stimuli, including just-detectable differences, also depend on the state of chromatic adaptation.

Among the experimental measures used to evaluate the way the visual system performs with respect to the discrimination of small color differences are wavelength-discrimination data. Figure 9 summarizes some of these results. They are obtained by presenting an observer with a bipartite field that contains the same wavelength in the two halves and at the same energy level. The test field looks essentially like a full uniformly colored moon. The observer is then asked to adjust the wavelength in one half-field until he just detects a perceptible difference between the two half-fields. Once a difference is seen, the observer varies the energy of the light in the changed field to see whether he or she can restore the equality between the two half-fields. If so, he or she then varies the wavelength to introduce a perceptible difference again. The light energy is again adjusted and this procedure repeated until a point is reached where an adjustment for brightness does not eliminate the color difference introduced by the wavelength manipulation. In such a set of measurements we see that there are two minimal points where discrimination is best

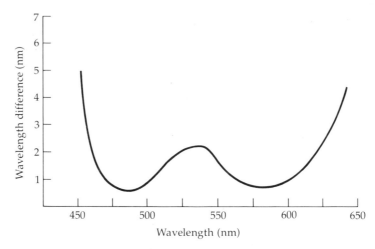

9 WAVELENGTH DISCRIMINATION RESULTS. The wavelength difference necessary to produce a just noticeable difference between two fields is shown on the ordinate as a function of the wavelength at which sensitivity is tested. Several different experiments are included.

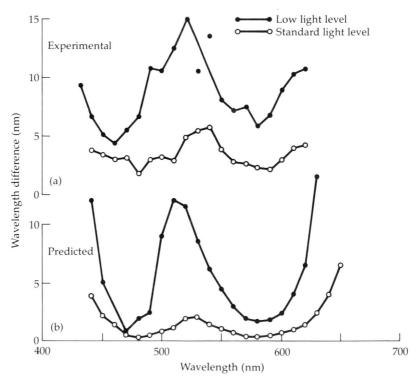

10 WAVELENGTH DISCRIMINATION RESULTS obtained at two different light levels. (a) Experimental results. (b) Theoretical calculations derived to fit the experimental data.

(470 nm and 580 nm) and that discrimination is relatively poorer both in the midspectral region (about 535 nm) and at the spectral extremes.

In Figure 10a, results of an experiment of this sort carried out at two different light levels are shown. In Figure 10b theoretical calculations are shown that seek to explain these discriminations. The calculations are based on using a combination of the average observer's sensitivity to both a small hue and saturation change at each of two light levels. The values that enter into the computation are based on the hue and saturation coefficients described earlier.

Precisely the same experimental wavelength discrimination procedure has been used to evaluate color sensitivity for different chromatic adaptation conditions. Results of such an experiment are given in Figure 11 for

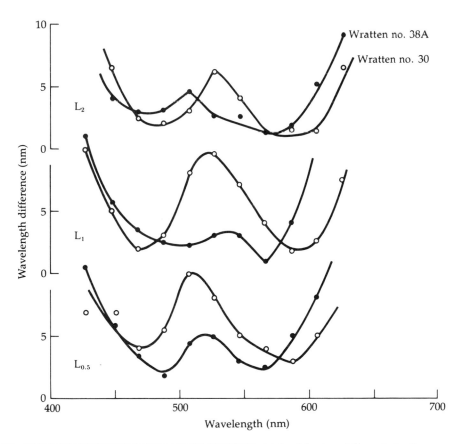

11 WAVELENGTH DISCRIMINATION RESULTS obtained for two different adapting surrounds, one a yellowish red (Wratten filter no. 30) and the other a bluish green (Wratten filter no. 38A). In all three panels the test stimuli are of the same moderate light level, but the ratio of test to background light level changes. (L_2) test: surround = 2:1; (L_1) test: surround = 1:1; ($L_{0.5}$) test: surround = 0.5:1.

two different adaptation conditions, one where a yellowish-red was the surround adapting field (Wratten no. 30) and the other where a bluish-green adapting surround field (Wratten no. 38A) was used. The discrimination functions, like those obtained without adaptation surrounds, have minima in two wavelength regions. But the effect of chromatic adaptation is to displace the curves relative to each other for the different adaptations.

Notice that with the yellowish-red surround (no. 30) the discrimination is poorer in the midspectral region (larger $\Delta\lambda$), but in the long-wavelength region the $\Delta\lambda$ tends to increase less rapidly than it does with the bluish-green (no. 38A) surround. What this implies is that with reddishness induced in the test areas, discriminations become more difficult at the long wavelengths. Conversely, with more green induced in the midspectral region by the yellowish-red background, midspectral discrimination becomes worse. This means that we are more likely to distinguish slightly different reds in an overall reddish scene than when the same slightly different reds are seen against green backgrounds.

As the ratio of test to adapting surround varies, striking changes in the *shape* of the wavelength discrimination functions accompany the changes in the functions' amplitudes. Notice that the difference between the discrimination functions for the two different adaptations are least at the high test levels. To interpret these results in a meaningful way it becomes necessary to incorporate a contrast induction factor of the sort already discussed. The result (Figure 11) is consistent with the view that the inductive effects produced in a test area by a surround of constant light level are progressively less significant as the focal stimulation is increased in magnitude relative to that of the inducing stimulus. As we saw, a low-reflectance stimulus takes on a hue complimentary to that of the illuminant, but with an increase in reflectance of the test stimulus, the constant size induction from the surround is imperceptible. It is clear from all the considerations that the adaptation process is one that involves both "multiplicative" receptor sensitivity changes and induced "incremental" neural changes. It is best referred to as a "two-process" interpretation of color adaptation.

In Chapter 11 we wrote three expressions that linked the achromatic and chromatic responses at the opponent-process neural level to the photopigment absorbance functions. If these response expressions, which correlate with our perceptions, are to have a more general applicability, they must incorporate a factor that takes account of the induced or contrast responses. To do this we can write the following three equations:

$$w_\lambda - bk_\lambda = f_1[e_\lambda(a_{11}\alpha_\lambda + a_{12}\beta_\lambda + a_{13}\gamma_\lambda)] + i_{w-bk}$$

$$r_\lambda - g_\lambda = f_2[e_\lambda(a_{21}\alpha_\lambda + a_{22}\beta_\lambda + a_{23}\gamma_\lambda)] + i_{r-g}$$

$$y_\lambda - b_\lambda = f_3[e_\lambda(a_{31}\alpha_\lambda + a_{32}\beta_\lambda + a_{33}\gamma_\lambda)] + i_{y-b}$$

These generalized equations tell us that in the case of each response function the outcome is dependent on the three photopigment absorbances (α_λ, β_λ, & γ_λ), the specific weightings assigned to these absorbances (a_{11}, a_{12}, . . .), the nature of the light source (e_λ), and the incremental changes in achromatic or chromatic response (i_{w-bk}, i_{r-g}, and i_{y-b}). A change in chromatic adaptation that alters α, β, and γ to α', β', and γ' by a coefficient rule also alters i_{w-bk}, i_{r-g}, and i_{y-b} to i'_{w-bk}, i'_{r-g}, and i'_{y-b}.

Some of the details of the opponent-induction or contrast effects were examined in earlier chapters. What we need to recognize here is that both the simultaneous and successive contrast effects serve to keep the visual system in a highly responsive state, because they prevent the "fatigue" of any of the component neural sensitivities. Continued "redness" excitation, for example, could conceivably exhaust the "redness" response. However, the "greenness" reaction built up during the "redness" action process sets the stage for a restoration to an equilibrium condition as soon as "redness" action is halted. This occurs when the "greenness" response rebounds.

The presence of a multiplicity of objects and fields of different sizes, shapes, and "adjacencies" acts in a similar way in the spatial domain. The multiplicity of neural interactions keeps the system in a perpetual tug-of-war between action and reaction processes in adjoining retinal areas and in the presence of eye movements prevents the excitatory processes from "running down hill," as it were, and creating a general washout effect of the sort we turn to now.

The adaptation we have been discussing up to this point may be characterized as "partial." Complete color adaptation cannot ordinarily be achieved because the eyes are always in motion and the visual field contains a multiplicity of many differently colored forms. If the eyes could be held perfectly still for a long period and stimulation kept uniform over a large area, however, it is possible that the action/reaction process discussed in Chapter 14 could reach a zero-equilibrium condition. Thus, as shown in Figure 12, the action process moves toward a baseline condition, which in turn entrains a progressively smaller reaction process, and ultimately there is a zero difference between the two processes.

It is extremely difficult to maintain rigorous fixation for any extended period as described in the previous paragraph because eye movements are a necessary functional part of our visual mechanisms. Without them, our visual perceptions would soon lose any useful function for commerce with the world of objects about us. This is emphasized by considering a class of experiments that involves stimulating the eye with a uniformly illuminated homogeneous field. A visual stimulus field can be produced that remains unchanged on the retina in spite of the continuous motion of the eye. In such an experiment we place in front of each eye with the lid open one half of a ping-pong ball that forms a diffuse translucent hemisphere

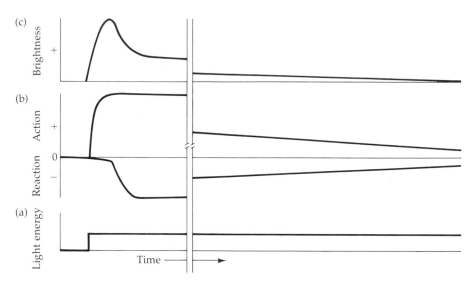

12 EQUILIBRIUM CONDITION represented as situation in which stimulation is uniform and both the action/reaction processes reach a balanced-zero condition.

around the outer part of the eyeball. Each hemisphere is then uniformly illuminated by shining an external light source on it, and the observer's whole retina is uniformly illuminated by the light coming through the hemisphere. Since the ping-pong ball itself is uniformly illuminated, movements of the eye behind it produce no change whatsoever in the stimulation of any part of the retina. When the light is turned on under these circumstances, the subject initially sees a uniformly colored field, and as exposure to the same unchanged retinal stimulation continues, the total field gradually decreases in brightness, and finally, after some time, the subject no longer perceives any light stimulation at all. Some observers suspect that the experimenter has gradually turned off the stimulus light. The effect of continued, really unchanging stimulation on the retina therefore becomes equivalent, in terms of useful visual perceptions, to having no stimulation at all. Now, in order to reactivate the visual system, the experimenter can either increase or decrease the light on the ping-pong ball—cast a shadow or a small intense spot of light on it—and once again the observer is able to see something as a result of the *change* in visual stimulation. This must be emphasized because the reason for the stimulus disappearance in these experiments is not that the visual system has become so insensitive that the stimulus level has to be increased in order to produce an effect; *any change* will be effective whether it be an increase or a decrease in the level of stimulation.

It must be emphasized that the homogeneous field may be illuminated with a broad-band colored stimulus or a highly saturated spectral stimulus. After some short lapse of time there is a complete loss of the hue experience and the observer will report a uniform field of overall darkness or grayness—the steady-state balanced equilibrium point—the point at which the action/reaction processes are in balance.

When we have a stimulus field that is not uniformly illuminated, but contains, for example, light and dark areas, or various colored areas, it is still possible to achieve a state of equilibrium, a stationary state in which there is a balance of the action/reaction events, both focally and with adjacent peripheral areas. The easiest way to demonstrate this is as follows.

Make a small pencil mark in the center of a sheet of uniformly illuminated white paper. With one eye closed fixate the mark steadily, and then hold the pencil in a fixed position above and near the edge of the paper so that it casts a dim shadow at the edge of the white paper while you continue to look as steadily as possible at your fixation mark. The intensity of the shadow stimulus is, of course, lower than the unshadowed light level of the white paper. Since this is true, we know from our earlier discussion that, in time, this shadow area will increase somewhat in apparent brightness as contrasted to its brightness on initial appearance. What will the steady brightness of the shadow area become?

If you do this demonstration experiment carefully (don't wiggle the pencil!) and if you are able to fixate very steadily, in time you will find that the shadow in the periphery of your field of view eventually disappears completely: the shadow area finally reaches the same apparent brightness as the remainder of the field of view provided by the white paper. As soon as you shift your fixation away from the pencil mark, however, the shadow will reappear. This is very simply because when your eyes move, the lower light level of the shadow area now represents a change in stimulation for the part of your retina that had just been in equilibrium with respect to the level of stimulation from the white paper surround, and consequently the change in stimulation is again registered as a change in the brightness response. If you were to hold your eyes steadily in the new fixation direction established by moving the eyes away from the original fixation point, the same gradual disappearance of the shadow would be repeated once more. Similar effects occur with colored targets. Except when we are staring vacantly into space and not really "looking" at anything, this sort of fading of external objects or differently illuminated areas does not normally occur. In everyday viewing, our eyes are constantly in motion, and we are continuously shifting our fixation from one part of the field of view to another. Our retinas are therefore constantly subjected to *changes* in stimulation.

Other techniques for eliminating the effects of eye movements in producing shifts of the pattern of stimulation on the retina involve special optical devices. These devices are designed in such a way as to cause the location of the light image on the retina to depend upon the position of the eye itself. One such technique involves the use of a contact lens on the eye with a mirror attachment which is used to alter the direction of the stimulus light path as the eye is moved (Figure 13a). Since the alterations in the direction of the incident light are almost perfectly correlated with the eye movements by such a contact lens and mirror device, the image continues to fall on precisely the same part of the retina as the eyeball moves from one position or orientation to the next. A related technique involves placing a small stalk on a contact lens, with a miniature stimulus and imaging device located at the end of the stalk (Figure 13b). When the eye moves and the contact lens with it, so does the stalk and the image forming device, and thus the image remains painted, as it were, on the retina even though the eyes are able to continue in constant motion. In all of these instances the perceptions after continued viewing are the same as those we have already described for the homogeneous field produced with the illuminated ping-pong balls. With continued exposure to

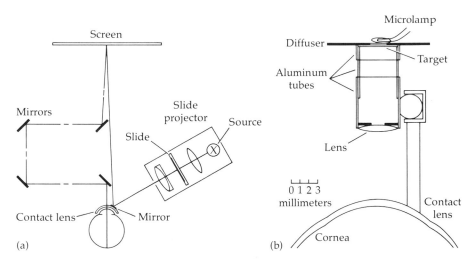

13 ARRANGEMENTS TO STABILIZE TARGETS on the retina. (a) Mirror arrangement. The target in the slide projector is imaged on a mirror mounted on a contact lens. As the eye moves, the object is reflected from this mirror to a screen and by means of mirrors (and prisms that are not shown) through a path length that is twice the distance of the eye from the screen. The target then moves by an amount that exactly matches the eye movement. Consequently, no target motion is perceived. (b) Stalk arrangement on contact lens to stabilize target on retina. The stalk holds what is effectively a miniature projector. The contact lens, stalk, and projector all move with movements of the eye. Consequently, no target motion is perceived.

light stimulation that falls on the same part of the retina in an unchanging way, in time a complete equilibrium state is reached—there is no differential brightness or hue perception and no perception of an image delineated by contours of different brightness or hues. The two opposite processes of action and reaction that occur as a result of visual stimulation are clearly demonstrated when any of these special techniques is used to maintain the local stimulation of the retina constant in time which allows these two opposite processes to reach equal magnitude and thus cancel their relative contributions to apparent brightness or hue.

Why do we not see the macula pigment that surrounds the fovea or for that matter the network of retinal blood vessels? We do not see them because they are, so to speak, permanent shadow casters. We are ordinarily not aware of them at all because, like the pencil shadow when our fixation was steadily maintained, their retinal shadows are constant and our eyes are completely adapted to them. Only early in the morning when we are adapted to darkness after a night's sleep can we get a glimpse of the diffuse macular pigment shadow on a white ceiling at the instant we first open our eyes. Another way to make the macula visible is to quickly shift the kind of illumination entering the eye. These changes prevent adaptation from setting in. One way to do this is to look at the blue sky with one eye open and hold close in front of it a filter half of which is picked to look neutral and about as bright as the other half, which is a purple. If this filter is rapidly moved back and forth (about ½-second exposures to each filter half), the macula will appear as a diffuse, darker, somewhat irregular blob.

Strong illumination directed from the side through the semiopaque wall of the eyeball will reveal the entoptic phenomena produced by the blood vessels in the eye. With the lids shut (preferably in a darkened room), rapidly jiggling a small pencil flashlight up and down at the outside corner of the eye will make the retinal blood vessels and capillaries visible (Figure 14). Fortunately, these shadows do not vary in position with eye movements, and consequently they do not interfere with our useful visual perceptions.

In concluding this chapter we should call attention to the use of adaptation experiments to isolate the three photopigment absorbance functions. We have discussed the long history of failure of the chemical extraction techniques to isolate the cone photopigments and the rather recent success that came with microspectrophotometric methods. Color-adaptation experiments have also long been used to attack this problem.

One of the classical ways of studying visual mechanisms makes use of threshold methods. In seeking to determine the properties of selected retinal areas, observers are asked to detect the presence or absence of test

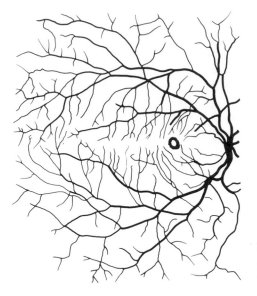

14 RETINAL BLOOD VESSELS seen when the eye is illuminated at its edge by a small pencil flashlight which is rapidly jiggled. The distribution of arteries and veins are those in the retina of an adult rhesus macaque. The small dark ring is the central fovea.

lights in the presence of backgrounds of different light levels. Experiments of this sort have usually been carried out using broad-band "white" stimuli, and are called intensity discrimination, increment threshold, or contrast threshold experiments. From an analysis of the psychophysical data, which show that an increase in light level of the background requires in general a proportionate increase in the test stimulus energy for the observer to report its detection (Weber's law), conclusions can be drawn about the response properties of the visual system.

The British investigator W. S. Stiles has extended this classical discrimination experiment to include background lights and test stimuli that are of different spectral composition or colors. This is called the TWO-COLOR THRESHOLD TECHNIQUE. Stiles sought to isolate and reveal the individual color mechanism components by selectively reducing the sensitivity or influence of competing mechanisms. To do this he used one wavelength for the background or adapting field and a different wavelength for the test flashes. With the use of a variety of different spectral backgrounds and a large number of test fields also of different spectral qualities, the results were initially analyzed to show the presence of three differently selective spectral mechanisms called π mechanisms. They are usually interpreted by most people to be different cone mechanisms. Stiles himself has recognized that the situation is more complicated than this, but a discussion of the details of this research effort is beyond the scope of this book.

In an extension of the Stiles increment threshold technique, increment thresholds have been determined in the presence of single highly intense selective bleaches or adaptation rather than against a series of increasing levels of adaptation. The assumption in these experiments is that there are three photopigments present, and by choosing bleaching or adaptation lights so as to depress as fully as possible the contribution of, say, two of them, the detectibility of threshold flashes of various spectral lights, when measured against the background of the adaptation light, gives us results that are presumably mediated by the photopigment that is not inactivated by the selective bleach. With the use of different strong adaptation lights the threshold data permit us to draw inferences about the peak loci and forms of the photopigment absorbances. Electrophysiologists also frequently use selective chromatic adaptation to analyze the receptoral inputs to the single cells from which they record.

Depressing or "knocking out" the contributions of one or two of the photopigments is connected in some researchers' minds with the notion that this is directly comparable to the situation that color deficients are in. In "color-blindness" cases, however, it is assumed that the photopigment is lost or inactivated because of inherent genetic factors. The deficiency is innate. We turn now to a discussion of the color-deficiency problem.

Background Readings

Burnham, R. W., Evans, R. M., and Newhall, S. M. 1952. Influences on color perception of adaptation to illumination. *J. Opt. Soc. Amer. 42*: 597–605.

Helson, H. 1938. Fundamental problems in color vision. I. The principle governing changes in hue, saturation, and lightness of non-selective samples in chromatic illumination. *J. Exp. Psychol. 23*: 439–476.

Hering, E. 1920. *Grundzüge der Lehre vom Lichtsinn.* Springer-Verlag, Berlin. (*Outlines of a Theory of the Light Sense.* Translated by L. M. Hurvich and D. Jameson. Harvard University Press, Cambridge, Mass., 1964.)

Hess, C. 1890. Ueber die Tonänderungen der Spectralfarben durch Ermüdung der Netzhaut mit homogenem Lichte. *Graefes Arch. Ophthalmol. 36*: 1–32.

Hochberg, J. E., Triebel, W., and Seaman, G. 1951. Color adaptation under conditions of homogeneous visual stimulation (Ganzfeld). *J. Exp. Psychol. 41*: 153–159.

Hurvich, L. M., and Jameson, D. 1958. Further development of a quantified opponent-colours theory. In *Visual Problems of Colour. II,* Chap. 22, pp. 691–723. Her Majesty's Stationery Office, London.

Hurvich, L. M., and Jameson, D. 1961. Opponent chromatic induction and wavelength discrimination. In R. Jung and H. Kornhuber (eds.),

The Visual System: Neurophysiology and Psychophysics. Springer-Verlag, Berlin.

Hurvich, L. M., and Jameson, D. 1966. Temporal Aspects of Brightness Perception. In *Perception of Brightness and Darkness,* Chap. 2. Allyn and Bacon, Boston, Mass.

Jameson, D. 1972. Theoretical Issues of Color Vision. In D. Jameson and L. M. Hurvich (eds.), *Handbook of Sensory Physiology, 7/4, Visual Psychophysics,* Chap. 14. pp. 381–412. Springer-Verlag, Berlin.

Jameson, D., and Hurvich, L. M. 1951. Use of spectral hue-invariant loci for the specification of white stimuli. *J. Exp. Psychol. 41:* 455–463.

Jameson, D., and Hurvich, L. M. 1956. Some quantitative aspects of an opponent-colors theory. III. Changes in brightness, saturation, and hue with chromatic adaptation. *J. Opt. Soc. Amer. 46:* 405–415.

Jameson, D., and Hurvich, L. M. 1972. Color Adaptation: Sensitivity, Contrast, After-images. In D. Jameson and L. M. Hurvich (eds.), *Handbook of Sensory Physiology, 7/4, Visual Psychophysics,* Chap. 22. pp. 568–581. Springer-Verlag, Berlin.

Judd, D. B. 1940. Hue, saturation, and lightness of surface colors with chromatic illumination. *J. Res. Natl. Bur. Stand. 24:* 293–333.

Krauskopf, J. 1967. Heterochromatic stabilized images. A classroom demonstration. *Amer. J. Psychol. 80:* 634–637.

Ladd, G. T. 1899. A new color illusion. *Psychol. Rev. 6:* 173–174.

McCree, K. J. 1960. Colour confusion produced by voluntary fixation. *Opt. Acta 7:* 281–290.

Polyak, S. L. 1941. *The Retina.* University Chicago Press, Chicago, Ill.

Pritchard, R. M., Heron, W., and Hebb, D. O. 1960. Visual perception approached by the method of stabilized images. *Can J. Psychol. 14:* 67–77.

Riggs, L. A., Ratliff, F., Cornsweet, J. C., and Cornsweet, T. N. 1953. The disappearance of steadily fixated visual test objects. *J. Opt. Soc. Amer. 43:* 495–501.

Stiles, W. S. 1978. *Mechanisms of Colour Vision.* Academic Press, New York.

von Kries, J. 1905. *Die Gesichtsempfindungen.* In W. Nagel (ed.), *Handbuch der Physiologie der Menschen,* pp. 109–282. Vieweg, Brunswick.

Wald, G. 1964. The receptors of human color vision. *Science 145:* 1007–1017.

Weale, R. A. 1951. Hue-discrimination in para-central parts of the human retina measured at different luminance levels. *J. Physiol. 113:* 115–122.

Wright, W. D. 1969. *The Measurement of Colour.* Van Nostrand Reinhold, New York.

Yarbus, A. L. 1967. *Eye Movements and Vision.* Translated by B. Haigh. Plenum Press, New York.

Further Readings

Cicerone, C. M., Krantz, D. H., and Larimer, J. 1975. Opponent-process additivity. III. Effect of moderate chromatic adaptation. *Vision Res. 15*: 1125–1135.

Eichengreen, J. M. 1976. Unique hue loci: induced shifts with complementary surrounds. *Vision Res. 16*: 199–203.

Helson, H. 1964. *Adaptation Level Theory.* Harper & Row, New York.

Jameson, D., Hurvich, L. M., and Varner, F. D. 1979. Receptoral and postreceptoral visual processes in recovery from chromatic adaptation. *Proc. Natl. Acad. Sci. USA. 76*: 3034–3038.

Loomis, J. M. 1972. The photopigment bleaching hypothesis of complementary after-images: a psychophysical test. *Vision Res. 12*: 1587–1594.

Pugh, E. N., Jr., and Mollon, J. D. 1979. A theory of the π_1 and π_3 color mechanisms of Stiles. *Vision Res. 19*: 293–312.

16
Color Deficiencies: Anomalous Trichromats

UP to this point we have been discussing normal color vision. Normal color perceptions vary along three major dimensions, red/green, yellow/blue, and white/black, and for the normal population we can state precisely the relations between the external physical stimulus and the colors that are seen. We are able also to state some general rules about the way colors appear when stimuli are intermixed and the way colors vary with a change in state of the organism (i.e., with adaptive changes). We have also seen that this adaptive property plus the contrast mechanism are important for the perception of a "stable" color world. We have also considered a theoretical model that organizes and explains the varied phenomena. Moreover, the way I have conceptualized the organization of the nervous system is consistent with the data of neurophysiology.

But almost everyone has at one time or another run into an individual whose color perceptions differ from the normal, or at least knows of somebody, often somebody in one's own family, who is said to be "color blind." This is not especially surprising, since some 8 or 9 percent of the population (almost exclusively male) has some sort of color defect.* First it should be explained that all normals do not necessarily experience precisely the same color for a given fixed stimulus and set of viewing conditions. Just as with almost any physical or psychological property there is for color perception some variability within the normal population. Normal individuals come in a variety of heights, weights, and abilities; similarly with color experience. In a group of 50 individuals, most of them will select a wavelength of about 503 nm as the one that corresponds to a green that is uniquely green; that is, it is not yellowish or bluish green (for a neutral state of adaptation). But if we examine Figure 1 we see that some individuals must see this 503-nm wavelength stimulus as bluish, since they select, say, a 515-nm stimulus as uniquely green. To others the 503-nm stimulus apparently looks yellowish, since they select a 490-nm

---

* This percentage value varies with the population sampled (see Table I in Chapter 19).

stimulus as a unique green. These extremes are accepted as falling in the normal category, which is a statistical concept. Our concern in this and the following chapters is with individuals who deviate from what are accepted as the color norms, with the sort of individual who instead of seeing green at, say, 490 nm or 503 nm may see this region of the spectrum as white or gray. We are not concerned here with individuals suffering from disease or injury or from poisoning with alcohol, tobacco, or some other toxic agent, but rather with healthy individuals whose color vision has been defective from birth.

All color defects are not the same. In fact, color-vision defects take a variety of forms and it is useful to consider a number of them in turn, starting with what I will call "shifted" or "displaced" color systems.

There are some persons whose color vision is anomalous even though on the whole it is very much like that of normals. These individuals tend to use the same color names that the normal does for the many objects they both see in their common environments. On rare occasions, however, these individuals do not agree with the color name that a normal applies to a given colored object (and vice versa). For example, a normal person looking at the color circle in Plate 1-2 may see and call the chip at the 3 o'clock position, "yellow." The rare individual I have in mind may, on the other hand, call the same chip at the 3 o'clock position "greenish yellow" because it looks greenish yellow to him. Or the slightly reddish-yellow chip just above the normal's yellow may look yellow to this deviant individual. This is not a problem of misnaming. Precise laboratory tests

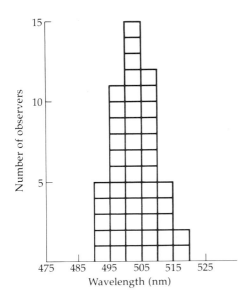

1 FREQUENCY DISTRIBUTION showing the unique green locus for 50 observers. Measurements made in a neutral state of adaptation.

leave no question that these individuals perceive reds, greens, yellows, blues, blacks, and whites, apply color names properly to what they see, and have excellent color discrimination. Moreover, they are very sensitive to slight color differences. It is as if their visual systems had a slightly different calibration from the normals as far as wavelength and perceived color are concerned. For example, the blue, the green, and the yellow that both they and the normal see in the spectrum are probably identical. However, the *wavelengths* that produce the same color experiences, the blue, the green, and the yellow, are, in the two instances, somewhat different.

When tested in the laboratory for the precise locations of the three unique hues, it becomes obvious how the chromatic systems of such an individual are shifted relative to normals. Thus an observer of this sort may have chromatic and achromatic response systems that look like those on the bottom of Figure 2.

Since both chromatic response pairs (red/green and yellow/blue) are shifted toward longer wavelengths compared to the normal ones, the spectral locus of unique blue may occur at 490 nm, of unique green at 520 nm, and of unique yellow at 595 nm instead of at the normal average values 475, 500, and 580 nm. The achromatic "whiteness" function for such an individual will also peak at a wavelength that is longer than the average wavelength at which the normal's spectral luminosity function* peaks. This may be in the region of 580 nm.

It should be emphasized that this shifted anomalous observer will disagree with the normal about color appearance only on rare occasions (anomalous = observer with anomalous color vision; normal = observer with normal color vision). Most reddish-yellow or greenish-yellow objects of the sort used here for examples are not at critical transition points; they are not yellows that are just barely green or just barely red to the normal observer. Therefore, in most cases where a normal says that an object is greenish yellow or reddish yellow (the same applies to greenish and reddish blues) there is no reason for the anomalous observer to disagree. A precise comparison may enable us to decide that the degree of redness or greenness is greater or less for the anomalous than for the normal, but for most practical purposes this is not of such a magnitude as to produce a seriously different color experience. Both see, let us say, reddish yellow but the anomalous may see it as slightly less reddish yellow. Therefore, both would use the same common descriptive term, "reddish yellow." Only in cases where there is a critical need to have very precise color

* This is the technical phrase used in the visual literature to designate the "whiteness" function (see Chapter 5).

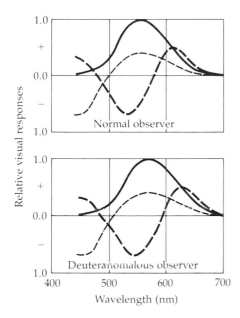

2 SPECTRAL DISTRIBUTIONS of the opponent response processes for a normal observer and for an observer with chromatic and achromatic response functions that are shifted toward longer wavelengths. This is a "shifted deuteranomalous" individual.

judgments, as in industrial and commercial situations where color tolerances are important from what will ultimately be someone's financial point of view, do such minor differences turn out to be of significance. For example, a color-anomalous observer who selected a given dye as a blue one might create problems if the normal population universally reported it to be greenish blue.

A priori there is no reason why we should anticipate that the chromatic and achromatic response functions are displaced in only one direction from the location of the normal curves. In fact, it appears that there are instances where the different "calibration" between color experience and wavelength involves a shift in the opposite direction. Such individuals who are excellent color discriminators might look at the yellow at 3 o'clock in Plate 1-2 and see it as slightly reddish yellow. The chip they see as yellow will be the one the normal sees as slightly greenish yellow. Their color vision is deviant from normal, or anomalous.

The chromatic and achromatic response curves of an observer who shows a shift toward the *short*-wavelength directions compared to the normal ones are shown in Figure 3. These functions and those shown in Figure 2 are theoretical curves. However, the achromatic and chromatic response functions of anomalous observers have been measured in the laboratory using the cancellation technique (see Chapter 5). This type of shifted anomalous may show a unique blue spectral locus at about 460 nm, a unique green at 490 nm, and a unique yellow at 560 nm. His spectral

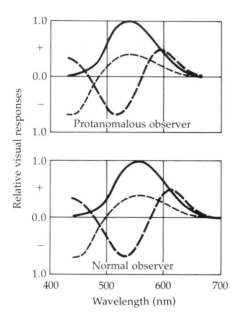

3 SPECTRAL DISTRIBUTIONS of the opponent response processes for a normal observer and for an observer with chromatic and achromatic response functions that are shifted toward shorter wavelengths. This is a "shifted protanomalous" observer.

luminosity function will peak at shorter wavelengths, say, 540 nm. To differentiate the two types of anomalous individuals, each of these two classes has been given a distinctive name. The reasons for the particular names that were chosen are now of historical interest only, but individuals whose response curves are displaced toward longer wavelengths (as compared with the normal) are called DEUTERANOMALOUS, those whose response curves are displaced toward the shorter wavelengths are called PROTANOMALOUS. Thus we have "shifted deuteranomalous" and "shifted protanomalous."

We have discussed at length the fact that the chromatic and achromatic response functions can be used to analyze and interpret stimulus color-mixture curves (Chapter 9). We saw that one set of curves can be transformed into the other. Since we have just seen that the chromatic and achromatic response functions of the shifted anomalous differ in spectral location from those of the normals, it follows that the spectral color-mixture curves of these observers must also differ from the normals, and they do. The anomalous observers just like normal observers who require three stimuli to make complete color matches throughout the spectrum, also require three mixture stimuli, hence they are TRICHROMATS. But the stimulus proportions that they use in making color matches differ from those of the normal trichromats, hence they are known as "anomalous trichromats." The two subgroups, deuteranomalous and protanomalous, are included in this superordinate category; both the deuteranomalous and protanomalous are anomalous trichromats.

When large numbers of these observers are tested, not all the observers within one group, for example the deuteranomalous, use the same proportions of the mixture stimuli for matches to spectral stimuli. In relation to the response curves this means that for individual deuteranomalous observers these curves are shifted by different amounts toward the long wavelengths. The same is true of shifted protanomalous observers. Their functions are shifted in the short-wavelength direction away from the normals but within this group the response functions of individual observers are shifted by different amounts.

Fortunately, it is not necessary to measure a complete set of color-mixture functions in order to differentiate observers who have normal response functions from those whose response functions are displaced in the spectrum. A single spectral color match or equation suffices to distinguish anomalous trichromats from normal observers. This fact was uncovered by Lord Rayleigh in 1881 and the color equation is still called a RAYLEIGH EQUATION. The color match so designated is between a mixture of the wavelengths 670 and 535 nm on one side of a color field and 589 nm on the other side of the split field.

We can represent this color equation as

$$v(535 \text{ nm}) + w(670 \text{ nm}) \equiv q(589 \text{ nm})$$

Plate 16-1a shows the way the field looks to a normal when 589 nm is on the bottom and 535 nm on the top, Plate 16-1b when 589 nm is on the bottom and 670 nm on the top, and Plate 16-1c when the mixture proportion between 535 and 670 nm on the top is such that it looks like the 589-nm test field on the bottom.

Many different instruments have been used to determine the 670 nm/535 nm proportions to match 589 nm, but the best known of these, the NAGEL ANOMALOSCOPE, is a simple, direct vision spectroscope, named after the visual scientist who designed it. What we find when a large population of observers is measured is that there are observers who require considerably more of the 535-nm stimulus compared to the normal, whereas certain others require considerably more of the 670-nm stimulus. When we use a measure like the ratio of 670 nm/535 nm to compare different individuals, we get three discrete populations of observers. These distributions are shown in Figure 4 and are representative of results obtained with protanomalous, normals, and deuteranomalous.

Let us return to our chromatic and achromatic response functions to see if we can analyze why the ratios of 670 nm/535 nm needed to match 589 nm differ for the three classes of observer. The Rayleigh equation is commonly described as a hue match made to a homogeneous yellow by a mixture of homogeneous red and green stimuli. This shorthand description is, however, far from an accurate one. (We have discussed this in

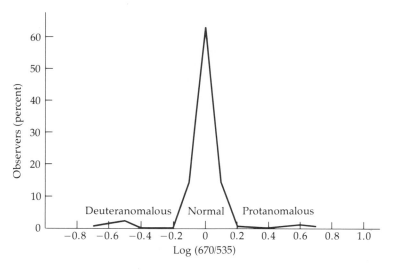

4 DISTRIBUTION OF MIDPOINT MATCHING RATIOS (670 nm/535 nm) that differentiate three groups (normals, protanomalous, and deuteranomalous) in a population of 864 males.

Chapter 6, p. 68.) If we look at the chromatic response functions of the normal observer in Figure 1 in Chapter 6 we see that the 535-nm stimulus looks yellow-green, 670 nm looks yellow-red, and 589 nm is a slightly reddish yellow. Of course, each of these three wavelengths also excites the achromatic white process. As our analysis of color mixing using the opponent-process concept has already made clear, when an observer varies the ratio of the 670- and 535-nm stimuli in one half of a bipartite visual field so that the mixture will match the slightly reddish 589-nm stimulus, he is canceling the excessive green in the yellow-green 535-nm stimulus with the opponent red excitation provided by the 670-nm yellow-red stimulus. The yellow of the 589-nm stimulus is matched by the yellow of the two mixture stimuli. The redness of the 589-nm stimulus is matched by a small additional increase in the amount of the long-wavelength 670-nm stimulus, which evokes red as well as yellow.

Suppose that a normal observer sets a color match between the test field halves of the Nagel anomaloscope. Now we ask a deuteranomalous observer (Figure 2) to look into the instrument's eyepiece. The deuteranomalous observer will report that the bottom, 589-nm stimulus looks greenish and that the upper, mixture field looks reddish (see Plate 16-2). To understand this anomalous color perception we have to compare the normal and deuteranomalous spectral response functions (Figure 2). When we look at these response functions we see that the wavelength 589 nm intercepts (i.e., stimulates) the green and *not* the red limb of the red/green response curve of the deuteranomalous.

Note also that the green and red responses evoked by the 535- and 670-nm stimuli also differ from those of the normals. But if 589 nm evokes a greenish-yellow hue instead of a reddish-yellow one, we begin to see why these deuteranomalous observers have to introduce more of the 535-nm green-yellow stimulus and less of the 670-nm reddish-yellow stimulus to match the 589-nm stimulus. It is ironic but nevertheless true that individuals of this sort are among those who have long inappropriately been called "green weak," because of the fact that they require relatively more of the 535-nm greenish-yellow light to make the Rayleigh color match.

The reverse is true for observers whose functions are shifted toward shorter wavelengths. We see in the upper panel of Figure 3 that 589 nm excites proportionally more of the reddish system than it does for the normal (lower panel of Figure 3). The red/green system also responds differently to the other two wavelengths and the need to match the redder 589-nm stimulus causes these observers to use proportionately more of the long-wavelength 670 nm in their color match. Because these particular individuals use more of the long-wavelength yellowish-red-appearing 670-nm stimulus, they have conventionally been labeled "red-weak."

Both the shifted deuteranomalous and shifted protanomalous observers can make essentially complete color matches in the anomaloscope. But after the shifted deuteranomalous has adjusted the proportions of 670 nm/535 nm for a complete color match for his eye, the normal observer looking into the eyepiece of the Nagel instrument sees a reddish-yellow field (589 nm) on the bottom and a greenish-yellow field on the top. After the shifted protanomalous has made a match that he finds satisfactory, a normal looking into the instrument sees a reddish-yellow field on the bottom and a yellowish-red field on top. Observers in any one group reject the equations of observers in any of the other groups.

How can we explain the fact that the neural response functions of anomalous observers have spectral locations that differ from the normals? We do not know the answer for a certainty, but a reasonable assumption is that their three photopigment absorption functions do not have precisely the same forms that normal ones do and that they tend to peak at somewhat different spectral loci than do those of the normal. This, in turn, would lead to deviant chromatic and achromatic response systems.

We have seen that light does not excite neural tissue directly. It must first be absorbed by photopigments in the receptors. Absorption in these photopigments triggers neuroelectric events and in some way these find expression in what we have called the chromatic and achromatic responses. We saw that the available psychophysical and physiological data permit us to express the relation between the photopigment absorption and the chromatic and achromatic response in a precise mathematical formulation. If the three photopigments in the human eye are shifted along the spectrum, possibly because of a genetic difference, and if we assume that the linkages between the cone absorptions and nervous tissues remain the same as those we have outlined (see chapter 11), we can expect some observers to show shifted chromatic and achromatic response curves. There is no reason, a priori, to anticipate that all the photopigment shifts will be precisely of the same degree or in the same direction compared with the spectral peak loci of the normal photopigment absorptions.

Data from lower organisms support the assumption of shifted photopigments. For example, the photopigment peaks of different species of marine fish are found to range over a considerable spectral region. Freshwater fish have quite different photopigments from saltwater fish because their photopigments are based on a different vitamin A. Furthermore, some fish are known to have pigments whose peaks shift during their life cycle and with changes in the waters they inhabit. More recent work on frogs has also documented the fact that even with the same species and a constant environment, a given type of photopigment will have its peak absorption at a somewhat different wavelength for different individuals. It is not a large step to assume that a similar situation prevails among human beings and that genetic variations as yet unknown and unspecified lie at the root of these photopigment variations.

Figure 5 presents the results of individual Rayleigh matches made by

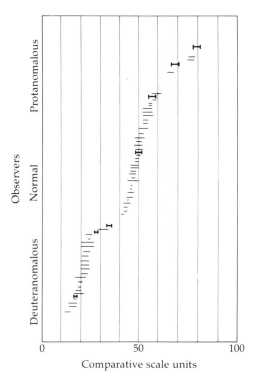

5 RAYLEIGH-EQUATION RATIOS for a group of observers with normal strength red/green chromatic response systems. Each thin line represents the results of an individual observer and the data are arbitrarily ordered in terms of increasing Rayleigh equation midpoint values (percent). The width of each line expresses the range of acceptable 670 nm/535 nm ratios that match 589 nm. The heavy bars represent theoretical calculations for seven different hypothetical observers.

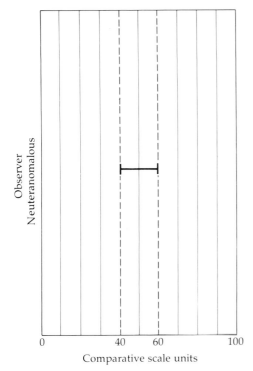

6 RAYLEIGH-EQUATION RATIOS for an observer with a red/green opponent response process of decreased efficiency. The matching midpoint is adjusted to fall at 50 percent (i.e., 50 percent of 535 nm and 50 percent of 670 nm). Matches are acceptable over a range of ratios that varies from 40 percent to 60 percent.

a number of deuteranomalous, protanomalous, and normal observers. Each line in the figure presents the results of a single observer and gives the ratio of 670 nm/535 nm stimuli used by the observer for a match to the 589-nm stimulus. These ratios are expressed in percentage terms, where 50 percent is the average value (midpoint of Rayleigh match) of the entire group of normals tested and the entries are arbitrarily ordered in terms of increasing Rayleigh-equation midpoint values.

If we look closely at the results in Figure 5 we see that the matching data of these individuals cover a rather small range of 670 nm/535 nm ratios. This small range of settings reflects the precision with which these individuals are able to detect a difference between the two matching half-fields (i.e., between 670 nm/535 nm vs. 589 nm). A small change in either the amount of 670-nm stimulus or 535-nm stimulus upsets the match. In Figure 6 are graphed the results of one individual who makes matches to 589 nm with ratios of 670 nm/535 nm that vary over the total extent of the horizontal line shown. Whether the ratio is 40 or 60 percent the match is still acceptable (provided that the 589-nm stimulus is adjusted to be equal in brightness to the combined 670 nm/535 nm lights).

Analyzing these data carefully we see that this individual tolerates the different mixture proportions of 670 nm/535 nm to match 589 nm because he seems not to be overly sensitive to the increase in redness and increase in greenness that is produced by using larger amounts of 670 or 535 nm. In terms of our chromatic and achromatic response systems we can assume that this individual lacks sharp discrimination of the red and green hue qualities because the opponent process red and green system is operating at a very much lower level of efficiency. This implies that a unit of stimulus energy does not evoke as much "redness" or "greenness" response as it does in the case of the normal. This is shown in Figure 7. Measurements of the unique hue loci in the spectrum of such an individual locates them in the same average positions as those of normals, but the blue and yellow loci can be measured only with great difficulty and imprecision, for as we see in the graphical representation of the chromatic response curves, the red/green curve is relatively flat, which makes it more difficult to detect a shift from, say, red to green or even the change within the single color quality red or green as wavelength is changed.

Since these functions are not displaced in the spectrum, we are justified in assuming that there is no photopigment shift for such observers. The relations between photopigments and neural excitation are presumably the same as for the normal. The only difference between the normal and this individual is in the degree of excitability of the nervous tissue. It is not as responsive as the normal's neural tissue. A name that we might apply to this nonshifted but less efficient type of color system is NEUTERANOMALOUS.

Two types of variation from normal are possible: (1) shifts or displacements of the peaks of the photopigment maxima and (2) reduced responsiveness or efficiency of the red/green chromatic systems. These properties are independent of each other and each may occur in an indefinite number of degrees. Thus we may find any degree of displacement associated with any degree of decreased responsiveness in the red/green system.

Figure 8 illustrates the sort of Rayleigh-equation matching data that would be obtained for both a deuteranomalous and protanomalous observer who have shifted photopigment functions and red/green response

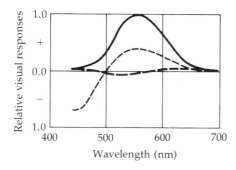

7 SPECTRAL DISTRIBUTIONS of the opponent response process for an observer whose red/green function is 10 percent efficient, compared to the normal 100 percent. No photopigment shift is present. This observer may be called "neuteranomalous."

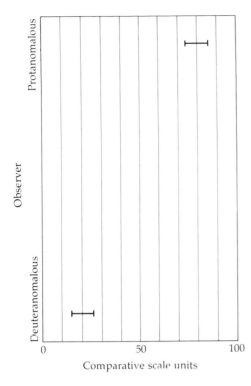

8 RAYLEIGH-EQUATION RATIOS for both a deuteranomalous and a protanomalous observer. The photopigments of the deuteranomalous are assumed to be shifted toward longer wavelengths, and those of the protanomalous toward shorter wavelengths. The range extents are related to the fact that in each instance the red/green function is assumed to be 10 percent efficient.

function operating at, say, 10 percent of normal efficiency (like the neuteranomalous of Figure 7). The response functions for each of these individuals, together with those of the neuteranomalous, are shown in Figure 9. Only a single photopigment shift in each direction is illustrated in Figure 8. This shift can, however, be of many degrees, as already noted, and the experimental data for a group of observers are shown in Figure 10. Presumably each individual's data relate to a separate set of response functions of the sort shown in Figure 9.

Figure 11 shows still another group of observers whose matching ranges are on the whole even greater than those shown in Figure 10. These observers are assumed to be operating with a red/green chromatic system that is about 3 percent efficient as compared with the normal's 100 percent efficiency. Although the relative efficiency of the yellow/blue chromatic response system probably varies in the various anomalous observers, it does not enter as a determinative factor in the setting of Rayleigh matches and thus can be left out of consideration in explaining these data.

Figure 12 is a summary graph that contains the Rayleigh-equation data of 134 individuals. The important points to note are: (1) all individuals are trichromats, (2) the midpoint of the Rayleigh-equation setting deviates

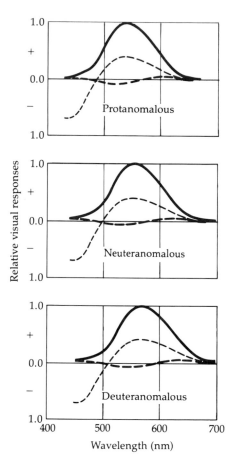

9 SPECTRAL DISTRIBUTIONS of the opponent response functions for an observer with nonshifted photopigments, and for each of two other observers with shifted photopigments. The red/green response function is 10 percent efficient compared to the normal 100 percent.

in either of two directions and to different degrees, and (3) range variations and midpoint settings vary independently. As a result of this independent variation in range and midpoint, there are anomalous observers with strong deviations from normality who are extremely keen color discriminators, and there are also individuals whose midpoint Rayleigh-equation matches fall in the normal range but who have very weak red/green chromatic response systems.

We have already discussed briefly the color perceptions of deuteranomalous and protanomalous persons with displaced photopigment functions. But as we have now seen, so many different combinations of displacement and relative efficiency of the response functions are possible that it is difficult to offer a single generalization about the perceptions of all anomalous observers. Assuming that we know the spectral distributions and magnitudes of the response functions, we can, of course, proceed to calculate hue and saturation coefficients for any anomalous ob-

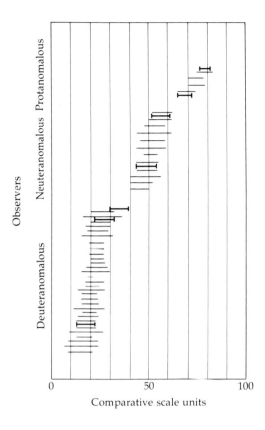

10 RAYLEIGH-EQUATION RATIOS for a group of observers with red/green response functions that are 10 percent efficient. Each thin line represents the results of an individual observer, and the data are arbitrarily ordered in terms of increasing Rayleigh-equation midpoint values. The width of each line expresses the range of acceptable 670 nm/535 nm ratios that match 589 nm. The heavy bars represent theoretical calculations for seven different hypothetical observers.

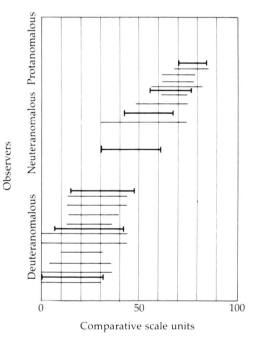

11 RAYLEIGH-EQUATION RATIOS for a group of observers with red/green response functions that are 3 percent efficient. Each thin line represents the results of an individual observer and the data are arbitrarily ordered in terms of increasing Rayleigh-equation midpoint values. The width of each line expresses the range of acceptable 670 nm/535 nm ratios that match 589 nm. The heavy bars represent theoretical calculations for seven different hypothetical observers.

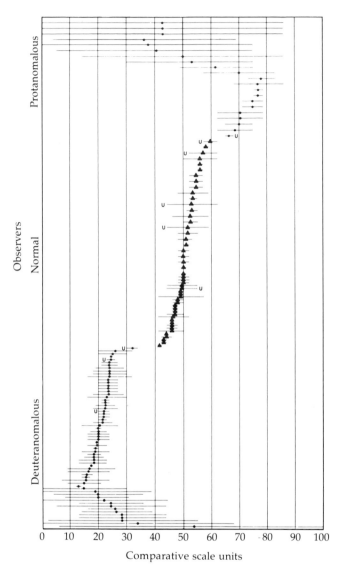

12 RAYLEIGH-EQUATION RATIOS for 134 individuals measured on the Nagel anomaloscope.

server just as we can for normals. This has been done for one type of protanomalous and one type of deuteranomalous observer, and the results for each are shown compared to those of a normal in Figures 13 and 14. Notice that the spectrum is dominated in each anomalous instance by blue and yellow hues with a minute percentage of red and green entering except at the "green" transition point near 495 or 505 nm. But notice also

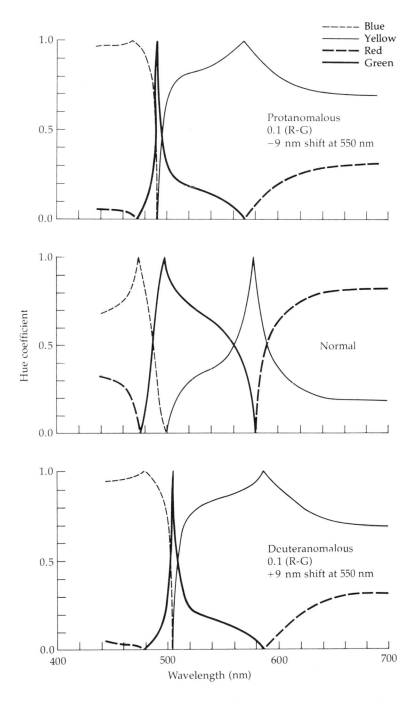

13 THEORETICAL SPECTRAL HUE COEFFICIENTS for a normal, a protanomalous, and a deuteranomalous observer. The anomalous observers are assumed to have red/green chromatic response functions that are 10 percent of the normals in efficiency.

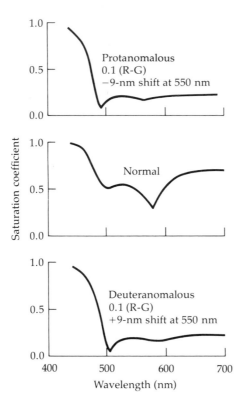

14 THEORETICAL SPECTRAL SATU-RATION coefficients for a normal, a pro-tanomalous, and a deuteranomalous observer. The anomalous observers are assumed to have red/green chromatic response functions that are 10 percent of the normals in efficiency.

that except for the short-wavelength region the spectrum is highly desaturated for these individuals and that the green point near 490 and 505 nm has almost zero saturation. These theoretically computed hue and saturation coefficients have been compared with the verbal reports of a deuteranomalous individual whose color-vision defect was confined to one eye. He was able, since he had a good normal eye, to report on the colors seen by his defective deuteranomalous eye with good assurance. These reports are in high agreement with the theoretically computed numerical values. For example, where he reports a pure yellow at 590 nm seen with the color-defective eye, the theoretical computation was 98 percent yellow and 2 percent red. At 535 nm, to cite another example, the abnormal eye is reported as seeing a yellow with a slight shimmer of green. The computation gives 83 percent yellow and 18 percent green; and so on.

Just as with normals, we can also specify how objects will "appear" to anomalous observers. Integration of the response functions weighted by specified light sources and color samples enables us to determine hue and saturation coefficients that correlate highly with what the given type of observer sees.

Because of the many varieties of anomalous trichromatic color vision, it is extremely difficult to devise simple and relatively inexpensive color-vision tests that will effectively screen and diagnose them. The Nagel anomaloscope, which does this very effectively, is an expensive laboratory instrument that costs many thousands of dollars. Often with a single screening test these defective individuals are passed as normals and just as often they are incorrectly diagnosed as dichromats, people who have another and quite different color-vision defect (see Chapter 17).

The anomalous observers we have characterized as protanomalous, neuteranomalous, and deuteranomalous manifest primarily some change in the red/green system of responses, whether the problem is a spectral shift, a decrease in responsiveness, or a combination of a shift and decrement. The everyday difficulties of these observers become manifest especially in relation to the red/green dimension of visual experience and hence are easily checked by measuring both the midpoint and range of the Rayleigh equation in a laboratory or clinic equipped with an anomaloscope.

There are other forms of anomalous trichromacies, however, that are not diagnosable with the use of the Rayleigh color match. These defects are called "tritanomaly" and involve the yellow/blue color dimension. They have a different inheritance pattern from the red/green defects, and are rarely reported. The diagnosis of this type of defect involves the use among others of short-wavelength lights (blue and blue-green), wavelengths of light that are strongly absorbed by the macula pigment. Since this pigment differs markedly from observer to observer, it is difficult to know whether differences in magnitude of response functions are being measured or whether the results obtained are due to differences in macula pigment absorption.

Background Readings

Allen, D. M., McFarland, W. N., Munz, F. W., and Poston, H. A. 1973. Changes in the visual pigments of the trout. *Can. J. Zool.* 51: 901–914.

Bowmaker, J. K., Loew, E. R., and Liebman, P. A. 1975. Variations in the λ_{max} of rhodopsin from individual frogs. *Vision Res.* 15: 997–1003.

Chapanis, A. 1944. Spectral saturation and its relation to color-vision defects. *J. Exp. Psychol.* 34: 24–44.

Dartnall, H. J. A., Lander, M. R., and Munz, F. W. 1961. Periodic Changes in the Visual Pigment of a Fish. In *Progress in Photobiology*. Elsevier, Amsterdam.

Engelking, E. 1925. Die Tritanomalie, ein bisher unbekannter Typus anomaler Trichromasie. *Graefes Arch. Ophthalmol.* 116: 196–244.

Hurvich, L. M. 1972. Color Vision Deficiencies. In D. Jameson and L. M. Hurvich (eds.), *Handbook of Sensory Physiology*, Vol. 7/4, *Visual Psychophysics*, Chap. 23, pp. 582–624. Springer-Verlag, Berlin.

Hurvich, L. M. 1973. Color Vision Deficiencies. In *Color Vision*, pp. 1–33. National Academy of Sciences, Washington, D.C.

Hurvich, L. M., and Jameson, D. 1964. Does anomalous color vision imply weakness? *Psychon, Sci. 1*: 11–12.

Hurvich, L. M., Jameson, D., and Cohen, J. D. 1968. The experimental determination of unique green in the spectrum. *Percept. Psychophys. 4*: 65–68.

Jameson, D., and Hurvich, L. M. 1956. Theoretical analysis of anomalous trichromatic color vision. *J. Opt. Soc. Amer. 46*: 1075–1089.

Pickford, R. W. 1951. *Individual Differences in Colour Vision.* Routledge & Kegan Paul Ltd., London.

Pickford, R. W., and Lakowski, R. 1960. The Pickford-Nicholson anomaloscope. *Br. J. Physiol. Opt. 17*: 131–150.

Rayleigh, Lord (J. W. Strutt). 1881. Experiments on colour. *Nature (Lond.) 25*: 64–66.

Romeskie, M. 1978. Chromatic opponent-response functions of anomalous trichromats. *Vision Res. 18*: 1521–1532.

Schmidt, I. 1955. Some problems related to testing color vision with the Nagel anomaloscope. *J. Opt. Soc. Amer. 45*: 514–522.

Willis, M. P., and Farnsworth, D. 1952. Comparative evaluation of anomaloscopes. Med. Res. Lab. Rep., 190. Bur. Med. Surg., U.S. Navy Dept., Washington, D.C.

Wright, W. D. 1947. *Researches on Normal and Defective Colour Vision.* Mosby, St. Louis, Mo.

Further Readings

Crescitelli, F. 1972. The Visual Cells and Visual Pigments of the Vertebrate Eye. In H. J. A. Dartnall (ed.), *Handbook of Sensory Physiology*, Vol. 7/1, *Photochemistry of Vision*, Chap. 8, pp. 245–363. Springer-Verlag, Berlin.

Dartnall, H. J. A. 1953. The interpretation of spectral sensitivity curves. *Br. Med. Bull. 9*: 24–30.

Hurvich, L. M., and Jameson, D. 1974. Evaluation of Single Pigment Shifts in Anomalous Color Vision. *Modern Problems in Ophthalmology.* Vol. 13, pp. 200–209. S. Karger, Basel.

Pokorny, J., and Smith, V. C. 1977. Evaluation of single-pigment shift model of anomalous trichromacy. *J. Opt. Soc. Amer. 67*: 1196–1209.

17
Color Deficiencies:
Dichromats

THE color confusions of some color deficients are often a source of puzzlement and sometimes amusement to normals. It is difficult to appreciate that there are individuals with otherwise perfect vision who cannot distinguish at any distance the ripe cherries on a tree, or strawberries from their leaves. The same is true of the red berries of hawthorn and holly, of flowers with red petals, and of scarlet poppies growing in a field of corn. Violet hues and cyan are not distinguishable from blues and chartreuse and oranges are not distinguishable in hue from yellow. To some color deficients dark reds look black. The anecdotes about the errors and color confusions that dichromats make are seemingly endless.

Can you imagine being a chemistry teacher who cannot tell that the litmus paper has changed from blue to red when dipped in acid and having to ask your pupils instead of telling them what the colors of precipitates are? Or complimenting your wife on her scarlet party dress only to have her tell you that it is bright green? An artist reported that he had a pupil-apprentice whom he "released from his engagement in consequence of finding him copy a brown horse in bluish-green, paint the sky rose colour and roses blue." In another instance a good draftsman is reported to have painted a head with the face muddy green. There are countless examples of dichromats who confuse reds with blacks, for example red ink with black ink or flakes of dry red paint with soot. On one occasion, a gentleman seeing a lady well known to him in church wearing what seemed to him "a *black* bonnet" asked her "for whom she was in mourning, and surprised her greatly by the question, for her bonnet was of crimson velvet." Can you imagine the plight of a tailor who could repair the elbow of a dark coat with a crimson patch and not know it?

The foregoing examples are taken from the book *Researches on Colour-Blindness* written in 1855 by George Wilson, a physician who was a professor of technology in the University of Edinburgh.

There is an increasing tendency in recent years to drop the use of the words "color blindness" or "color blind" to describe individuals who make confusions of the sort described. The simple reason for this tendency is the patently false connotation of the term "color blindness"—that these individuals see no color at all. In recent years the phrase "color defective" has been coming into more common use. Wilson raised this very issue in 1855 by noting that "the general character of the affliction . . . more frequently shows itself as an abnormal perception of colours, than as a total disability to discern them."

The color deficients referred to in the examples cited are DICHROMATS. Dichromats fail to discriminate colors along one of the two opponent chromatic response dimensions. Most frequently they fail to discriminate reds from greens, as in the instances cited (this becomes most evident, as we shall see, in the Rayleigh-equation test situation), and in some small percentage of cases they fail to discriminate yellows from blues. The red/green confusers, as they are often called, fall into two groups: deuteranopes and protanopes.* Note the resemblance of these two words to those used to categorize the two anomalous types discussed in Chapter 16—deuteranomalous and protanomalous. The single word DEUTAN has come into wide use to encompass both the deuteranomalous and deuteranopic color defectives and the single word PROTAN is used when referring to both the protanomalous and protanopic types.

The response functions that characterize a dichromat of the deuteranopic type are shown in Figure 1. The deuteranope's response functions are limited to a white/(black) one and a yellow/blue one. What we have here is a simple extrapolation from the deuteranomalous cases discussed in the last chapter. A series of red/green response functions of varying degrees of efficiency seemed to characterize various deuteranomalous observers and the specific degrees of red/green efficiency discussed in Chapter 16 were 100, 10, and 3 percent. Deuteranopes have red/green chromatic systems whose responsiveness is reduced to zero—there is no red/green system activation at any wavelength. As a result, the red/green system's efficiency may be said to be zero.

Since the spectral luminosity functions of most deuteranopes seem to approximate those of the normal, it may be assumed that all the photopigments of the normal are present in these color deficients and that the photopigments occupy the same spectral locus as do the normal's pigments. Absorbance of light in the photopigments may fail to activate the red/green neural system or it may have failed to develop because of some genetic factor. But since this color-vision defect arises from the absence of the red/green neural responses, we need only consider the yellow/blue

* These names were first proposed by von Kries and were related to the presumed loss of the first or second components of the three variable visual system. The word "tritanope" refers to the defect where the third component is lacking.

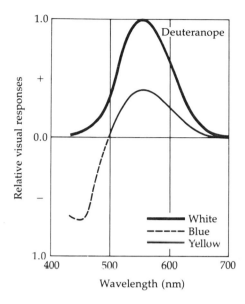

1 SPECTRAL DISTRIBUTIONS of the opponent response functions for the deuteranope. The spectral locus where the yellow/blue chromatic function crosses the 0.0 responsiveness level represents the neutral locus.

responses in relation to photopigment absorptions in order to evaluate the chromatic responses quantitatively. Thus

$$Y\text{-}B - \beta + \gamma - \alpha$$

The achromatic response, like that of normals, is

$$W\text{-}(Bk) = \alpha + \beta + \gamma$$

What would these spectral response functions lead us to believe a deuteranope sees? If we examine the curves of Figure 1 we see that starting in the short-wavelength region there is a small amount of whiteness and the beginning of the blue limb of the yellow/blue curve. As we move toward longer wavelengths, there is a progressive increase in the amount of whiteness response and a simultaneous decrease in blueness. At about 500 nm the yellow/blue curve takes on a value of zero. What, according to these functions, would we expect such an individual to see if stimulated with this wavelength? Since only the whiteness system is excited by 500 nm, the individual should experience a white or gray sensation that is neither blue nor yellow. As we move toward longer wavelengths, there is an increase in yellowness and whiteness followed by a diminution of both at the longest wavelengths.

Individuals with this sort of color system should see neither reds nor greens in the spectrum but only various saturations of blues and yellows separated by a white point at about 500 nm. There is little reason to doubt that the 500-nm spectral locus does indeed look white to such persons.

Our own experiences of dimly lit objects at night tend to grayishness and there is every reason to believe that color-defective persons see similar whites or grays at low illumination levels. Since the crossover neutral point is reported to be of the same general nature as the grayness of "night vision," we have a way of tying into this particular color experience of the color defective.*

A number of additional lines of evidence converge to argue that the red/green-deficient dichromat sees only yellows and blues in addition to white. One of these relates to "acquired" dichromacies or dichromacies that develop during the lifetime of an individual. We alluded to them in Chapter 16. These deficiencies, in contrast to the congenital types we are primarily concerned with, are usually the result of some disease entity or traumatic accident. Individuals of this sort know what the variety of hues available to the normal are. Up to the time when the disease strikes, or the toxic poison takes effect, these individuals are in fact normal. Following optic nerve atrophy, for example, whether caused by trauma, chronic intoxication, inflammation, or a neoplasm, these patients may lose their ability to discriminate "reds" from "greens" and usually report their color experiences as limited to blues, yellows, and whites. George Wilson, for example, reports the case of a "Mr. B," a lecturer in anatomy, who suffered an apparent concussion of the brain on being thrown from his horse. Following his recovery he has "found that his perception of colours which was formerly normal and acute, had become weakened and perverted; and it has continued so." On testing him Wilson says: "Bright blue and yellow he never mistook; red and green, I may say, he never knew; and he put aside, as incapable of definition, all the more mixed or composite colours." More recent literature on this sort of accident includes additional cases of such trauma and confirms this early description. These individuals must rely on their memories of the way things looked before they suffered the damage to their visual systems.

But there is also evidence concerning the color perceptions of dichromats that comes from the reports of those who are *unilaterally* deficient. Such individuals have normal color experiences and trichromatic color vision in one eye. Hence such an individual's color experience and color naming provide the base against which to evaluate the colors seen by the deficient eye. Individuals with a unilateral color defect are extremely rare; only 40 or so such cases have been reported.

In one instance of this sort, a series of spectral stimuli was presented to the defective eye of the observer, who varied the wavelength of light

* We put aside unanswerable questions of the type: "How can I know that my color experiences are like yours?" because these apply, of course, to the normals as well as to color defectives. See also previous discussion of the normal's peripheral color vision (Chapter 2).

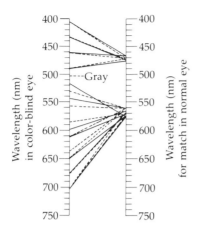

2 RESULTS OF A HAPLOSCOPIC MATCHING EXPERIMENT for a unilateral color-deficient individual. The wavelengths seen by the color-deficient eye (left-hand scale) are matched by the wavelengths indicated for the normal eye (right-hand scale). Series 1 and 2 are indicated by a dotted line and a solid line, respectively.

reaching the normal eye until a match was achieved. The results of this experiment are shown in Figure 2. All wavelengths below 502 nm presented to the abnormal eye are matched by the wavelength 470 nm in the normal eye and all the wavelengths that were longer than 502 nm and seen by the abnormal eye were matched by wavelengths approximating 570 nm. Since the wavelength 470 nm was seen as blue and 570 nm as yellow by the normal eye, it is fair to conclude that the colors perceived by the abnormal eye are limited to yellows, blues, and white (and black). We can, of course, ask the observer to name the hues of each of the spectral stimuli presented to the color-deficient eye. The result is the same. The spectrum divides into a blue region and a yellow one separated by a neutral white or gray zone.

It should be added here that there have been a number of famous scientists and engineers and physicians with dichromatic vision, among them John Dalton and William Pole, both Britishers, and Heinz Ahlenstiel, a German. In all these cases their efforts to relate what they themselves experienced in relation to normal color vision convinced them that their own color systems were limited to yellows, blues, whites, and blacks.

Figure 1 makes it clear that a dichromat needs only two spectral stimuli in order to make color equations throughout the entire spectrum. One short-wavelength stimulus, say 460 nm (blue), and one long-wavelength stimulus, say 650 nm (yellow), and their mixture are all that are necessary to achieve color matches throughout the spectrum. Just as for the normal (see Chapter 5), mixtures of yellow-appearing and blue-appearing stimuli produce cancellation of the antagonistic hues, leaving a white remainder. These mixture results are summarized in Figure 3.

Rayleigh-equation data are reproduced in Figure 4 for two groups of dichromats. These Rayleigh-equation results indicate that there are indi-

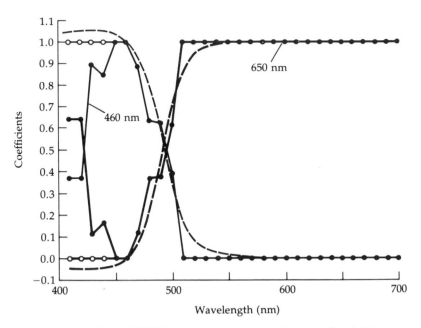

3 SPECTRAL MIXTURE CURVES in percentage values for the color-deficient eye of a unilateral color-deficient individual. The mixture of primaries are 460 nm and 650 nm.

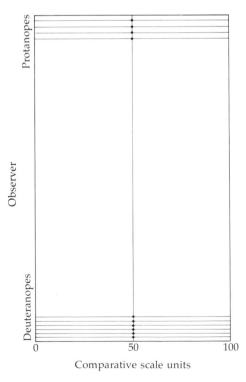

4 RAYLEIGH-EQUATION RATIOS (670 nm/535 nm) as measured on protanopes and deuteranopes. These individuals will match a 589-nm stimulus with 100 percent of 535 nm, 100 percent of 670 nm, or with any mixture ratio of 670 nm/535 nm. The results for each group are arbitrarily located on the graph. Those labeled protanopes are placed adjacent to the protanomalous data; those labeled deuteranopes, next to the deuteranomalous data (see Figure 6).

viduals who, in contrast to normals and anomalous (see Figure 12 in Chapter 16), will make a match to the 589-nm stimulus with either 100 percent of the 535-nm stimulus or 100 percent of the 670-nm stimulus; and therefore, of course, with any mixture ratio of 670 nm/535 nm. The match is a complete one if the observer adjusts the 589-nm stimulus so that its brightness is equal to that produced by the mixture stimuli. If the matching light level of the 589-nm stimulus is plotted against the 670 nm/535 nm stimulus ratios used to make the Rayleigh match, the results for the deuteranopes are as shown in Figure 5.

The dichromat behaves as he does on the Nagel anomaloscope because all wavelengths of about 500 nm and longer evoke only yellow and white sensations. Consider the 589-nm stimulus, which evokes a yellow (and white). If 670 nm is placed in the top half of the anomaloscope and the relative brightnesses of these two stimuli (589 and 670 nm) are adjusted, the individual sees them as essentially identical. Now replace 670 with 535 nm. It, too, looks whitish yellow and merely by adjusting the brightnesses of 535 nm and 589 nm, a complete equation is achieved. Since the intermixture of 535 and 670 nm can obviously only generate a yellowish (white) end product, this color-deficient observer will accept any stimulus ratio of 670 nm/535 nm as a match to 589 nm provided that a brightness adjustment can be made between the two halves of the equation. This result is, of course, reflected in the match ranges shown in Figures 4 and 5. The midpoint of the match is taken as the value that bisects the range. This is arbitrary and has no particular significance.

We have dealt so far only with spectral stimuli. Excitation by broadband stimuli of the chromatic and achromatic response functions is treated in the same way for the color-deficient as it is for normals (see Chapter 7). For a stimulus with an energy distribution that covers a broad spectral region, we need only evaluate the output of the yellow/blue chromatic and white/black achromatic systems integrated over wavelengths in the

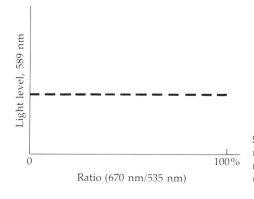

5 RAYLEIGH-EQUATION RATIOS (670 nm/535 nm) for an average deuteranope matched in light level to the 589-nm stimulus.

stimulus. When this is done for all the usual light distributions of objects that we encounter in our daily lives, the calculations show the deuteranopes' color world to be limited to yellows and blues of different saturations. The yellows of the normal are, of course, seen as such; so are the blues. But lacking redness, the normal's oranges also look yellow to the deuteranope; and lacking greens, the cyans look blue.

One point that should be emphasized is that the extraspectral red of the normal (i.e., the unique red seen by the normal that is composed of a mixture of, say, 440 + 640 nm) is for the deuteranope exactly equivalent to the sensation that corresponds to 500 nm: a white or gray. If we recall the chromatic and achromatic responses of the normal (see Chapter 5), the 440-nm stimulus evokes red and blue, and the 640-nm stimulus evokes red and yellow. When we adjust the energies of these two wavelengths so that the opponent yellow and blue just cancel each other, the remaining excitations are red and white; hence we are left with a unique or pure red sensation for the normal observer. Note that if the same two wavelengths are used for the deuteranope, one excites blue responses, the other yellow responses (plus white in each instance). Depending upon the relative energies of the two stimuli, the observer may see yellow or blue. When the excitation ratio is such that an exact balance or antagonism exists between yellow and blue, we have only the remainder excitation—the white that each wavelength excites independently.

Directly comparable to the deuteranopes there is another type of dichromat who lacks the red/green chromatic response system, but these individuals are called protanopes. The available evidence suggests that, like the deuteranopes, they see only yellow and blues and white and blacks and that when their discrimination functions* are measured they behave pretty much like those of the deuteranope. They differ from the deuteranope with respect to the luminosity or achromatic function, which peaks at a shorter wavelength, and their yellow versus blue chromatic spectral response function is on the average also shifted toward shorter wavelengths. Figure 6 summarizes these facts.

Statistically speaking, the location of the neutral locus in the spectrum, the region that looks white or gray, is displaced for the protanopes relative to the deuteranopes toward shorter wavelengths, say, to 495 nm. However, in individual instances the neutral point of a deuteranope may fall at a shorter wavelength than some of the protanopes. The fact that the luminosity curve is displaced toward shorter wavelengths implies that the protanope responds less efficiently to long wavelengths or light as compared to the deuteranope. Long wavelengths of light which will still be

---

* Wavelength and saturation discrimination functions.

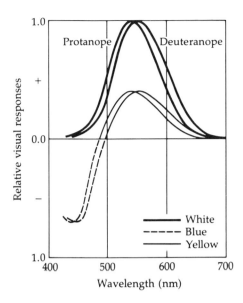

6 SPECTRAL DISTRIBUTIONS of the opponent response functions for the protanope and the deuteranope. Compared to the deuteranope's functions, both the chromatic yellow/blue and achromatic response functions of the protanope are displaced toward shorter wavelengths.

seen as yellows by the deuteranope will look darker to the protanopes (if the same stimulus energy of long-wavelength light is used) and may be confused with dark gray or blackish colors.

Since normals see these long wavelengths as reds (slightly yellowish) the protanope has long been inappropriately named "red-blind." We are agreed that he does not see reds. But what is more important is that protanopes like deuteranopes do not see greens either. Thus protanopes and deuteranopes lack *both* red and green experiences. If we insist on retaining the word "blind," both deuteranopes and protanopes could be more appropriately called "red *and* green blind."

Protanopes behave the way deuteranopes do with respect to color matches (i.e., they are dichromatic). With proper mixtures of one wavelength from the short-wavelength end of the spectrum and another from the long-wavelength end, they can match all spectral stimuli. However, since the chromatic and achromatic response functions are displaced toward the short wavelengths, the proportions of the two mixture stimuli that the protanope uses to match the series of spectral lights are not the same as those used by the deuteranope. The fact that the protanope's luminosity function is displaced from the deuteranopes is also reflected in the matches made with the Nagel anomaloscope. Although like the deuteranope, the protanope will accept matches to 589 nm with 100 percent of the 535 or 670-nm stimulus, the energy values of the 589-nm stimulus adjusted to match these stimuli (or varying proportions of them) differ from the deuteranope's. The summary data on these matches are given in

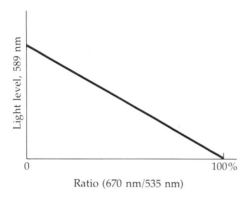

7 RAYLEIGH-EQUATION RATIOS (670 nm/535 nm) for an average protanope matched in light level to the 589-nm stimulus (compare with Figure 5).

Figure 7. This function should be contrasted with that shown in Figure 5.

It may be assumed that like the normal (and deuteranope), the protanope has three photopigments. However, we must assume that the protanopic photopigment functions are displaced toward shorter wavelengths. As we have seen, the location of the photopigment maxima control the way the response functions are distributed in the spectrum. It is the photopigment shift that is responsible for the displaced response functions of the protanope toward shorter wavelengths.

As in the case of the normal observer, a change in prevailing illumination from, say, daylight to incandescent excites the longer-wavelength pigment to a greater degree than either the middle- or short-wavelength pigment and a relative desensitization occurs which is directly related to the degree of excitation. These changes, in turn, modify the forms of the chromatic and achromatic response curves. Exposure to incandescent light or candlelight leaves an observer less sensitive to stimulation by long-wavelength lights and more sensitive to stimulation by short-wavelength lights. But, as in the case of normals, the relative desensitization that occurs does not necessarily compensate for the change in the stimulus itself. An object of a given fixed reflectance provides a different stimulus to the eye, depending on its illumination.

It is not surprising to find, therefore, that dichromats who confuse certain reds and greens in daylight illumination note a difference between the objects if yellowish incandescent or gas light is the illuminant. Thus a scarlet geranium confused with its leaves in daylight is seen as distinct from its leaves in incandescent light. Scarlet and greens or blues and purples for the normal eye which are indistinguishable from each other in daylight become strikingly different in illuminants whose spectral distributions are more heavily weighted in the long wavelengths.

What procedures or tests can be used to detect color deficiencies? The

Nagel anomaloscope is the instrument par excellence for detecting and analyzing the varieties of red/green color deficiency I have been describing. Figure 8 shows in summary fashion the color match midpoint and ranges acceptable to the average normal observer, a typical protanope, deuteranope, a sharply discriminating protanomalous, and a deuteranomalous observer as well as an instance of each type of anomalous color vision with less sharp discrimination. Because this optical instrument is expensive, its use is limited mainly to the research laboratory, but it is occasionally found in the clinic or office of a practicing ophthalmologist.

However, using other techniques, hundreds of thousands of individuals have been tested for color-vision defects—a recent study, for example, reports data on color-vision deficiencies among 29,985 young Greeks. These large populations have traditionally been tested with what are called "pseudoisochromatic plates." These tests come in booklet form usually, are relatively inexpensive compared to an optical instrument, and are easy to administer. There are many versions of this type of screening test, one of the best known of which is the Ishihara. In this form of test, numerical characters made up of dots of varying size and color are superimposed on backgrounds made up of similar dots. The various dots that make up the figure have the same distribution of brightnesses as those that make up the background and in general the figures or numerals are yellowish red and the backgrounds yellowish green, or vice versa. Normals distinguish the figures from the background as hue differences. For a color deficient,

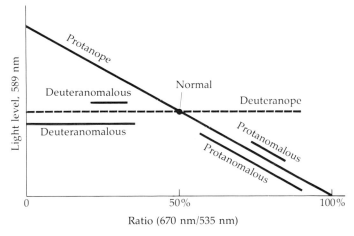

8 RAYLEIGH-EQUATION RATIOS (670 nm/535 nm) for an average normal, an average protanope, and average deuteranope and two illustrative instances of each of the types deuteranomalous and protanomalous. Only two ranges of acceptable matches are illustrated for the latter two types. See Figure 12 in Chapter 16 for the varieties of ranges actually measured.

say, a deuteranope who cannot discriminate reds from greens, the dots of equal brightnesses provide no differentiating cues and hence the numeral fuses with the background. Diagnoses are based on an arbitrary criterion of number of items "passed" and "failed." Since the response systems of protanopes and deuteranopes differ, these tests usually contain plates with somewhat different stimulus combinations in order to differentiate protanopes from deuteranopes.

A recent popular variant of this form of test is the American Optical Company Hardy-Rand-Rittler (AO H-R-R) set of plates. Instead of numerals, this test uses three different symbols (circles, triangles, and crosses) and instead of backgrounds made up of the "complementary" hues, the backgrounds are made up of dots of gray of varying brightnesses. As we have seen, dichromats who lack the red/green dimension experience a white or gray at the spectral locus where yellow and blue are in balance. Properly selected broad-band stimuli that are uniquely green and red under appropriate illumination can be expected to look like a set of grays to these color defectives and hence not discriminable from the gray dots that make up the background. In accordance with the displacement of the chromatic response functions relative to each other (Figure 6), the red and green stimuli that are confused with grays by the two types differ somewhat. Two plates from the AO H-R-R test are shown in Plate 17-1. The protanope would not be expected to see the triangle in Plate 17-1a nor the circle in Plate 17-1b, and it is anticipated that the deuteranope will fail to see the circle and the cross in these particular illustrative plates. This particular test also uses differently saturated stimuli in an effort to discriminate among anomalous individuals who have different degrees of discriminative capacity.

Another very widely used test is illustrated in Plate 17-2. This is the Farnsworth dichotomous (or D-15 panel) test. This test is composed of 15 small colored chips (plus one reference chip for a total of 16) and the observers' task is to line up the series of chips sequentially so that they form a continuous color series in terms of similarity. For the normal the series starts with a reddish-blue chip and moves progressively through a series of hues that can be roughly described as blue, blue-green, green-blue, green, yellowish-green, yellow, yellow-red, and back to bluish red. They are all presumably equally bright. The normal can set these chips in proper order in a minute or two. A dichromat who lacks the red/green sense orders these chips in a different fashion. Since neither "red" nor "green" provides a differentiating clue, he first alternates chips that are blue and red with chips that are blue and green. As the series progresses he alternates between the normal's green-yellow and red-yellow chips since neither red nor green is detected here either. In short, where the

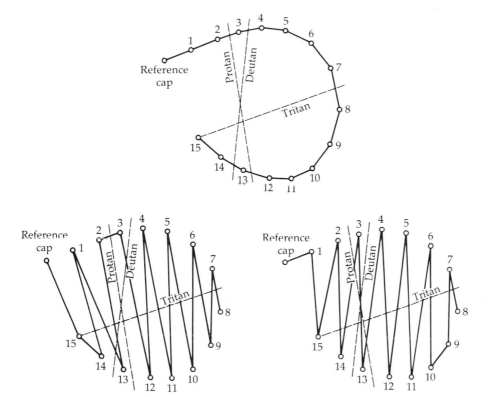

9 FORMAT FOR FARNSWORTH DICHOTOMOUS TEST (The Psychological Corporation, New York) for color deficiency. Upper figure shows similarity ordering of normal trichromats. Dashed lines are protan, deutan, and tritan confusion axes. Lower left figure shows similarity ordering of protanope; lower right shows deuteranope.

normal's choices can be graphed in a circular form like the hue circle of Plate 1-2, the choices of the dichromat criss cross the graph because the similarities for this observer are among common blues and the common yellows. Here, too, the protanope and deuteranope select different stimulus sequences as forming a continuous pattern, and this difference in sort is used to differentiate between them. Typical normal, protanopic, and deuteranopic sortings are illustrated in Figure 9. Slight deviations from these typical sortings, do, of course, occur but rarely interfere with the diagnosis.

We have discussed at length that changes occur in color appearance with changes in illumination and that a change from daylight illumination to incandescent may flip a given stimulus from blueness to yellowness for deuteranopes and protanopes.* It should be obvious therefore why the

* See the discussion of metamers for normals in Chapter 15.

various pseudoisochromatic plates and D-15 test that have been designed for use with daylight illumination must under no circumstances be used with nonstandardized illuminants (particularly fluorescent lights) if meaningful data are to be obtained.

There are many screening tests of the foregoing sort. Their design is not perfect and in the manufacture of the tests, design criteria may not be precisely met, since color printing is variable. In addition, dyes fade in time. It is not surprising, therefore, that in some small percentage of cases, color deficients are diagnosed as normals and normals as color deficient. But if their shortcomings are recognized and the tests are administered as the designers intended them to be, they are extremely valuable instruments.

In addition to protanopia and deuteranopia another form of dichromatic color vision is also known: tritanopia. This very rare dichromatic deficiency corresponds to the trichromatic anomaly of the same root name mentioned in Chapter 16. But instead of having the reduced yellow/blue response system of the tritanomalous observers, tritanopes are totally lacking the yellow/blue sense. These individuals perceive only greens, reds, and whites and blacks.

Observers of this type have spectral luminosity functions that approximate the normal's curve and appear to have only one spectral neutral point, which approximates the normal's yellow locus at 580 nm. If one assumed a loss of the normal's yellow/blue chromatic response functions for this type of dichromat, a second short-wavelength neutral locus would be anticipated at about 475 nm, but it seems to be lacking,* and we do not find a red region from 400 to 475 nm. The only red that seems to occur in the short-wavelength spectral region is relatively weak and it appears only at the extreme short-wavelength end of the spectrum in the region of 400 or 410 nm.

This type of observer's response functions are given in Figure 10. The equations that can be used to relate the chromatic and achromatic functions of the tritanope to the photopigment curves are the following:

$$R\text{-}G = \gamma - \beta$$
$$Wh\text{-}(Bk) = \beta + \gamma$$

What is assumed here is not only a loss (or inactivation) of the yellow/blue neural response function but also a loss of the short-wavelength absorbing photopigment. Comparisons of various discriminative capacities based on the theoretical response functions have been made to experimentally measured functions and the fits between the two are reasonably

* Occasional reports of two spectral neutral points have appeared in the literature. Individuals of this sort have been labeled "tetartanopes."

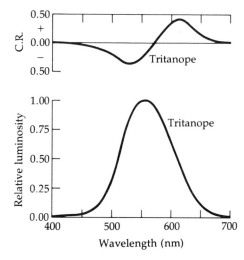

10 SPECTRAL DISTRIBUTIONS of the opponent response functions for the tritanope. The spectral locus where the red/green chromatic function crosses the 0.0 responsiveness level represents the neutral locus.

good. There is no simple optical device to measure and diagnose these rare forms of congenital color defect, and both the pseudoisochromatic plates described and the D-15 test are used for this purpose.*

In discussing the more common forms of dichromacy, protanopia and deuteranopia, we have assumed that the α, β, and γ photopigments are all present and that the color-vision defect rests exclusively on the absence of the red/green neural response mechanisms. We have just seen that it is possible to assume for tritanopia the loss of the α photopigment as well as a loss at the neural level of one of the chromatic response systems.

In directly comparable fashion we can assume that the protanope lacks the long-wavelength photopigment, γ. The loss of this pigment would account for the peaking of the protanope's spectral luminosity function at shorter wavelengths than the normals and the relative darkness of the long-wavelength spectral region.

If we express the chromatic response functions in the usual normal form,

$$R\text{-}G = \alpha + \gamma - \beta$$
$$Y\text{-}B = \beta + \gamma - \alpha$$
$$Wh\text{-}(Bk) = \alpha + \beta + \gamma$$

and then examine the consequence of eliminating the long-wavelength photopigment, we have

$$R\text{-}G = \alpha - \beta$$
$$Y\text{-}B = \beta - \alpha$$
$$Wh\text{-}(Bk) = \alpha + \beta$$

* A special plate designed by Farnsworth is also used.

The R-G and Y-B functions are simple mirror images of the same form and hence these individuals manifest only one chromatic response function as well as the white (black) achromatic response.

The situation is the same in principle if we assume a loss of the midwave β photopigment for the deuteranope. Now we have

$$R\text{-}G = \alpha + \gamma$$
$$Y\text{-}B = \gamma - \alpha$$
$$Wh\text{-}(Bk) = \alpha + \gamma$$

There is a single form of chromatic response function plus an achromatic response function just as in the case of the protanope. The (R-G) and Wh-(Bk) functions are the same.

This view, that the loss of the red/green response function is directly related to the loss of one of the photopigments, is in fact the view that is most widely held. However, when red/green deficiencies occur because of injuries to the higher nervous centers, it is, of course, unlikely that anything has happened at the photopigment level.

Can someone with one of the various deficiencies we have been discussing be "cured?" This question arises time and again and if the deficiency is not an acquired one (arising from toxins or disease), the answer is always the same: no. Some of the acquired color deficiencies that derive from toxins are sometimes reversible. In the older literature on color deficiencies, we can read that "temporary color blindness resulting from congestion, hepatic derangement, and dyspepsia' disappear under appropriate treatment." But congenital color deficiencies of the sort described in Chapter 16 and in this chapter and the monochromacies to be discussed in Chapter 18 are inherited in specific ways and cannot be cured. They cannot be cured in the sense that an individual who lacks the red/green sense from birth cannot in some miraculous way have this neural capacity or photopigment lack restored by any known drug or treatment which will ultimately enable him to experience reds, blues, greens, cyans, yellows, and oranges as the normal does.

But a number of techniques may enable the color-deficient person to discriminate among colors which he would otherwise confuse. We have already seen that some greens and reds that are indistinguishable by daylight are seen as different if the illumination is switched to incandescent or candlelight. When the illuminant changes, they are seen not as red and green but probably as being of different brightness or even as being yellow and gray rather than two grays. This is admittedly useful.

Still another maneuver involves the use of colored filters. This technique was first used in 1817—one hundred and sixty years ago—and by many others thereafter. Thus a red/green-deficient observer who fails to see one of the green symbols on the gray background of Plate 17-1 will, on looking at them through a red filter, see both of them as dark symbols on a lighter background; or, if a green filter is used, both of the red symbols will be seen against a lighter background. This is the essence of the way normals can penetrate camouflage where an object is masked by a paint of similar appearance so that the object will blend or fuse with the background.*

James Clerk Maxwell proposed around 1854–1855 that a "spectacle frame" be constructed with one red glass and one green one so that one eye always looked through one glass and the other eye through the other glass. Red objects look brighter than greens seen through the red glass and green objects look brighter than reds when seen through the green glass. "The colour blind party using them must know from independent authority which of the eye-pieces is red and which green," wrote George Wilson—still a solid piece of advice.

A device of this sort may be helpful in specific instances, and with the development of contact lenses, such devices are being marketed commercially. (Linksz, 1965). But we must not lose sight of the fact that discrimination thus facilitated never brings with it the full experiential color world of the normal. "Mr. B.," the gentleman who had normal vision before he suffered the cerebral accident, "knows what he loses by his colour-blindness . . . the colours which he saw are not only effaced, but are replaced by tints most unlike those which they once bore." (Wilson, 1855, p. 40).

Background Readings

Ahlenstiel, H. 1951. *Rotgrünblinheit als Erlebnis.* Musterschmidt Wissenshaft, Göttingen.

Cameron, R. G. 1967. Rational approach to color vision testing. *Aerosp. Med. 38*: 51–59.

Dalton, J. 1798. Extraordinary facts relating to the vision of colours. *Mem. Lit. Phil. Soc.* (Manchester) 5: 28–45.

Farnsworth, D. 1943. The Farnsworth-Munsell 100-hue and dichotomous tests for color vision. *J. Opt. Soc. Amer. 33*: 568–578.

Graham, C. H., and Hsia, Y. 1958. Color defect and color theory. *Science 157*: 675–682.

---

* Materials used to camouflage the object of interest are paints, foliage, and other objects that have the same appearance. Almost invariably we are dealing with a metameric match. Since the object and the camouflage material have different spectral distributions, by looking through selectively transmitting filters, the difference between the object and the masking material is immediately revealed.

Hardy, L. M., Rand, G., and Rittler, M. C. 1954. H-R-R polychromatic plates. *J. Opt. Soc. Amer. 44*: 509–523.

Hecht, S. and Shlaer, S. 1936–1937. The color vision of dichromats. II. Saturation as the basis for wavelength discrimination and color mixture. *J. Gen. Physiol. 20*: 83–93.

Hurvich, L. M. 1972. Color Vision Deficiencies. In D. Jameson and L. M. Hurvich (eds.), *Handbook of Sensory Physiology,* Vol. 7/4, *Visual Psychophysics,* Chap. 23, pp. 582–624. Springer-Verlag, Berlin.

Hurvich, L. M., and Jameson, D. 1955. Some quantitative aspects of an opponent-colors theory. II. Brightness, saturation, and hue in normal and dichromatic vision. *J. Opt. Soc. Amer. 45*: 602–616.

Hurvich, L. M., and Jameson, D. 1974–1975. On the measurement of dichromatic neutral points. *Acta Chromat. 2*: 207–216.

Judd, D. B. 1945. Standard response functions for protanopic and deuteranopic vision. *J. Opt. Soc. Amer. 35*: 199–221.

Linksz, A. 1964. *An Essay on Color Vision and Clinical Color-Vision Tests.* Grune & Stratton, New York.

Linksz, A. 1965. Colored lenses and color vision. *Amer. J. Ophthalmol. 60*: 1135–1136.

Maxwell, J. C. 1855. Experiments on colour, as perceived by the eye, with remarks on colour-blindness. *Trans. R. Soc. Edinb. 21*: 275–298.

Murray, E. 1943. Evolution of color vision tests. *J. Opt. Soc. Amer. 33*: 316–334.

Murray, E. 1945. Alleged cures of color blindness. *Amer. J. Psychol. 58*: 253–261.

Pitt, F. H. G. 1935. *Characteristics of Dichromatic Vision,* Gt. Br. Med. Res. Counc. Rep. 200. Her Majesty's Stationery Office, London.

Pole, W. 1893. On the present state of knowledge and opinion in regard to colour-blindness. *Trans. R. Soc. Edinb. 37*: 441–479.

Wilson, G. 1855. *Researches on Colour-Blindness.* Sutherland and Knox, Edinburgh.

Wright, W. D. 1947. *Researches on Normal and Defective Colour Vision.* Mosby, St. Louis, Mo.

Further Readings

Verriest, G. (ed.). 1972. *Modern Problems in Ophthalmology,* Vol. 11, *Acquired Colour Vision Deficiencies.* S. Karger, Basel.

Verriest, G. (ed.). 1974. *Modern Problems in Ophthalmology,* Vol. 13, *Colour Vision Deficiencies II.* S. Karger, Basel.

Verriest, G. (ed.). 1976. *Modern Problems in Ophthalmology,* Vol. 17, *Colour Vision Deficiencies III.* S. Karger, Basel.

Verriest, G. (ed.). 1978. *Modern Problems in Ophthalmology,* Vol. 19, *Colour Vision Deficiencies IV.* S. Karger, Basel.

18
Color Deficiencies: Monochromatism

IN discussing anomalous color deficiencies we have noted that the red/green and/or yellow/blue chromatic response systems may show various degrees of neural response efficiency, varying from 100 percent to minimal values, say, 3 percent. In discussing the dichromacies we have seen that one pair of the chromatic responses may, in given instances, be totally lacking, thus giving rise to red/green or yellow/blue types of "color blindness." By simple extension, if *both* the red/green and yellow/blue response mechanisms are lacking simultaneously, we have what is commonly called "total color blindness" or MONOCHROMACY.

In all the recorded literature on this type of color deficiency there are reports of about 500 or so cases. In many instances there are associated other visual symptoms and complications (see below) that have led to a variety of different kinds of classifications of these defects. It seems to be true, however, that there are monochromats of a simple uncomplicated type that are easily understood in relation to the color model we have used in this book.

First, what do such individuals see? They see a world of objects that are differentiated only by lightness, like our whites, grays, and blacks. What they see is limited to what normal individuals can see when they look at ordinary black-and-white photographs or a black-and-white television screen.

When taken into the laboratory to check their matches to various regions of the spectrum with selected spectral comparison stimuli, we find that they can do this with ease using only a *single* spectral stimulus for the matches to *all* other spectral stimuli. They require only that the single spectral stimulus be adjustable in its relative energy. And any spectral stimulus from any part of the spectrum can be used for the match, since these observers discriminate no hues whatsoever: the individual spectral test stimuli are all apparently achromatic, and so is the variable comparison stimulus.

Observers of this sort who have good foveal vision, no central blind

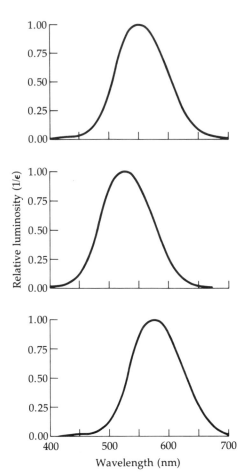

1 SPECTRAL DISTRIBUTIONS OF ACHROMATIC response functions of cone monochromats. These functions of cone monochromats peak at different spectral loci. These observers have no measurable chromatic response functions.

areas or scotomata, normal acuity, and no nystagmus* or photophobia† have photopic luminosity functions. Furthermore, in line with what we have said about various anomalous trichromats and types of dichromatic vision, the measured luminosity functions of these "cone monochromats," as they are called, can be similar to the spectral luminosity of the protanope, to that of the normal or to that of the deuteranope. There have been relatively few precisely measured functions, but instances of each of these types are reported in the literature. These response functions are illustrated in Figure 1. In cases of this sort there are no chromatic response functions and once again we need only assume that the cone photopigment functions of the normal spectral locus may be displaced somewhat toward the short- or long-wavelength directions in different instances.

* Nystagmus is a rapid involuntary oscillation of the eyes.
† Photophobia is a condition where an individual has an extreme and even painful sensitivity to high light levels.

Since these absorption functions determine the white/black neural response, the luminosity function is displaced accordingly. Various measures of the accommodation, selective adaptation, and electrical responses made on the eyes of observers of this type support the view that their cone mechanisms are intact and that the color losses are postreceptoral (i.e., neural).

Just as was true for dichromatic vision, however, there is an alternative explanation for cone monochromacy. The most widely held view as far as dichromats is concerned is that there are specific receptor and photopigment losses for each type. Protanopes have presumably lost the γ photopigment, deuteranopes the β photopigment, and tritanopes the α photopigment. To account for the cone monochromats on a receptoral-photopigment basis it is only necessary to assume that although they have cone vision they have lost two of the normals' three photopigments. An opponents-type neural signal cannot be generated by a single type of photopigment acting in isolation. Depending on which photopigment type is spared, moreover, we may expect corresponding displacements of the luminosity functions of the sort reported.

Cone monochromacy occurs only rarely and the evidence points to different mechanisms in different cases. There have also been cases to which the name "pseudomonochromacy" has been applied. To all intents and purposes these individuals are also monochromatic and see nothing but whites, grays, and blacks. However, careful analysis reveals trace amounts of color response, for example a trace of yellow/blue response. Such individuals might more appropriately be referred to as dichromats.

There is a different form of monochromacy from the one described. The more frequently occurring cases of monochromacy is rod monochromacy (Figure 2). The individuals are named "rod monochromats" or "typical achromats" and these deficiencies are more difficult to understand. Researchers have disagreed and continue to disagree very sharply about these individuals, whose condition is also sometimes called "congenital achromatopsia."

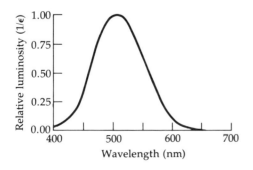

2 SPECTRAL DISTRIBUTION of achromatic response function of typical rod monochromats.

The typical achromats are likely to have low visual acuity, pupillo-motor symptoms, central blind spots, nystagmus, and photophobia. Not all individuals exhibit all of these associated defects, but many of them are present in most cases. What does characterize all these persons is that they have a scotopic spectral luminosity function that peaks at about 505 nm and hence have poor vision in daylight. It is for this reason that these individuals, who also see only whites, grays, and blacks, are called "rod monochromats." But whether or not these individuals have only rod receptors to the exclusion of cones is a much debated issue. Some investigators believe they do have cones but that the photopigment in their cones, like that in the rods, is rhodopsin, the pigment that is normally associated exclusively with rods and night vision.

Background Readings

Alpern, M. 1974. What is it that confines in a world without color? *Invest. Ophthalmol. 13*: 648–674.

Alpern, M., Falls, H. G., and Lee, G. B. 1960. The enigma of typical total monochromacy. *Amer. J. Ophthalmol. 56*: 996–1011.

Blackwell, H. R., and Blackwell, O. M. 1961. Rod and cone receptor mechanisms in typical and atypical congenital achromatopsia. *Vision Res. 1*: 62–107.

Fincham, E. F. 1953. Defects of the colour sense mechanisms as indicated by the accommodation reflex. *J. Physiol. Lond. 121*: 570–580.

Francois, J., Verriest, G., and De Rouck, A. 1955. L'Acromatopsie congénitale. *Doc. Ophthalmol. 9*: 338–424.

Gibson, I. M. 1962. Visual mechanisms in a cone-monochromat. *J. Physiol. Lond. 161*: 10–11.

Glickstein, M., and Heath, G. G. 1975. Receptors in the monochromat eye. *Vision Res. 15*: 633–636.

Hurvich, L. M. 1972. Color Vision Deficiencies. In D. Jameson and L. M. Hurvich (eds.), *Handbook of Sensory Physiology*, Vol. 7/4, *Visual Psychophysics*, Chap. 23, pp. 582–624. Springer-Verlag, Berlin.

Ikeda, H., and Ripps, H. 1966. The electroretinogram of a cone-monochromat. *Arch. Ophthalmol. 75*: 513–517.

Jaeger, W. 1951. Angeborene totale Farbenblindheit mit Resten von Farbempfindung. *Klin. Monatsbl. Augenheilkd. 118*: 282–288.

Sloan, L. L. 1946. A case of atypical achromatopsia. *Amer. J. Ophthalmol. 29*: 290–294.

Sloan, L. L. 1954. Congenital achromatopsia: A report of 19 cases. *J. Opt. Soc. Amer. 44*: 117–128.

Weale, R. A. 1953. Cone-monochromatism. *J. Physiol. Lond. 121*: 548–569.

19
Color Deficiencies:
Heredity and Incidence

THAT color deficiencies "run" in families has been known for at least 200 years. There is, for example, a report made in 1777 on a family of seven children. Two brothers and a sister were normal, as were the parents, but four brothers could only distinguish yellow from blue. A few years later a family tree was described in which there were three successive generations of red/green color defects, and John Dalton, whom I mentioned earlier, had a color-defective brother, as well as a normal brother and sister.

Among the many pedigrees that began to be published thereafter is one of Horner's, a Swiss ophthalmologist. This particular pedigree, covering eight generations of the descendants of a color-normal woman born in 1642, is shown in Figure 1. The pattern of red/green-color-deficient males in every second generation is clear-cut.* Grandchildren seem to inherit the deficiency from their grandfathers via daughters who are color-normal. Alternatively stated, the deficiency is inherited by sons of normal daughters whose fathers were color-defective.

The genetic basis of this pattern of inheritance is of great interest to geneticists and vision researchers. To the former, the inheritance patterns provide the data that will ultimately help solve the many unresolved issues of gene transfer from generation to generation; for the latter, the inheritance pattern may illuminate the mechanisms of normal as well as abnormal color vision.

Despite the accumulation of many pedigrees it was not until 1911 that this form of transmission (which is also characteristic of haemophilia) was related to the new discoveries then being made about heredity. The transmission of the red/green deficiencies was analyzed at that time as a recessive sex-linked Mendelian type of inheritance, clarifying what had previously been so puzzling. The puzzles were the disappearance of the defect

---

* There is a single exception. One color-deficient man had a color-deficient son, but this man had married a distant cousin.

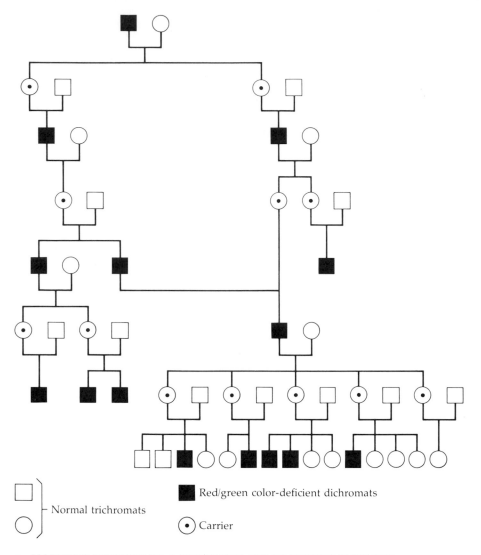

1 HORNER'S PEDIGREE OF A RED/GREEN-COLOR-DEFICIENT FAMILY.

for one or two generations, that children of color-deficient men were almost never color-deficient, and that there were so many more color-deficient men than color-deficient women.

The genes that control inherited traits and qualities that are transmitted from generation to generation are borne on chromosomes that reside in the nuclei of the cells in the human body. There are 23 pairs of chromosomes, of which one pair is the sex chromosome pair.

In the human body the two sex chromosomes that characterize the female are identical and known as XX. The two sex chromosomes in the male are dissimilar. One of these is like those in the female and is therefore called an X chromosome. The other, smaller and of different shape, is called the Y chromosome. Thus the male's sex chromosome pair is an XY pair. The other 22 pairs of chromosomes, which are structurally similar in both males and females, are called autosomes.

Most of the genetic material found on the male's X chromosome does not also appear on the Y chromosome because of the Y chromosome's smaller size. Thus most genes present on the X chromosome are not found on the Y chromosome. Such genes are said to be sex-linked because females would have duplicate sets of such genes (one set on each chromosome) but males would have only one set (on the single X chromosome).

Assume that a gene that controls color vision is located on the X chromosome. This gene has alternative forms called alleles. In its normal form it leads to normal color vision, but in some alternative form it may lead to defective color vision. The normal form or allele is dominant, whereas the gene form for the red/green deficiency is recessive. Hence with one normal and one defective gene for color vision, color vision would still be normal. Since the male has an XY constellation of chromosomes, if the gene for color vision that resides on X is normal, the male is normal. However, if the gene is defective, since the male has only one X chromosome, he would be color-defective.

Females, as we have seen, have an XX constellation of chromosomes. Therefore, only if both X chromosomes carry the defective gene for red/green deficiency will a female be color-defective. This is a very rare occurrence. If only one X chromosome is affected and the other X chromosome carries the dominant gene for normal color vision, these females will be normal in the expression of this property (phenotype) but will carry an abnormal gene. They are known as carriers.

Figure 2 shows in summary form how the red/green deficiencies are transmitted for matings between normal fathers and mothers who are either carriers or color-deficient, and for matings between color-deficient fathers and mothers who are normal, carriers, or color-deficient.

There is also another rule that seems to operate. There appears to be a dominance relation among the different types of defective color vision in the sense that just as the gene for normal color vision predominates over the gene for color deficiency, genes for minor defects seem to be dominant relative to genes for more serious ones. Thus an anomalous trichromatic condition is presumably less serious than a total loss of the red/green sense, and we know that anomalous color vision occurs more frequently than red/green dichromacy. A female who is assumed to carry

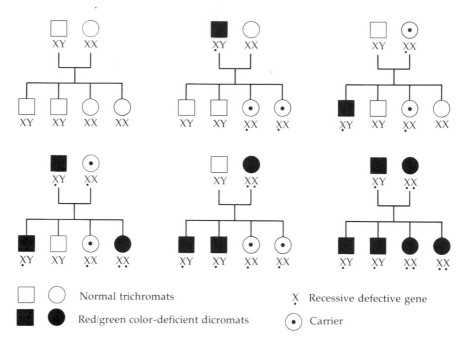

2 X-CHROMOSOMAL HEREDITARY RECESSIVE TRANSMISSION of red/green deficiencies.

an anomalous X gene and an X gene for complete red/green deficiency will be phenotypically anomalous (i.e., the anomalous gene will be manifest rather than the one for the full deficiency).

The sex linkage of the inheritance of color deficiency accounts for the fact that there are more color defectives among males than among females. The occurrence of a *pair* of defective genes is patently less likely than the occurrence of one such gene. If we assume that no selective mating occurs for color deficiencies (i.e., no genetical determined trait influences the selection of a spouse), then since there are approximately 8 percent color defectives among the males in Caucasian groups (see Table I) and 8 percent of the females are assumed to be carriers, the population ratio of females who are color-defective may be expected to be $0.08 \times 0.08 = 0.0064$, or 0.64 percent. The anticipated ratio of color-deficient females is the square of the proportions of color-defective males.

The actual occurrence of female red/green deficiencies has been found to be closer to 0.40 percent than to 0.64 percent. This finding has led in turn to the idea that the alleles for the protan defects (protanomalous plus protanope) and for deutan defects (deuteranomalous plus deuteranopes) are on different locations on the X chromosome. Calculations that treat the male protan and deutan defects separately were found to give values for the occurrence of female deficiencies that are very close to the observed value, 0.40 percent.

But this problem is far from resolved. Some authorities doubt the validity of the TWO-LOCUS THEORY. In fact, as Table I shows, the incidence of color deficiency among males is not the same for all racial types studied, yet the female incidence figures do seem to be essentially the same for all groups.

These data are based on approximately 50 separate studies and include measures on more than 600,000 individuals. They deal mostly with red/green color deficiencies. Although different measuring techniques (anomaloscope versus pseudoisochromatic plates) are a factor, males of the white races have a significantly higher incidence of color-vision deficiencies than do Asiatic males and those of the other racial groups.

There are also some puzzling facts about the way the various types of red/green deficiencies are distributed. In almost all statistical analyses, 50 percent of males with red/green defects are deuteranomalous. The deuteranomalous percentage is even greater, relatively speaking, for the small population of females who are red/green-deficient.

The percentage of the Caucasian population with the specified defects are given in Table II.

The information on types of color deficiency other than red/green ones is much more meager. There are many fewer cases of yellow/blue defects and monochromatism, but the values given in Table II are the best approximations we have. There are also fewer pedigrees and they tend to be incomplete. However, this situation has been improving in recent years (Cole et al., 1965; Schmidt, 1970).

Table I Incidence of color deficiency

	Incidence in Males	Incidence in Females

Caucasians
  Northern European
  American
  Australian
	8.08 ± 0.26%	0.74 ± 0.11%

Asiatics
  Japanese
  Chinese
  Others (e.g., Korean,
    Philippino)
	4.90 ± 0.18%	0.64 ± 0.08%

Other racial groups
  American Indian
  Mexican
  American Blacks
  Eskimo
	3.12 ± 0.40%	0.69 ± 0.07%

Table II Visual defects in the Caucasian
population

	Male	Female
Protanopes	1.0	0.02
Protanomalous	1.0	0.02
Deuteranopes	1.1	0.01
Deuteranomalous	4.9	0.38
Tritanopes	0.0001	0.001
	(0.002?)	
Monochromats	0.003	0.002

The inheritance of yellow/blue color-vision defects is an issue that is far from settled. Some investigators believe that all the yellow/blue deficiencies that have been detected may be acquired rather than congenital. Others believe that the gene for tritan defects is carried on a third locus on the X chromosome. Still another view is that tritanopia may be due to an incompletely dominant *autosomal* gene. This would mean that it is carried on a chromosome that is not a sex chromosome (see above). Some investigators believe that tritanomaly, on the other hand, which is less severe than tritanopia, could be associated with a sex-linked recessive gene. Others argue against this (Schmidt, 1970). In any event, the incidence figures do suggest a different hereditary mechanism for the red/green and yellow/blue deficiencies.

The rod and cone monochromats appear to be unrelated to each other as far as genetic factors are concerned. One detailed genetic family study (Crone, 1956) supports the idea that in cone monochromats either protan or deutan defects are combined with tritan deficiencies. The protan or deutan defects appear to be related to the X chromosome and the tritan defects seem to behave autosomally.

The data for rod monochromats or congenital achromatopsia indicate that 70 percent of all cases are familial. Parents were related in 30 percent of the cases studied and females were affected as often as males. Congenital achromatopsia must follow a mode of inheritance that differs from the red/green defects. Since it is transmitted autosomal-recessively, the largest pedigrees are found in inbreeding situations.

More information is needed on these varied genetic problems. We have seen, for example, that the category "anomalous" cannot be treated as a single grab bag. It seems likely that separate genetic controls will be shown to produce shifts in photopigment peak loci, to account for the loss of certain photopigments in some cases, and to account for degrees of neural loss in other instances. A solid data base on the inheritance of specific qualities needs to be established.

Background Readings

Cole, B. L., Henry, G. H., and Nathan, J. 1965. Phenotypical variations of tritanopia. *Vision Res. 6*: 301–313.

Crone, R. A. 1956. Combined forms of congenital colour defects. A pedigree with atypical colour blindness. *Br. J. Ophthalmol. 40*: 462–472.

Gray, R. D. 1943. Incidence of green-red blindness. *Arch. Ophthalmol. 28*: 446–448.

Grutzner, P. 1972. Acquired Color Vision Defects. In D. Jameson and L. M. Hurvich (eds.), *Handbook of Sensory Physiology,* Vol. 7/4, *Visual Psychophysics,* Chap. 25, pp. 643–659. Springer-Verlag, Berlin.

Horner, J. F. 1876. Die Erblichkeit des Daltonismus. Ein Beitrag zum Vererbungsgesetz. *Amtlicher Bericht über die Verwaltung des Medizinalwesens des Kantons Zürich vom Jahr 1876,* pp. 208–211.

Iinuma, I., and Handa, Y. 1976. A consideration of the racial evidence of congenital dyschromats in males and females. In G. Verriest (ed.), *Modern Problems in Ophthalmology,* Vol. 17, *Colour Vision Deficiencies III,* pp. 151–157. S. Karger, Basel.

Jaeger, W. 1972. Genetics of Congenital Colour Deficiencies. In D. Jameson and L. M. Hurvich (eds.), *Handbook of Sensory Physiology,* Vol. 7/4, *Visual Psychophysics,* Chap. 24, pp. 625–642. Springer-Verlag, Berlin.

Kalmus, H. 1955–1956. The familial distribution of congenital tritanopia. With some remarks on some similar conditions. *Ann. Hum. Genet. 26*: 39–56.

Kherumian, R., and Pickford, R. W. 1959. *Hérédité et fréquence des anomalies congénitales du sens chromatique* (dyschromatopsies). Vigot Frères, Paris.

Linksz, A. 1964. *An Essay on Color Vision and Clinical Color-Vision Tests.* Grune & Stratton, New York.

Schmidt, I. 1970. On congenital tritanomaly. *Vision Res. 10*: 717–743.

Scott, J. 1778. An account of a remarkable imperfection of sight. In a letter from J. Scott to Mr. Whisson of Trinity College, Cambridge. *Phil. Trans. R. Lond.,* pp. 611–614.

Wilson, E. B. 1911. The sex chromosomes. *Arch. Mikrobiol. Anat. 77*: 249–271.

Further Readings

Waardenburg, P. J., Franceschetti, A., and Klein, D. 1961. *Genetics and Ophthalmology.* Royal van Gorcum, Assen, Netherlands.

20
Color Specification

THE discussion of color-vision deficiencies in the last four chapters has made it amply clear how varied they are. Such extreme variations from normal may have important consequences in many circumstances. This is particularly true in highly industrialized and technologically oriented societies. Could we, for example, tolerate airline pilots who see as red what most of us call yellow light? Or someone who sees the same color as green? Remember that our discussion of anomalous color vision shows this to be a real possibility for sharp discriminators. Can anyone in electronics be trusted with color-coded resistors or capacitors if his color vision differs markedly from normal? When the whole world is in "living color" there are countless occupations where color deficiency may be a serious handicap. But we must keep in mind that even normal color vision (see Figure 12 in Chapter 16) varies from individual to individual and may, on occasion, lead to minor disagreements about hue identification. However, in most of their exchanges about colors, normals fortunately have little difficulty communicating with each other. But what happens when the color distinctions we want to talk about become more subtle than those that can be expressed by words such as "red," "blue," "violet," "emerald," "turquoise"?

When Robert Louis Stevenson was living in the Samoan Islands in the early 1890s he wanted a particular kind of wallpaper to decorate a room. He wrote to a friend in England and described, or, more accurately, tried to describe the color he wanted. This is what he wrote: "For a little work-room of my own at the back, I should rather like to see some patterns of unglossy—well, I'll be hanged if I can describe this red—it's not Turkish and it's not Roman and it's not Indian, but it seems to partake of the two last, and yet it can't be either of them because it ought to be able to go with vermillion. Ah, what a tangled web we weave—anyway, with what brains you have left chose me and send me some—many—patterns of this exact shade." The way Stevenson was specifying the color he wanted was in relation to other familiar colors that were presumably known to his correspondent, Sidney Colvin, in England.

If we turn to the dictionary to seek out color "definitions" we begin more fully to appreciate that color definition is largely a matter of denoting or pointing to other known colored objects or stimuli. Thus blue is "a color whose hue is that of the clear sky or that of the portion of the spectrum lying between green and violet"; green is "a color whose hue is somewhat less yellow than that of growing fresh grass or of the emerald or that of the part of the spectrum lying between blue and yellow"; red is "a color whose hue resembles that of blood or of the ruby or is that of the long-wave extreme of the visible spectrum"; and yellow is "a color whose hue resembles that of ripe lemons or sunflowers or is that of the portion of the spectrum lying between green and orange." If we are going to convey the "meaning" of blue, green, yellow, or red to someone ignorant of the terms (that is, of course, difficult to imagine), we had better be prepared to have clear sky, fresh grass, emerald, blood, lemons, or sunflowers at hand or—lacking any of these the physical means of generating a spectrum!

Suppose that we read in a novel that the color of an object is "celadon." Celadon? Like any intelligent reader we appeal to a dictionary. "Celadon" it says, is "a grayish yellow green that is paler and slightly yellower than average sage green, yellower and lighter than palmetto and greener and lighter than mermaid." Not having any sage green, palmetto, or mermaid at hand, we pursue the dictionary trail. "Sage green," we learn is "a variable color averaging a grayish yellow green that is greener and deeper than mermaid, stronger and very slightly yellower than palmetto, and deeper and slightly greener than celadon." Logically, mermaid and palmetto seem necessary to describe celadon. Mermaid, we are told, is "a grayish yellow green that is yellower and paler than average sage green or palmetto and yellower and darker than celadon, and palmetto "a grayish yellow green that is less strong and very slightly greener and darker than average sage green, greener and deeper than mermaid, and greener and darker than celadon."

This is a series of internally consistent statements that places the four colors in relation to one another along the hue, brightness/darkness, and saturation dimensions. But without some denotable objects at hand they can leave one woefully ignorant of the appearance of each and every one of the four colors mentioned. Surprisingly, the same sort of relational description is used for color definitions throughout *Webster's Third New International Dictionary*.

The obvious way out of the difficulty that Stevenson faced would have been for him to paint or color a small piece of paper or cardboard with the color he had in mind by mixing a few paints or pastels or crayons and to have mailed it on to England, where it could have been matched directly. There is little doubt, however, that the match would have been a metameric match (i.e., the spectral reflectances of Stevenson's home-made sample and the wallpaper forwarded to him would have been different). If we recall the way metameric matches may change with changes in illumination, the wallpaper he received by return steamer might or might not have been precisely what he expected, but in any event, what Stevenson would have been resorting to is the use of a MATERIAL STANDARD.

Material standards are what paint stores provide us with when we ask, usually in vague terms, for a desired paint. We select the sample we want from a color chart and the salesperson provides us either with a can or cans that match the sample we have selected in the color chart. Or he or she may proceed to mix a number of paints in some way that is specified by the paint manufacturer so that the end product matches the material standard we selected.

Any collection of object colors may be used as a material standard to help specify or grade color samples in any area of art, commerce, industry, or research for any specific purpose the user has in mind. There are collections that serve as standards for "fabrics, plastic, fibers, paint, printing inks, architectural materials, soils, ceramics, fruits, flowers, vegetables, electrical wiring, plumbing, petroleum, vegetable oils, animal tallows, and grasses." There are even standards for eye and skin color that are used by anthropologists. These standards, however useful, tend, of course, to be limited in their application.

Material standards can be organized systematically to cover a broad range of colors and because they are convenient, easy to handle, and can be carried from place to place (usually in loose-leaf binders), their use is widespread. In most instances they are arranged to cover the entire hue gamut as well as broad ranges of lightness/darkness and saturation.

Different principles may be used to construct a material standard. Consequently, different standards do not provide the same number of samples or identical samples, nor are the perceived differences among the available samples the same.

There are essentially three ways to go about constructing a material standard. Colorant mixtures, additive color mixtures, or appearance criteria may be used to generate material standards. The paint standards mentioned above are an instance of the colorant-mixture approach. In one system of this kind (the Nu-Hue Custom System) 1000 painted cards were generated by systematically varying the proportions of eight basic paints, six chromatic ones, one near-black one, and one white one. Since each sample in the standard set is made by mixing the eight base paints in known amounts by weight and volume, a satisfactory match can be made to any one of the samples in the standard by using the same proportions

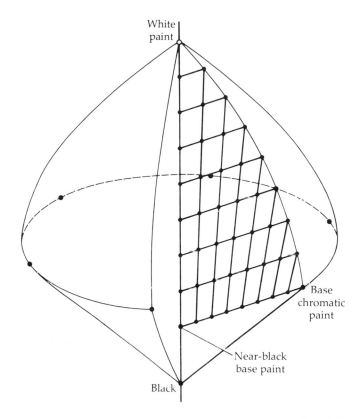

White paint

Base chromatic paint

Near-black base paint

Black

1 COLOR SOLID that shows schematically the organization of the colors derived from one of the six basic chromatic paints of the Nu-Hue Custom Color System by the mixture of black-and-white paints. This is an example of a colorant-mixture system.

of the base paints for a customer's use. The organization of this system is shown schematically in Figure 1 for just one of the base chromatic paints. This is only one of many such colorant-mixture systems. Another is the Pittsburgh Paint Company's Designa Color System.

Additive color-mixture standards are derived by selecting a limited number of lights (or colored papers for use on a Maxwell disc) and combining them in systematically varied proportions. The colors thus generated are then copied either by painting or printing them on paper or plastic base chips. In the printing process the colors of the chromatic inks, the black ink, and the white of the paper on which the printing is done are imaged as small dotlike patterns that mix in pointillist fashion on the retina. The Ostwald Color System is the classical example of this type of color-mixture system, and some years ago a color manual made up of 943 individual chips was issued that was based on this approach. It was called the *Color Harmony Manual* and was issued "to promote the knowledge and study of color harmony and color coordination in design." Because the colors are produced by color mixture, the system becomes organized around the variables that are associated with colorimetry: dominant wavelength, excitation purity, and chromaticity coordinates.

A third type of material standard is one that is prepared on the basis of some visual appearance criterion. Material charts of this sort, like the others, cover a broad color gamut, but in these charts the individual chips or samples are ordered along specific perceptual dimensions. They may also be chosen to satisfy a given perceptual criterion. Thus we could generate an appearance system in the form of a set of materials by putting together a large set of samples that followed the schematization outlined in Chapter 1. The perceptual dimensions are hue, whiteness/grayness/blackness, and saturation. We could impose a further restriction: that each perceptual step between individual chips be equal.

In a general way the Munsell Color System, originally devised in 1905

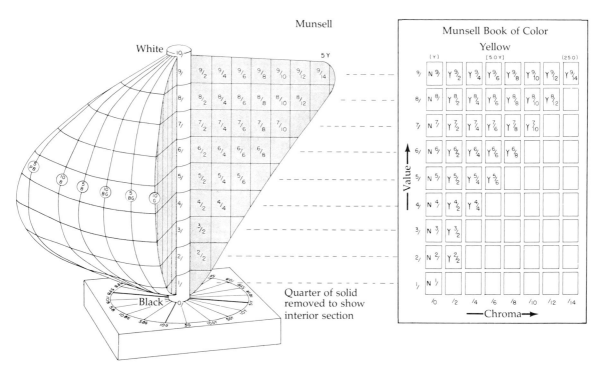

2 MUNSELL COLOR SYSTEM. This is an appearance system for specifying colors on scales of hue, value, and chroma. Hues are arranged in equal angular spacing around the central axis and a section of the solid is removed (right) to show a plane of constant Munsell hue (Yellow, 5Y). Chroma is the distance from the central axis, and planes of constant value intersect this axis perpendicularly.

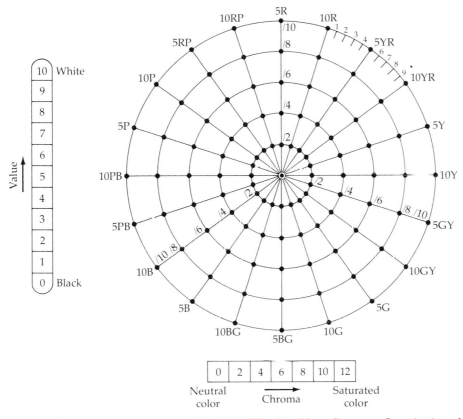

3 HUE, VALUE, AND CHROMA COORDINATES of the Munsell system. Organization of the colors of constant Munsell value in the *Munsell Book of Color* is shown in the radial chart.

by A. Munsell, an artist and art teacher, approximates such an appearance system. The individual chips are ordered into a three-dimensional color solid with a vertical black-to-white axis. HUES are arranged in equal angular spacing around the central axis and CHROMA (saturation) is the distance of a chip from the central axis at any given VALUE (lightness) level (Figure 2). The coordinate system is shown in Figure 3.

In its present form the samples are included in the *Munsell Book of Color,* where they are ordered on the basis of equal hue, value, and chroma. In the most recent two-volume edition, there are 1600 glossy color paint chips. They are organized in 40 constant-hue charts and in each chart there is a value scale of 10 equally spaced brightness intervals (Figures 2 and 4). At each value level a series of equally spaced chromas are stepped off. The number of chroma steps varies with the hue and the specific value scale level. To specify a given item in Munsell terms, one merely finds the Munsell chip that most closely approximates the sample

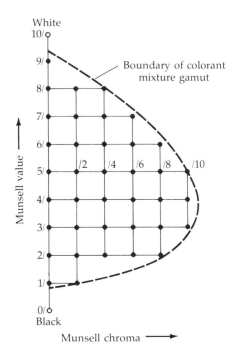

4 ORGANIZATION OF THE COLORS of constant Munsell hue in the *Munsell Book of Color*.

at hand. Since each Munsell chip has a three-symbol specification, one for hue, such as 5R, 2.5 YR; one for lightness, where black is 0/ and white 10/; and one for chroma, which increases in steps of two, such as /2, /4, the sample specification is given as 5R 6/4, 10PB 8/2, and so on. The first number specifies the hue and the other two, Munsell value and Munsell chroma.

Numerous other color atlases of color appearance type are available. They are of different national origins, and the French, German, Swedish, Argentinian, and British versions of material standards tend, like the United States one, to find their greatest use in the country of their origin.

It should be noted that object-color standards need not necessarily be constructed on the basis of a single principle, such as colorant mixture or an appearance criterion. Standards such as the *Maerz and Paul Dictionary of Color* and the *Methuen Handbook of Colour* (described briefly in Chapter 1) are, for example, produced by screen-plate printing processes. One series of colors in such a method is produced by juxtaposing small dots unresolved by the eye (pointillist type of color mixture; see Chapter 8) and another series by overlapping the printing inks (colorant mixtures). Thus this system illustrates the use of two methods to generate a color system. The *Maerz and Paul Dictionary of Color* contains 7056 different samples and an alphabetical list of 4000 color names with keys to the location of these names in the printed charts. The Methuen book contains about 600 color names and also gives a series of 30 locator charts with color names.

We should also call attention to *The Inter-Society Color Council–National Bureau of Standards* (ISCC-NBS) *Method of Designating Colors and a Dictionary of Color Names* (National Bureau of Standards Circular 553, 1955).* It is not a color specification system in the sense of those already discussed but was developed to enable people who work in different areas of color and who use different color names to communicate more efficiently.

What was done in this particular systematization, based on color naming, was to compile some 7500 individual color names and translate them into the ISCC–NBS system by simple descriptive hue designations. The hue names and their abbreviations are given in Table I. Appropriate modifiers are applied to the hue terms to indicate both brightness and saturation variations. Modifiers are pale, moderate, strong, brilliant, deep, medium, and dark and the word "very." Terms that combine two modifiers are also used: for example, the words pale (light weak), brilliant (light strong), deep (dark strong), and vivid (very strong). Figure 5a illustrates this scheme in relation to Munsell chroma and value.

This logical system of naming colors subdivides the color solid into 267 compartments (Figure 5b). Each compartment can be represented by a CENTROID COLOR and 250 of these are now available in the form of glossy paint samples on printed charts. This system makes it possible to translate from one color vocabulary to another and now, with the availability of material centroid charts, the value of the system is increased.

Table I Hue names and abbreviations used in the ISCC–NBS system

Color Name	Abbreviation	Color Name	Abbreviation
Red	R	Violet	V
Reddish orange	rO	Purple	P
Orange	O	Reddish purple	rP
Orange yellow	OY	Purplish red	pR
Yellow	Y	Purplish pink	pPK
Greenish yellow	gY	Pink	PK
Yellow green	YG	Yellowish pink	yPK
Yellowish green	yG	Reddish brown	rBr
Green	G	Brown	Br
Bluish green	bG	Yellowish brown	yBr
Greenish blue	gB	Olive brown	OlBr
Blue	B	Olive	Ol
Purplish blue	pB	Olive green	OlG

* Now superseded by National Bureau of Standards Special Publication 440, 1976.

Vivid					Munsell value
	Brilliant	Very light	Very pale	-ish white	White
		Light	Pale	Light -ish gray	Light gray
			Light grayish		
	Strong	Moderate	Grayish	-ish gray	Medium gray
	Deep	Dark	Dark grayish	Dark -ish gray	Dark gray
	Very deep	Very dark	Blackish	-ish black	Black

(a) Munsell chroma

5 MODIFIERS proposed for use in conjunction with the Munsell notation.

It may seem paradoxical at first glance, but the fact that there are many different systems of material standards available implies that whatever principles may underlie their construction (colorant, additive, etc.), they are fundamentally very similar. The standards sample the total gamut of colors in varying degrees, and some sort of unique designation is assigned to each chip in the set. Customers can, for example, select a given sample, provide a merchant or manufacturer with the specification,

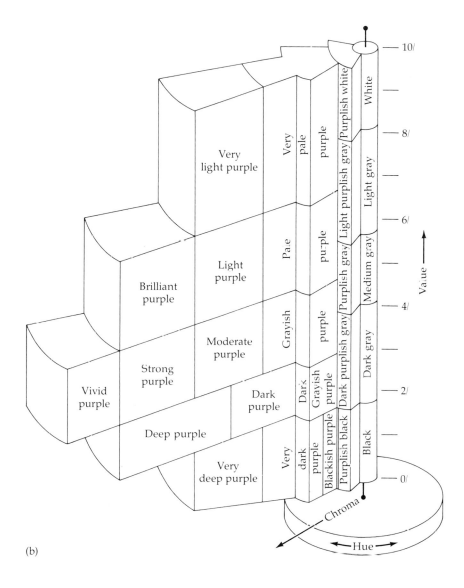

(b)

and expect the product to be available or producible in the wanted color. Why? Because the system provides a precise means of communicating about color. Had there been available in Samoa and England copies of the *Munsell Book of Color* when Stevenson wrote, he could have selected a Munsell chip, say, 6R 5/10, from the book, and could have expected to receive a wallpaper as close to this chip as his correspondent could find on the merchants' shelves in London.

As we noted in Chapter 1, there are probably millions of discriminable colors. It is therefore very unlikely that any material standard, even one with 800 to 1000 or more chips in it, will permit precise matches to be found between given samples and available chips in the material system. Furthermore, there are many situations that require more precise color specification than that permitted by material standards. Many examples can be cited: signal glasses used in traffic lights sometimes require national or even international agreement, many products need to be graded for quality, and color often plays an important part in quality evaluation. Industrial standards have to be set for the component parts of what ultimately becomes a single product, such as an automobile or a refrigerator. Lights must be specified with great accuracy and scientists often require precise stimulus specifications in many different sorts of experiments.

Can we improve on the color-specification procedures so far outlined and assure ourselves of more precise matches than material sample systems provide? The answer is "yes," and the way it can be achieved has already been foreshadowed in Chapter 9. Three appropriately selected stimuli enable us to make perfect color matches to any color stimulus whatsoever. The spectral color-mixture curves provide color specifications in terms of three arbitrarily selected primaries. The proportions of the three mixture stimuli used to match any sample provide the exact specification for a given illuminant and a given individual—the one who is making the match.

The instruments for color specification work that use the color matching procedure are called VISUAL COLORIMETERS. They make it possible to put the sample we want specified in one part of the visual field, and next to it a comparison field that contains the three stimuli whose ratios are varied to make a match to the sample.* The instruments discussed in connection with color matching in Chapter 9 can be used as visual colorimeters. They are relatively expensive instruments, however, and their major uses have been in research. For color-specification purposes, less expensive instruments with three color filters in the comparison field can be used. One such simple instrument is shown in Figure 6. No provision is made for desaturating the test samples in such instruments, and this limits the color gamut of samples that can be matched. One way out of this restriction is to introduce a larger number of comparison stimuli for carrying out the matches. One instrument of this type made use of six primaries.

Visual colorimeters tend to be insensitive compared to direct visual

* There are also commercially available subtractive colorimeters.

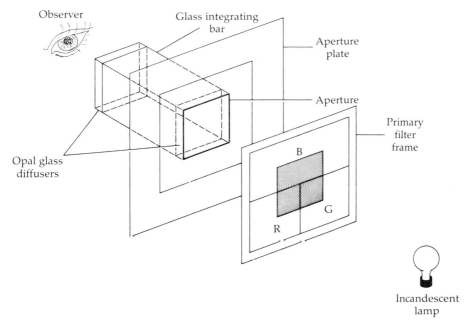

6 A THREE-FILTER COLORIMETER for color specification. Elements are an incandescent lamp, a three-color filter assembly, an aperture plate, and a glass integrating bar with opal glass diffusers. The back face of the integrating bar appears uniformly illuminated with the mixture of the primary stimuli. The proportions of the primaries are adjusted by horizontal and vertical movements of the filter frame behind the aperture plate. A second similar colorimeter assembly usually provides another visual field that is juxtaposed to the first field.

comparisons between the samples themselves, and in recent years, with rapid advances in both electronics and filter design, there is an increased use of electrical recording instruments that are intended to mimic the behavior of the human "eye." Instruments of this sort are called PHOTO-ELECTRIC COLORIMETERS and use combinations of three photocells and appropriate filters. The "sensitivities" of the combination correspond in a general way to the three presumed sensitivity functions of the normal observer's photopigments or linear transformations of them. The values that are recorded on instrument meters are in a general way directly comparable to those that would be made by a human observer using a standard visual colorimeter.

It should be noted, however, that nothing whatsoever is said about the appearance of any sample that is specified in numerical terms either with the use of the visual colorimeter by a human being or with the use of the photoelectric colorimeter. Since the photoelectric colorimeter is an electrical recording device that can only give us three meter readings, it is obvious that nothing is or can be reported by such an instrument about how a sample will look to a human being. The same thing is true of visual colorimeters. We must recall that visual colorimeters are null instruments. Three knobs are used to vary three stimulus proportions to match any sample that appears in a field adjacent to the comparison mixture field. When the two fields look matched, it is as if the single sample produced some integrated value of the three different photopigment sensitivities of the eye that matches precisely the integrated value produced by the mixture of the three separate stimuli. What the ultimate neural signals are and what the appearance of both the test sample and comparison field are is in a sense irrelevant. It is important to know only that they match and that we have the three numbers that are needed to specify the sample in a unique way.

Visual colorimeters have been useful in a limited way.* They once were used in a single factory or plant by a few individuals to make certain that a given product, say "white" paper, does not vary from roll to roll or from day to day (or more reasonably, and that the variations that do occur stay within certain agreed-upon limits). The same is true of dyes, printing inks, food products (e.g., butter) and color pigments used in paints or for packaging purposes. How much variation could the Eastman Kodak company tolerate in its "Kodak yellow" packaging and still maintain its instantly recognizable shelf color?

But what of industries and companies that have factories now scattered around the world, let alone throughout any one country? Would the color specification arrived at in one plant with one colorimeter by one observer possibly be comparable to that arrived at in a second plant with a similar but different colorimeter and a similar but different observer? The color specification would probably be approximately the same, but experience has shown that there are too many instrumental and human variables to give useful results. The variations in the colorimetric measurements usually exceed the variations in product color that are acceptable as matches by large groups of individuals.

This has led to the almost universal adoption by both the world of commerce and science of a method of specifying colors that is based on the principle of three-variable color mixture but which, by international agreement, is referred to the visual properties of a STANDARD OBSERVER.

To specify the color vision of the Standard Observer, the color-mixture results of a group of observers for a set of rigorously specified viewing conditions (2-degree field, dark surround) were averaged and smoothed and accepted in 1931 as representative of the color-matching properties of

* Photoelectric colorimeters, although precise, are not accurate in their present state of development. The specifications they provide differ from those obtained by calculation procedures. See below.

the average human eye by the Commission International de l'Éclairage (CIE) (International Commission on Illumination).*

We have already seen that the measured color-mixture functions have negative values, which reflects the fact that the mixture of any two stimuli to match the hue of a third stimulus tends to produce a desaturated mixture color relative to the single stimulus that is being matched. The latter stimulus has therefore to be "diluted" in order to achieve complete color matches. In the algebraic equations that represent color-mixture results, the "dilutant" takes on negative arithmetic values. But as we have seen, color-mixture curves can be transformed from one set of primaries to another by simple linear algebra.

To avoid negative values in the use of color-mixture functions when computing color specifications simply because the use of both positive and negative numbers would lead to more calculating errors, the CIE adopted for its color mixture curves a set of functions with all positive spectral tristimulus values $\bar{x}$, $\bar{y}$, and $\bar{z}$. The three functions are shown again in Figure 7. These curves give the relative amounts $\bar{x}$, $\bar{y}$, and $\bar{z}$ of the X, Y, and Z CIE primaries, respectively, that are needed by the Standard Observer to match the color of a given wavelength of unit energy. The tristimulus values are given for 10-nm steps in Table II.

Table II CIE 1931 tristimulus values $\bar{x}$, $\bar{y}$, and $\bar{z}$

Wavelength, (nm)	Color-Matching Functions			Wavelength, (nm)	Color-Matching Functions		
	$\bar{x}_\lambda$	$\bar{y}_\lambda$	$\bar{z}_\lambda$		$\bar{x}_\lambda$	$\bar{y}_\lambda$	$\bar{z}_\lambda$
400	0.0143	0.0004	0.0679	560	0.5945	0.9950	0.0039
410	0.0435	0.0012	0.2074	570	0.7621	0.9520	0.0021
420	0.1344	0.0040	0.6456	580	0.9163	0.8700	0.0017
430	0.2839	0.0116	1.3856	590	1.0263	0.7570	0.0011
440	0.3483	0.0230	1.7471	600	1.0622	0.6310	0.0008
450	0.3362	0.0380	1.7721	610	1.0026	0.5030	0.0003
460	0.2908	0.0600	1.6692	620	0.8544	0.3810	0.0002
470	0.1954	0.0910	1.2876	630	0.6424	0.2650	0.0000
480	0.0956	0.1390	0.8130	640	0.4479	0.1750	0.0000
490	0.0320	0.2080	0.4652	650	0.2835	0.1070	0.0000
500	0.0049	0.3230	0.2720	660	0.1649	0.0610	0.0000
510	0.0093	0.5030	0.1582	670	0.0874	0.0320	0.0000
520	0.0633	0.7100	0.0782	680	0.0468	0.0170	0.0000
530	0.1655	0.8620	0.0422	690	0.0227	0.0082	0.0000
540	0.2904	0.9540	0.0203	700	0.0114	0.0041	0.0000
550	0.4334	0.9950	0.0087				

* A new 1964 CIE Supplementary Standard Observer was later introduced to specify colors for fields that subtended more than 4 degrees of visual angle at the eye.

Another arbitrary but perfectly valid mathematical procedure that was adopted when these functions were accepted by international agreement was to give one of the three color-mixture curves, the $\bar{y}$ one, the form of the spectral luminosity function V_λ. When the product of the $\bar{y}$ curve multiplied by the spectral-light distribution for a given sample is summed across the spectrum, we obtain the integrated or total Y value, which is a measure of the sample's light level.

The match to the equal-energy light source is arbitrarily adjusted to represent a mixture of the three primaries in equal amounts. Thus the areas under the three curves in Figure 7 are equal, and summations of each of the tristimulus values $\bar{x}$, $\bar{y}$, and $\bar{z}$ for an equal energy stimulus (multiplied by unity in each case) across the spectrum to obtain X, Y, and Z are equal.

To specify any illuminated object or surface colorimetrically we only require the object's or surface's spectral reflectance or transmittance and the spectral-energy distribution (in relative terms) of the light source illuminating it. If the products of these two distribution curves at each wavelength are then multiplied by each of the three Standard Observer spectral tristimulus values at each wavelength and the resultant values for all wavelengths added separately, we obtain the three numbers needed to specify the color (Table III and Figure 8). These three summed values are called the X, Y, and Z tristimulus values. Given the stimulus spectral distribution function for any object (reflectance × light source, for example) and the standardized color-mixture functions of the 1931 CIE Standard Observer, anyone who uses the system will obtain precisely the same

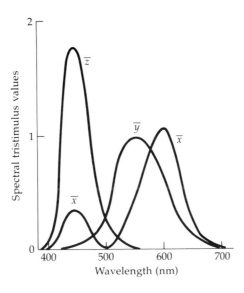

7 COLOR-MIXTURE FUNCTIONS for the 1931 CIE Standard Colorimetric Observer. The spectral tristimulus values of constant radiance stimuli for different wavelengths are specified by $\bar{x}_\lambda$, $\bar{y}_\lambda$ and $\bar{z}_\lambda$.

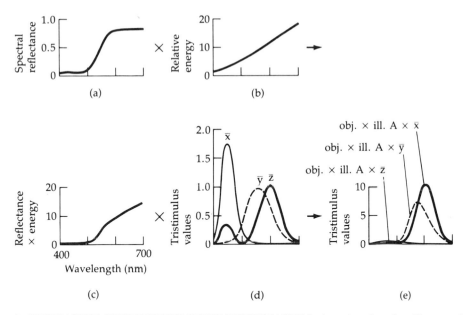

8 DERIVATION OF THE TRISTIMULUS SPECIFICATION of a colored surface illustrated graphically. (a) Spectral reflectance of the object. (b) Relative energy distribution of illuminant A. (c) The product of (a) × (b). (d) CIE tristimulus values. (e) The product of (c) × (d). The areas under these curves are the X, Y, Z tristimulus values of the colored surface.

three stimulus specification values, inasmuch as the procedure used is merely an arithmetic computation. In the practical situation, the only possible source of variation is instrumental error in the physical measurement of the spectral-light distribution.

Several points need to be emphasized. This system gives us a unique specification of a colored sample, and if anyone else duplicates this numerical specification for the given sample, we can be certain that the two test samples will match exactly for the specified viewing and illumination conditions evaluated by the Standard Observer. A real individual with normal color vision may find that two samples with the same X, Y, and Z values do not precisely match when they are looked at side by side under the specified conditions. Why? Because the color-mixture curves of any *individual* observer will in all likelihood differ from those of the Standard Observer, which are based on *averages* of the color matches of many individuals.

Note that stimuli do not have to have the same spectral distributions to generate the same X, Y, and Z tristimulus values any more than they have to have the same spectral distributions to match in a color-mixture experiment. For example, if we consider the spectral stimuli that constitute the Rayleigh match stimuli, a band that centers on 589 nm will have the

Table III CIE Standard Observer values and cross products

Wave-length	Object (Figure 5c in Chapter 4)	Illumination A (Normalized)*	CIE 1931 Standard Observer Spectral Tristimulus Values		
			$\bar{x}$	$\bar{y}$	$\bar{z}$
400	0.05	1.3651	0.0143	0.0004	0.0679
410	0.06	1.6407	0.0435	0.0012	0.2074
420	0.06	1.9488	0.1344	0.0040	0.6456
430	0.06	2.2894	0.2839	0.0116	1.3856
440	0.06	2.6634	0.3483	0.0230	1.7471
450	0.06	3.0708	0.3362	0.0380	1.7721
460	0.05	3.4633	0.2908	0.0600	1.6692
470	0.05	3.9783	0.1954	0.0910	1.2876
480	0.06	4.4776	0.0956	0.1390	0.8130
490	0.07	5.0028	0.0320	0.2080	0.4622
500	0.10	5.5550	0.0049	0.3230	0.2720
510	0.15	6.1304	0.0093	0.5030	0.1582
520	0.22	6.7280	0.0633	0.7100	0.0782
530	0.32	7.3433	0.1655	0.8620	0.0422
540	0.43	7.9762	0.2904	0.9540	0.0203
550	0.53	8.6220	0.4334	0.9950	0.0087
560	0.69	9.2800	0.5945	0.9950	0.0039
570	0.76	9.9463	0.7621	0.9520	0.0021
580	0.79	10.6200	0.9163	0.8700	0.0017
590	0.80	11.2965	1.0263	0.7570	0.0011
600	0.80	11.9749	1.0622	0.6310	0.0008
610	0.81	12.6524	1.0026	0.5030	0.0003
620	0.81	13.3279	0.8544	0.3810	0.0002
630	0.81	13.9970	0.6424	0.2650	0.0000
640	0.81	14.6605	0.4479	0.1750	0.0000
650	0.81	15.3148	0.2835	0.1070	0.0000
660	0.81	15.9579	0.1649	0.0610	0.0000
670	0.81	16.5899	0.0874	0.0320	0.0000
680	0.81	17.1151	0.0468	0.0170	0.0000
690	0.81	17.8111	0.0227	0.0082	0.0000
700	0.81	18.3985	0.0114	0.0041	0.0000

CIE 1931 tristimulus values: $X = 7.4750$, $Y = 5.8235$, $Z = 0.2339$.

CIE 1931 chromaticity coordinates: $x = \dfrac{X}{X + Y + Z} = 0.5524$, $y = \dfrac{Y}{X + Y + Z} = 0.4303$.

* Normalized means that the relative distribution curve is adjusted so that the sum across the spectrum of the cross products of the illuminant times $\bar{y}$ equals 100.

	Cross Products	
Object × Illumination × $\bar{x} =$	Object × Illumination × $\bar{y} =$	Object × Illumination × $\bar{z} =$
0.0010	0.0000	0.0046
0.0043	0.0001	0.0204
0.0157	0.0005	0.0755
0.0390	0.0016	0.1903
0.0557	0.0037	0.2792
0.0619	0.0070	0.3265
0.0504	0.0104	0.2890
0.0389	0.0181	0.2561
0.0257	0.0373	0.2184
0.0112	0.0728	0.1619
0.0027	0.1794	0.1511
0.0086	0.4625	0.1455
0.0937	1.0509	0.1157
0.3889	2.0256	0.0992
0.9960	3.2720	0.0696
1.9805	4.5468	0.0398
3.8067	6.3712	0.0250
5.7609	7.1963	0.0159
7.6876	7.2991	0.0143
9.2749	6.8412	0.0099
10.1758	6.0449	0.0077
10.2751	5.1550	0.0031
9.2238	4.1131	0.0022
7.2833	3.0045	—
5.3188	2.0781	—
3.5168	1.3273	—
2.1315	0.7885	—
1.1745	0.4300	—
0.6488	0.2357	—
0.3275	0.1183	—
0.1699	0.0611	—
Σ 80.5501	62.7530	2.5209
λ		

same X, Y, and Z values as does a matching pair of stimuli made up of appropriate proportions of 670 and 535 nm or even a different pair of stimuli, say 650 and 550 nm, that also matches a band centered on 589 nm. Different spectral distributions, such as those shown in Figure 8 in Chapter 15, which are metamers that match for specified illumination conditions, have precisely the same three valued specification. They have the same X, Y, and Z values.

All conceivable colors may be given a three-number specification in terms of the X, Y, and Z tristimulus values, which are the sums of the appropriately weighted *spectral* tristimulus values $\bar{x}$, $\bar{y}$, and $\bar{z}$. Alternative numerical specifications are also possible. We can, for example, determine what fraction or percentage any tristimulus value is of the total of all three tristimulus values and use these values for stimulus specification. Thus

$$x = \frac{X}{X + Y + Z}$$

$$y = \frac{Y}{X + Y + Z}$$

and

$$z = \frac{Z}{X + Y + Z}$$

where x, y, and z are called the CHROMATICITY COORDINATES of the color.

Since the CIE chromaticity coordinates are percentages and their sum is 100 percent (i.e., $x + y + z = 100$ percent), if we know any two chromaticity coordinates, the value of the third one is automatically given. (We need only subtract the sum of any two of them from unity to obtain it.) Instead of stating the CIE specification in X, Y, and Z tristimulus terms, we can therefore specify a color by using only two chromaticity coordinates, say, x and y. For a three-variable specification they may be used together with the Y tristimulus value, which, we recall, specifies the light level. If the x, y, and Y values are identical, the stimuli will appear identical (to the Standard Observer).

The two-number chromaticity specifications can be represented in a two-dimensional chromaticity diagram plotted in Cartesian coordinates, where x and y represent the two coordinates (Figure 9). This two-dimensional chromaticity chart is an outgrowth and refinement of the simple geometric figures long used to represent colors and their mixtures. Since the equal-energy light source, as we saw, represents equal total amounts X, Y, and Z, an equal-energy stimulus plots at the values $0.333x$ and $0.333y$. Reference to the CIE color-mixture curves allows us to calculate the chromaticity coordinates of any spectral stimulus, and these are plotted at the values of x and y shown in Figure 9. Table 2 can be consulted to

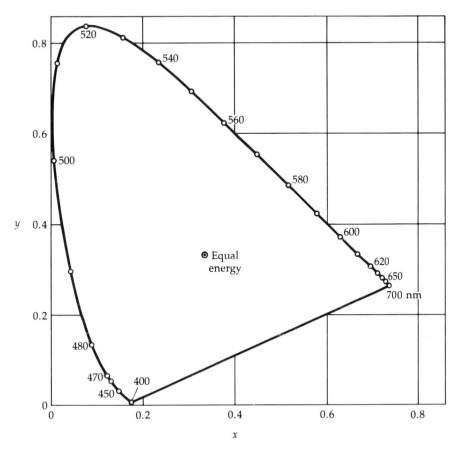

9 TWO-DIMENSIONAL CHROMATICITY DIAGRAM. This diagram permits the stimulus to be specified with two numbers in a Cartesian coordinate framework. The locus of the equal energy light stimulus is plotted at $x = 0.333$ and $y = 0.333$.

check a few of these spectral loci. All spectral wavelengths are located along the "horseshoe" locus shown in the figure. The straight line connecting the two spectral extremes (400 and 700 nm) is the locus of all mixtures of these two extreme stimuli. Most important, the calculated x and y chromaticity values of all real objects (opaque, transmitting, etc.) fall within the confines of the enclosed horseshoe-like figure.

Figure 10 shows the chromaticity loci of a number of different stimuli that have been discussed elsewhere in this book. In addition to the equal-energy illuminant E, the loci of a variety of illuminants and the stimuli of different color temperatures are plotted. The locus of the object whose reflectance curve is given in Figure 5c in Chapter 4 (in illuminant A) and the loci of the stimuli shown in Figures 5 and 7 in Chapter 4 are also plotted in Figure 10.

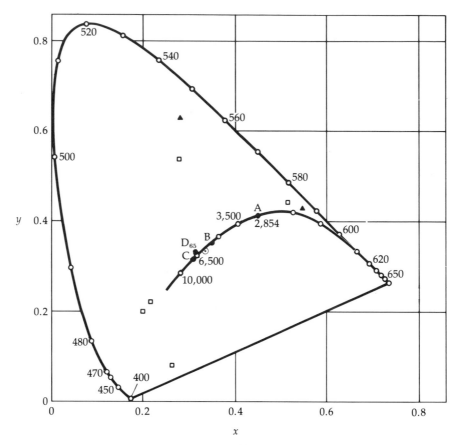

10 CHROMATICITY LOCI of a number of different stimuli discussed earlier in this book: equal energy illuminant E, (○); illuminants of various color temperatures as noted, (○●); and the five stimulus distributions shown in Figure 5 in Chapter 4 (□). An object with the spectral reflectance curve of Figure 5C in Chapter 4 in illuminant A has x, y chromaticity coordinates $x = 0.55$, $y = 0.43$ (▲). An object with the narrower spectral reflectance curve of Figure 7 in Chapter 4, in equal energy illumination, has x, y chromaticity coordinates $x = 0.27$, $y = 0.62$ (▲).

A fundamental property of chromaticity diagrams, including the CIE chromaticity diagram, is that additive mixtures of stimuli that are represented by any two points in the chart always lie on the straight line connecting them. (See the extraspectral line above.) These straight lines always lie on the spectrum locus or within it and the results of all possible additive light mixtures that match any given point can be determined. In Figure 11a, for example, points A and B represent the mixtures of known proportions of the three mixture primaries X, Y, and Z. The stimulus that results from a mixture of A and B lies at point D on the straight line connecting them. The exact point at which D lies depends on the ratio of

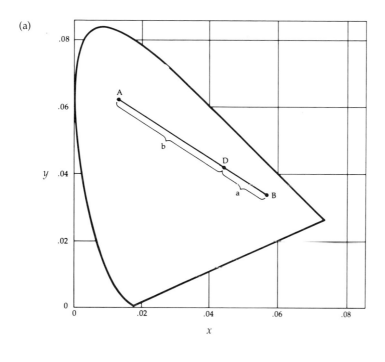

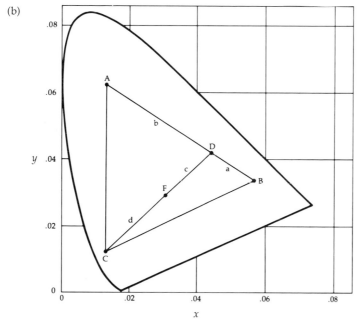

(b)

11 CHROMATICITY DIAGRAMS. (a) Additive color mixtures are located along the straight line that connects the two mixture stimuli. (b) The stimulus gamut provided by the mixtures of three stimuli lies within the confines of the triangular area delimited by the chromaticity coordinates of the three mixture stimuli.

the amounts of the two stimuli A and B, and its location is inversely related to the relative amounts of A and B that make up the mixture. (A center-of-gravity analysis is basic to the "straight-line rule," as it is called.)

Given this property, the chromaticity diagram is extremely useful in defining stimulus gamuts. For example, if we select any three points that do not lie on a straight line (see Figure 11b), a triangular area, determined by interconnecting the three points, includes all the chromaticities that can be matched by real mixtures of the three selected stimuli. Three component mixtures are located by first locating the mixture point produced by two of the stimuli, and then combining this outcome with the use of the third stimulus.

Any chromaticity can also be specified by its dominant wavelength (λ_d) and excitation purity (p_e) (Figure 12). If we connect an illuminant point, say, CIE Illuminant C and the chromaticity locus of any stimulus by a straight line and project the straight line until it intercepts the spectrum locus, the wavelength of this intercept is the dominant wavelength of the stimulus.* The stimulus so designated is matchable by a mixture of the specified spectral stimulus and the given illuminant. The position of the stimulus on this line is given by the ratio of the distance from the reference illuminant to the total distance between the illuminant and the spectrum locus. This is called the EXCITATION PURITY of the stimulus and excitation purity varies from 0 at the illuminant reference point to 1.0 at the spectrum locus. If the reference illuminant is CIE Illuminant A instead, notice that both the dominant wavelength and excitation purity values of the stimulus will not be the same.

It should be clear from this discussion that the CIE system provides us with an alternative way of specifying complementary stimuli that match a reference broad-band illuminant like an equal-energy source or illuminant C. (See Chapter 4 on determining complementaries by a perceptual criterion.) If we draw a straight line from a spectrum locus through the reference illuminant and allow this line to intercept the spectrum locus on the other side of the illuminant point, the two spectral stimuli of the specified dominant wavelengths will, if mixed in the proper ratio, plot precisely on the locus of the reference illuminant and therefore match it. Thus 670 nm and 472 nm, for example, constitute such a match on an equal-energy stimulus. Indeed, an indefinite number of pairs of stimuli fulfill this requirement. This family of straight lines provides us with an alternative way of specifying complementary wavelengths in terms of

---

* If the extraspectral line is intercepted, the line connecting the extraspectral locus and the reference illuminant is projected backward until the spectral locus is intercepted. This intercept specifies what is called the complementary dominant wavelength (λ_{dc}).

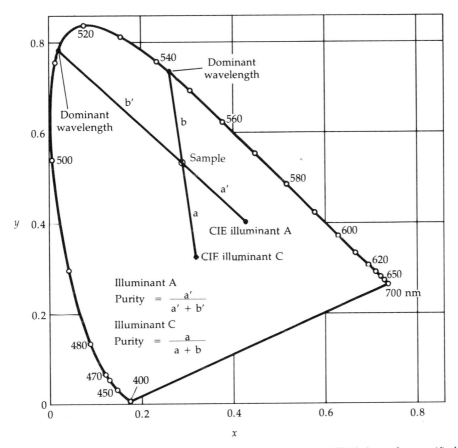

12 DOMINANT WAVELENGTH (λ_d) AND EXCITATION PURITY (p_e) can be specified graphically as illustrated. Note that both dominant wavelength and excitation purity differ for the same sample, depending on the illuminant used.

stimulus matches, and they can be represented on the rectangular hyperbola mentioned in Chapter 4.

The CIE chromaticity diagram is sometimes used to characterize the major color-vision deficiencies. The way it is used for this purpose is to plot on the CIE chart the chromaticities of stimuli that are confused by an observer with a deficiency of a given type and to link these chromaticities by connecting them with straight lines. These lines are called CONFUSION LINES or confusion loci, and Figure 13a shows the protanopic confusion loci.

Different patterns of confusion lines emerge for the different types of color deficiency, and Figure 13b shows the deuteranopic confusion loci. The tritanopic confusion loci are shown in Figure 13c. These plots of confusion chromaticities accord completely with what we already know

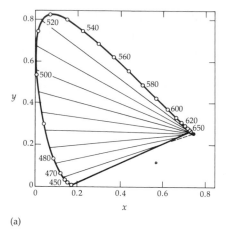

(a)

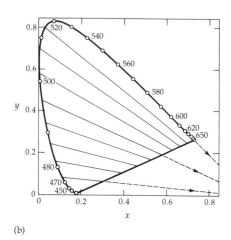

(b)

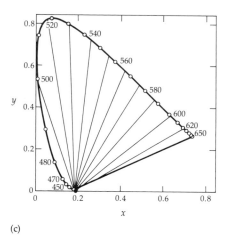

(c)

13 MAJOR COLOR-VISION DEFICIEN-CIES defined in terms of chromaticity confusions made by three types of dichromats: (a) Protanopes; (b) deuteranopes; (c) tritanopes.

about the different kinds of dichromats. We saw in Chapter 17 that the deuteranope, for example, has a neutral point at about 500 nm in the spectrum. We also saw that the unique red of the normal, composed of the mixture of, say, 440 and 650 nm, evokes the same neutral sensation for the deuteranope that 500 nm does. If we connect these two points, the confusion line passes through that region of the chart where the broad-band reference illuminants are plotted. Thus the confusion line connects a series of stimuli that are indistinguishable from each other. (Information from other sources—unilateral defects, for example—tells us that all these stimuli are neutral.) All the confusion lines that lie above and below this midline also connect stimulus chromaticities that the deuteranope finds indistinguishable.

The neutral locus in the spectrum of the protanope is located at

495 nm on the average, and inspection of the chromaticity confusions of this type indicates that a different series of chromaticities are confused by this type of color-deficient individual. These average results accord with the chromatic and achromatic response functions of these two types of dichromatic observer and with their sorting results on the Farnsworth D-15 test.

All the lines on each of the graphs in Figure 13 form a family, and in each family the lines intersect in a common point outside the "horseshoe" diagram that represents real stimuli. These intersection points have been interpreted as representing the primary color that each type of dichromatic system lacks, but this is an issue that is far from resolved and it is one that is too complex to pursue here.

These plots of the chromaticity confusion loci of the different types of dichromats tell us nothing about the *appearance* of the stimuli that are confused with each other. They only identify stimuli that look alike to the dichromat.

For that matter the CIE colorimetric specification of a color stimulus in X, Y, Z terms, however precisely stated, provides us with no information about color appearance beyond the information about identity for the prescribed conditions, even for the normal observer. We need only recall the two strips in Plate 2-2. If we were to obtain spectrophotometric reflectance curves for each of the narrow strips in the figure, they would be identical. If, for some illuminant, say, D_{65}, we calculated the X, Y, Z values based on the $\bar{x}$, $\bar{y}$, $\bar{z}$ spectral tristimulus values of the CIE Standard Observer, they would be identical in the two instances. Nevertheless, any real observer, even one whose color-mixture functions happened to be exactly those of the average Standard Observer, would see the narrow strips as yellowish, or reddish in Plate 2-2, depending on its surround. As we have already seen, perceived color is not definable if we ignore the adaptive and inductive aspect of the viewing situation (Chapter 15).

By introducing colored surrounds we have, of course, violated the conditions described at the outset for specifying color matches in CIE terms. But one more caveat with respect to color appearance that does not involve the introduction of different surrounds relates to spectral stimuli. We need only remember that every spectral stimulus has fixed chromaticity coordinates. Nevertheless, as we saw in Chapter 6, changing the lightness level of spectral stimuli (the CIE Y value) changes their appearance. They become bluer or yellower at higher light levels and redder and greener at lower energies. This is called the Bezold-Brücke phenomenon. The fixed positions of spectral stimuli on the CIE chromaticity chart give no hint of this.

The CIE chart is also used to specify visual tolerances. But since it is not a perceptual chart, equal stimulus distances in it do not represent equal perceived differences. This can be seen by referring to Figure 14, where a series of Munsell chips of different hues and chromas are plotted. The Munsell steps are presumably equal, but note that very different line lengths separate equal steps of hue and chroma in different parts of the chart. The CIE chromaticity distances are poor indicators of the stimulus differences needed for color discrimination. Many attempts have consequently been made to convert the CIE chart by changing its projection (tilting it, say, in a variety of ways) to give the required "uniform spacing." These efforts have not been fully successful and this is the reason for the increased concern of the CIE with ADVANCED COLORIMETRY which deals with *perceived* color differences.

Only by converting stimulus values to "perceptual values" for direct comparison with samples spaced in accordance with the way we judge their hue, saturation and lightness to vary, are we likely to achieve "uniform spacing". Examples of such a perceptual chart based on a 1956 report by Dorothea Jameson and me are shown in Chapter 7. The CIE has

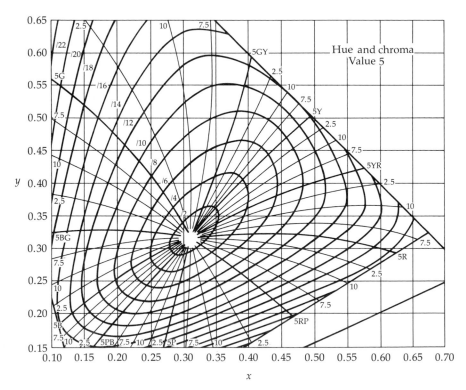

14 CHROMATICITY LOCI of Munsell colors of constant hue and chroma (and constant value 5). Note the unequal spacing of these presumably equally spaced visual steps.

recently recommended (1978) the CIELAB system to represent uniform color space for surface colors. It too is based on a conversion of stimulus values to perceptual scales.

In the discussion of material standards we touched briefly on a number of ways they can be prepared. To complete this volume we will discuss at somewhat greater length the ways in which colors are produced in a variety of situations, such as color photography, color printing, color televison, and painting.

Background Readings

Billmeyer, F. W., Jr., and Saltzman, M. 1966. *Principles of Color Technology.* Wiley, New York.

Birren, F. 1979. Color identification and nomenclature: A history. *Color Res. Appl.* 4: 14–18.

Burnham, R. W. 1952. A colorimeter for research in color perception. *Amer. J. Psychol.* 65: 603–608.

CIE (Commission International de l'Éclairage). 1971. *Colorimetry; Official Recommendations of the International Commission on Illumination.* Pub. CIE 15 (E-1.3.1) (Suppl. 2, 1978). Bureau Central de la CIE, Paris.

Committee on Colorimetry, Optical Society of America. 1953. *The Science of Color.* Crowell, New York.

Donaldson, R. 1947. A colorimeter with six matching stimuli. *Proc. Phys. Soc. Lond.* 59: 554–560.

Foss, C. E., Nickerson, D., and Granville, W. C. 1944. Analysis of the Ostwald Color System. *J. Opt. Soc. Amer.* 34: 361–381.

Hardy, A. C. 1936. *Handbook of Colorimetry.* MIT Press, Cambridge, Mass.

Hurvich, L. M., and Jameson, D. 1956. Some quantitative aspects of an opponent-colors theory. IV. A psychological color specification system. *J. Opt. Soc. Amer.* 46: 416–421.

ISCC-NBS Centroid Color Charts. [1958] Standard Sample 2106. Office of Standard Reference Materials. National Bureau of Standards, Washington, D.C.

Jacobsen, E., Granville, W. C., and Foss, C. E. 1948. *Color Harmony Manual,* 3rd ed. Container Corporation of America, Chicago.

Judd, D. B., and Wyszecki, G. 1975. *Color in Business, Science and Industry,* 3rd ed. Wiley, New York.

Kelly, K. L., and Judd, D. B. 1955. *The ISCC-NBS Method of Designating Colors and a Dictionary of Color Names.* National Bureau of Standards, Circ. 553. Washington, D.C.

Kelly, K. L., and Judd, D. B. 1976. *Color. Universal Language and Dictionary of Names.* Nat. Bur. Stand. (U.S.) Spec. Publ. 440. Washington, D.C.

Kornerup, A., and Wanscher, J. H. 1967. *Methuen Handbook of Colour*, 2nd ed. Methuen, London.

MacAdam, D. L. 1971. Geodesic chromaticity diagram based on variances of color matching by 14 normal observers. *Appl. Opt. 10*: 1–7.

Maerz, A., and Paul, M. R. 1950. *A Dictionary of Color*. McGraw-Hill, New York.

Munsell, A. H. 1905. *A Color Notation*, 1st ed. Ellis, Boston. (2nd ed., 1971. Munsell Color Co., Baltimore, Md.)

Munsell Color Company. 1976. *Munsell Book of Color*, Glossy ed. Munsell Color Co., Baltimore, Md.

Nickerson, D. 1961. *Munsell Color System*. Newsletter 156, Nov.-Dec. Inter-Society Color Council, Rochester, N.Y.

Ostwald, W. 1931. *Colour Science*. Translated by J. S. Taylor. Winsor and Newton, London.

Webster's Third New International Dictionary. 1965. Unabridged. Merriam, Springfield, Mass.

The Works of Robert Louis Stevenson. Vailima ed., Vol. 23. Letters, IV, 1891–1894, pp. 151–152. AMS Press, New York, reprinted 1974. [*The Letters of Robert Louis Stevenson*, Sidney Colvin, (ed.), Scribner, New York, 1923.]

21
Color Reproduction: Photography, Printing, Television, and Painting

I BEGAN this book by describing the colored objects I saw as I looked out of my study window near the ocean's edge. I wrote that our visual world is made up of differently formed colors and that the objects we see are colors of different kinds and forms. With this as the starting point, the remainder of the book presents an account of the structure and neural organization of visual system to enable us to understand what lies at the basis of our manifold color experiences. I have tried to explain how the system functions and how, via the contrast and adaptation mechanisms, individuals with normal vision manage to see a world of approximate color constancy despite large and varied light changes. To do this the physics of light, the reflectance and transmittance of various objects, and the interaction of light with the organism have all been considered. The data of color cancellation and color-mixture experiments were analyzed at length, as were the photopigments in the eye and the known relevant facts of electrophysiology. Contrast and adaptation were reviewed. I also discussed a variety of color-deficient visual systems whose color gamuts are limited and gave an account of the whys and wherefores of these types of defects. And in Chapter 20 I discussed color specification.

But is this not a rather limited view of our world of color? If I stop gazing out of my study window and settle back to look at my desk, or walk over to my bookshelves, or open a desk drawer, or look at the study walls, I am confronted by a totally different sort of world of color. Now I have before me colored reproductions of figures in color-vision texts and biology books, colored reproductions of well-known paintings, an original painting by a local artist, colored advertisements in magazines, some colored photographic transparencies and prints of people and faraway places, as well as a few rolls of Super-8 colored movie film. To complete the picture I should not overlook a color television set that will be available for my use in the evening.

How closely do these various kinds of two-dimensional reproductions approximate the original scenes, objects, and people they represent? (We leave original artworks aside, because the artist, except for the trompe l'oeil efforts, is rarely concerned with precise duplication.) Were those Bermuda skies, seas, and sands in the color transparencies and color film really that blue, that green, or that pink? Does the reproduction of Matisse's "Interior with Egyptian Curtain" (1948) really reproduce faithfully his painting in the Phillips collection in Washington? The plethora of magazine ads and mail-order catalogs may be of trivial interest, but are there really people with faces that are pink, or green, or pale, or whatever the case may be? Are there gins that are really that yellow? In short, do color reproductions faithfully mimic the originals? If they do not, why not? To answer questions of this sort, we must first raise another question: How are color reproductions made? Once we have answered this basic question we may begin to investigate the limitations of color reproduction. Considering what we have learned about the way the visual mechanism functions, we may begin to see why color reproductions, however excellent they may be, can never fully duplicate the originals.

We explored at length in Chapter 9 the fact that any color can be perfectly matched in the laboratory by an appropriate combination of three appropriately selected spectral stimuli. Whether the stimulus mixture is of an additive or subtractive type, as long as the chromatic and achromatic activities evoked in the neural system by some combination of the three spectral variables are precisely those produced by, say, a single broad-band stimulus, both the mixture and the stimulus with the broad-band distribution look identical. And the principles of color mixture lie at the heart of all color reproduction, whether we are dealing with colors reproduced on photographic film, on the printed page, or on the television screen.

In the discussion of colorimetry we have seen that we can provide a tripartite specification of any colored stimulus with the use of visual or electronic colorimeters. In industry and commerce a single test sample or stimulus is usually evaluated in these instruments as the need arises. Suppose, however, that the sample contains a variety of colors, say a woman wearing a green sweater and a white shirt, with a reddish kerchief tied over her hair, standing in a wheat field with a blue sky as "backdrop." By making a colorimetric scan in discrete steps, we can obtain a three-part colorimetric record for every area of interest in this scene: the clothes, the woman's face, the background, and so on. However fine we make these steps, at each point in the scene I have just described we will register a record in triplicate—a record of the three matching stimuli.

This is precisely what happens in color reproduction. A triplex record is made of each point in the scene but it is not made in numerical terms (i.e., in amounts of matching stimuli). It is made in the form of three separate colored records. Let us consider color photography first.

Almost everyone knows that the black-and-white photographic process provides us with a NEGATIVE that records the relative amounts of light in the original scene. Where there is an appreciable amount of light, we get, after developing our film, heavy silver deposits and hence dense black areas in the negative. Where there is little light, there is relatively little reaction in the film, the silver deposits are therefore small, and hence the negative tends to be clear or transparent. Areas with moderate amounts of light react as we would anticipate on the basis of the extreme reactions. In short, the amount of silver deposit varies with the degree of light exposure. If we print a positive from the negative, the dark areas are reproduced as light, and vice versa. The original scene is thus reproduced appropriately as far as its lightness and darkness aspects are concerned.

If we were to look at the same scene through a colored filter, the relative lightnesses of the different surfaces would be changed, and the same thing is true if we were to place the colored filter in front of the camera lens. Without moving the camera or anything in the scene, suppose we take three successive black-and-white pictures of the woman in the wheat field. Now we introduce, in turn, three differently colored filters (taking-filters) in front of the camera lens. For the first exposure, let us use a filter with a short- and midspectral-wavelength cutoff. This allows only the long wavelengths of light to register on the black-and-white film and only those aspects of the scene that look yellow, orange, and reddish to our eyes will register on the black-and-white negative. The areas in the original scene that we see as blue and green are excluded by the cutoff filter and will not be recorded on the film. These areas will accordingly be transparent in the negative. The second and third exposures are each made on a separate black-and-white negative, one with a filter that has a short- and long-wavelength cutoff, thus registering midspectral light only, and the other with a filter that has a mid- and long-wavelength cutoff to register the short-wavelength light.

From each of the three negatives, three POSITIVE black-and-white transparencies or slides are now made. If we place each positive transparency in a separate slide projector and place in front of each projector the same filter that was used in making the particular exposure, we will see, on bringing the three images simultaneously in register on a screen, a fairly good reproduction of the original scene. A three-part record of each stimulus element in the original scene has been made in photographing it, and a three-part additive mixture of each element is formed on projection to reproduce the colors in the original scene. For each element in the original scene we have, in principle, a metameric match.

Once we have three black-and-white separation negatives, as they are called, we can make a photographic reproduction of the original scene in the form of a colored PRINT instead of the resorting to additive projection. To do this, each of the three negatives* is first placed in a different dye bath. The negative exposed through short-wavelength light only is placed in a dye bath to absorb a yellow dye, the negative shot through a filter that transmits only midspectral light is placed in a blue-red (magenta) dye, and the negative exposed through the long-wavelength-transmitting filter is placed in a blue-green (cyan) dye. Film areas that have had less light exposure and consequently less silver deposit in them absorb dyes to a greater degree than those that have more silver deposit. If each dyed negative is then positioned above a special white copying paper, with care to ensure proper registration, each dye is transferred one at a time by a "rolling pin" procedure from the negative to the white paper, and we end up with a DYE TRANSFER PRINT.

If we refer back to the original scene described above, we see that the negative that registered the greatest amount of light from the green sweater will be the most dense in this particular area; it will therefore absorb little, if any, of the magenta dye. The other two negatives with little exposure by midspectral light in the area of the green sweater will, on the other hand, each absorb relatively large amounts of yellow and blue-green (cyan) dye, respectively. Viewed in "white" light the three superimposed dye layers will be seen as green in the sweater area. Why? Because we are dealing with a *subtractive* light-mixture situation. The yellow and cyan dyes absorb all wavelengths but the midspectral ones, which are therefore reflected. And midspectral light, as we now know, is seen as predominantly greenish. A similar analysis can be made for the other elements in the original scene. We need only remember that the cyan dye controls the amount of long-wavelength light reflected or transmitted from the picture; the magenta dye controls the amount of midspectral light reflected or transmitted and the yellow dye the amount of short-wavelength light reflected or transmitted (see Chapter 8).

Instead of using the cumbersome additive light projection technique or the dye transfer print process, which requires professional skills of a high order, modern color photography relies mainly on subtractive color mixture as incorporated in what is called the INTEGRAL TRIPACK. The essence of the integral tripack is that it has three film layers that record three separate images from the different parts of the spectrum as described above for the separate negative taking filter combinations. The topmost layer is sensitive to short-wavelength light, the second to midspectral light, and the bottom layer is sensitive to long-wavelength light. This is the sort of color film most of us use in our own cameras. With a single

* The negatives are of a special "matrix" type.

light exposure three different images are recorded in the three layers of film. When the film is developed, dye-forming chemicals called dye couplers are released at each of the three layers, and the latent images originally recorded are changed to yellow, magenta, and cyan. (In some multilayer films the dye couplers are bound in the film emulsions themselves.) The analysis of why we see colors in the film appropriately colored in relation to the colors of the original scene is exactly the same as in the dye transfer print situation.

Color photography often gives us good reproductions of colored objects. (They can also be very bad.) But if the goal of color photography is to reproduce on film colors that match the colors of objects precisely, this is not achievable. The sensitivities of the three emulsion layers would, for one thing, have to be precisely those of the average eye and react to all energy distributions with the same response ratios as does the human eye. There is the further complication that the emulsion sensitivities would have to be converted into dye concentrations that would provide an observer with the same result that the theoretical ideal film emulsions do.

We need only reflect on the comparisons we made between observers with normal color vision and those with sharp but anomalous color-vision systems to appreciate the difficulties that are encountered with color film reproduction. With receptor sensitivities that differ from those of the normal observer, the anomalous observers do not "reproduce" the colors the normal sees. A normal observer's yellow may look greenish to a "sharp" deuteranomalous or reddish to a protanomalous individual with good color discrimination. If a scene is registered by a set of film sensitivities that differ from the set of normal photopigments in the human eye (assuming appropriate dye transformations in the film), a normal observer will report that the colors in an original scene are not matched by those he sees in the color reproduction.

Close analysis shows that despite generally good color reproduction, there are difficulties. Certain broad-band distributions that look different to the average eye often come out looking identical in color film. The film does not discriminate some color differences that are readily apparent to the eye. Furthermore, as we have noted, a given light distribution does not necessarily look the same in real life and in the film. Before the advent of instant films, comparisons of this sort were difficult to make. The guests were long gone, the visited vacation spot was far distant. But now, when we can take a completed photograph from an instant camera and compare it with the live subject, discrepancies are more easily judged. We can also see, without relying on memory, that objects that match visually in daylight but have different spectral reflectances (hence metamers under daylight illumination) fail to match in the film.

Several additional matters should be mentioned. One relates to the fact that film, unlike the human eye, has fixed sensitivities. Unlike the human visual system, which adapts to different types of illumination (see Chapter 15), balances among film emulsion sensitivities are adjusted for one type of illumination. Unless appropriate filters are used as recommended by the manufacturer for different illuminations, say, daylight versus incandescent, the film will record a scene that is differently illuminated at, say, different times of day, as very different. This is in contrast to the way the eyes and the visual system adjust and compensate to maintain approximate color constancy.

In viewing a small-scale reproduction of an original scene, even if the individual elements in the original and reproduction were exactly matched colorimetrically, it must be remembered that we are dealing with different sizes of the same item in the two instances. Not only will there be hue and saturation differences that depend on size differences (see Chapter 13), but the neural spatial interactions responsible for contrast effects will be different in the reproduction from what they are when we view the original scene. This is an important variable in achieving color constancy.

Nor can we ignore the additional fact that when any scene or subject is photographed, the field of view encompassed by ordinary cameras and recorded on film is only a fraction of the area seen by the photographer. The object or objects of interest in the real world are thus seen surrounded by relatively large fields, whereas there is relatively little surround area included in the print or transparency. Furthermore, the print is viewed in surroundings very different from those in the original scene. Instead of the extended sky, we have the viewer's tabletop or whatever.

The differences between real scenes and photographed scenes are well known to professional photographers and attentive amateurs. Various "tricks," which relate primarily to the manipulation of secondary light sources to create or eliminate shadows, are used to offset the differences between nature and the photograph, but a discussion of these is beyond the scope of this book.

One of the best reference volumes on photomechanical reproduction summarizes the uses of colored printing as follows: "Advertising and packaging use the greatest volume of color reproductions. Advertising takes many forms: magazines and newspapers, direct mail, catalogs, calendars, store displays, billboards, etc. Packaged goods, especially food, usually have color reproductions on the package or label. Illustrations in magazines and books are next in volume. Greeting cards come next, and finally there is a relatively low volume of fine arts reproductions." For these purposes, it is obvious that color printing usually involves making many copies of the same original.

Reproducing a color original by a printing process is based on the same principles as color photography. Three different types of photomechanical reproduction are generally used. These are (1) relief or letterpress printing; (2) planographic or lithographic printing; and (3) intaglio or gravure printing. The technical details and procedures differ in the three instances, but the common elements are that the original scene or material to be reproduced is usually in the form of a photographic color transparency (or a painting); the colored transparency itself is photographed to prepare printing plates; the printing plates are inked as required and the ink is transferred to the printed paper.

One aspect of the printing process that differentiates it from color photography is the use of HALFTONE SCREENS. In black-and-white printing it is possible with this technique to record and print black areas, white areas, and various intermediate grays. When the original photographic film is itself photographed to prepare halftone negatives, a finely meshed screen is interposed in the camera, which breaks up the image pattern into small dots. The final print contains a dot structure that depends on the degree of blackness, grayness, and whiteness of the original. The dots are large where the original is black, absent where it is white, and of intermediate sizes where there are grays. The dots are ordinarily too small to resolve with the naked eye and the ratio of black to whiteness in what is essentially a pointillist mixture situation (see Chapter 8) determines the appearance in the reproduction. With a preponderance of large dots we see black, and where the dots are all small we see light grays or white. Looking at any photograph in a newspaper, magazine, or book with a magnifying glass will reveal this dot structure.

In making color reproductions halftone negatives are also prepared, but now the process is repeated three times. Three differently selective filters are used in the camera, one that transmits mostly long-wavelength light, a second midspectral light, and a third short-wavelength light. The original transparency is photographed through a halftone grating screen and three printing plates are prepared, one dyed with cyan ink, a second with magenta ink, and a third with yellow ink. Similarly to the dye transfer process in photography, the three inks are transferred to the paper, the "printed" page.

The colors seen are primarily the result of the subtractive mixtures that occur in the overlap of the three dyes. But there is also a small additive element of the pointillist sort.

Nothing in this extremely brief summary account begins to convey the complexities of the color printing processes and the superb technological advances that have been made in the past few decades. Many of the advances are of an empirical sort. For example, it is known that color printing is improved by the addition of a black inked plate to the cyan, yellow, and blue ones, and a four-color printing process is used to obtain high fidelity. Technological and engineering skills are devoted to improving the photomechanical methods of reproduction since they play such a large role in commerce and business. These improvements concern the nature of the three-color separation negatives, methods of correcting and improving colored negatives, using computer controls to adjust color ink balances, and so on, and they are all concerned with manipulating the stimulus to be presented to the eye. However brilliant and ingenious, there is nothing to be learned from them about the workings of the eye.

Color television is based on additive color mixture that is both spatial and temporal. The spatial aspect is the pointillist or mosaic type (Chapter 8). The face of the color television cathode ray tube is covered with thousands and thousands of three-dot clusters of phosphors. If we examine the screen with a magnifying glass we find that these tiny phosphor dots, when activated to glow, are clusters of red, green, and blue phosphors. They are so small and so close that when they are focused on the retinal surface of the eye, they are not resolved. Even though they are separate points in space, they fall on what is effectively the same retinal locus and mix. The temporal aspect of color mixture in the television situation derives, of course, from the fact that at the same retinal positions there are extremely fast shifts among the different types of phosphor dots that are activated—so rapid, in fact, that fusion occurs.

If the colors on the screen are to mimic the colors of an original scene it is necessary that the television camera that records the original scene make an appropriate record of all the colors and that this record be transmittable over great distances. We need no more concern ourselves here with the technological and electrical "wizardry" that makes this possible than we concerned ourselves with the technical details of color photography and color printing. What we can expect is that the principles are the same, and they are.

The original scene is viewed essentially by three cameras, one camera sensitive to long-wavelength light, another to midspectral light, and the third to short-wavelength light. In practice, there is actually one camera, but by using beam-splitting mirrors the incoming light is fed through three spectrally selective filters to three camera tubes. The separate signals that are broadcast from the television station are picked up at the receiving end, where they are converted to three sets of small electrical voltages. These voltages control the emission of electrons from three separate "guns," each of which corresponds to one member of the set of selective filters. The guns are precisely directed and channeled so that the clusters of red, green, and blue phosphors on the face of the receiving tube are excited by electrons coming from the appropriate guns. Since the degree of phosphor excitation relates to the strength of the voltage signal, which in turn is dependent on the degree to which the three cameras of different wavelength selectivity respond to the original colored scene, we are ultimately dealing with a three-variable light mixture of the pointillist type in the reproduction.

For reasons of efficiency, the engineering of color television transmission uses the signal from one camera to record lightness or brightness and two difference signals to vary the voltages that control the ultimate hue records. The signal transmission is thus analogous to the way we envision the neural signals to be controlled following photochemical absorption in the human visual system. The similarity in design does not come about because visual theory influenced television design, or vice versa. Theoretical models of the visual system based on one achromatic signal and two chromatic difference signals were proposed long before engineers adopted this form of electronic signaling. The reasons for adapting these modes of signaling relate entirely to technical matters of signal bandwidth and the efficiencies of transmitting information electronically; they have nothing to do with knowing how the visual mechanism might operate.

Can the additive color-mixture system of color television provide us with reproduction of an original scene that is perfect from a colorimetric point of view? The answer is "no" and follows directly from what we now know about color mixture (see Chapters 9 and 20).

The three different phosphors used in color television have peak emittances in the spectral regions seen as blue, green, and red, respectively. More precisely, they are a somewhat desaturated blue, a somewhat desaturated yellow-green, and a yellow-red phosphor. As noted in Chapter 20, the triangle enclosed by the three primaries includes all possible chromaticities that can be matched by the phosphors now used. Note that this system can reproduce no spectral colors and no colors that lie beyond the boundaries of the mixture triangle.

It seems proper to ask why phosphors that appear green and blue and that lie close to the spectrum locus should not be sought out. The answer is that doing so would increase the stimulus gamut enclosed by the primaries, which could be done only at the cost of a loss in light level (not apparent from the diagram), since the closer the phosphor lies to the spectrum locus, the less broad is its spectral emittance curve. To increase the light level, more radiant energy would be necessary. This becomes too expensive—hence the use of relatively broad-band phosphors.

A second question is: How faithful is the reproduction of those colors that are enclosed in the available color gamut? Here the nature of the three spectral sensitivities of the television camera that control the ultimate output of the phosphors enters as a fundamental consideration. It turns out that for precise matching the three camera sensitivities would be required to have negative quantities (see the discussion of complete matching situation in Chapter 9). This is electronically impossible without the additional use of three more cameras. The difficulties are met to some extent, without adding cameras, by clever electronic circuitry. But still, at the extremes of the color gamut presently encompassed, the reproduced colors cannot precisely match the originals.

In color photography and color television there is also the question of how adaptation affects the reproduction as perceived by the viewer. Unlike viewing the final print in color photography, the picture on the television screen itself is not seen by reflection of room light, but is rather shielded from it. The controlling adaptation in viewing is, of course, determined by some combination of the light transmitted through the television screen itself and whatever room illumination is used. This is not necessarily the prevailing illumination in the original scene, whether a naturalistic one or one set up in a studio. If the viewing illumination is primarily yellowish, the whites seen in a reproduced studio scene could be satisfactory if the studio illumination is also yellowish. On the other hand, if the ambient room illumination is primarily bluish, the whites may seem excessively yellowish.

An additional factor is the overall level of surround illumination provided by the room light relative to the light level of the screen. Increasing the ambient light level in the room will, for example, make the television picture appear darker compared to the situation when the television set is in a darkened room. It is therefore not surprising to learn that observers looking at a dim picture on the television screen in a high surround illumination prefer that the screen light level be increased. In some newer television sets there is now automatic compensation of the screen light level for different ambient conditions of illumination.

The size problem is similar to that in color photography. Although relative sizes may remain the same as viewing distance changes, the contrast interactions among the stimulus elements in a given scene will obviously be size-dependent.

Despite all the difficulties, it is true that almost every baseball or football fan will prefer a color picture to a black-and-white one. Fidelity is less important than the increased discrimination the color picture offers. Viewers, particularly in bars, seem willing on occasion to accept baseball diamonds or gridirons that are reproduced as red rather than as their real or synthetic grass-green colors.

Faithful color reproduction may be one of the primary goals of artists whose main interest is in paintings of a "trompe l'oeil" type and those who do conventional portrait work. But most professional painters make individualistic, personal statements which more often than not bear only a slight resemblance to the "real" objects, persons, and scenes that the nonartist sees. In fact, it is obvious that the modern abstract expressionists, hard-edge painters, or pop artists are not usually concerned with or produce "subjects" that the lay person would regard as "real" objects. If we recall the variety of categories used to encompass and classify the output of painters in the last hundred years additional terms that come to mind are impressionism, postimpressionism, pointillism, expressionism, fauvism, cubism, pure abstractionism, surrealism, German expressionism, Dadaism, action painting, minimal art, and op-art, among many others. There is a lot of color production in the works of artists in these groups but very little faithful color reproduction of a representational sort. What we have in the abstract work, it has been said, are "images keyed to myth or unique individual crystallizations." Emil Nolde wrote "Colors, the materials of the painter; colors in their own lives, weeping and laughing, dream and bliss, hot and sacred, like love songs and the erotic, like songs and glorious chorals! Colors in vibration, pealing like silver bells and clanging like bronze bells, proclaiming happiness, passion and love, soul, blood and death."

But here we have a prosaic question: How do artists go about producing colors? This question leads into a consideration of various media. Are we, for example, dealing with watercolors, where one works in transparent washes on a white ground, or are we talking of oils? The media are important because mixtures of the same pigments will give different results if their "depth" of application is different. Nor are these two media the only ones. Another painting technique uses tempera emulsions. Dry pigments are mixed with water and egg yellow or waxes; in fresco painting powdered pigments are mixed with water and incorporated on freshly plastered walls. Encaustic paint is made by mixing beeswax with pigments and, after heating the mixture to liquify it, is applied with a pallette knife while still hot. There are also gouaches and pastels (or colored chalk), where pigments are mixed with water and gum solutions, and synthetic acrylic paints.

In view of the various media available and knowing that pigments "behave" differently in different situations, can we generalize about the way an artist produces various colors? Not easily. The mixture of paints to produce new colors is very complex. The outcome depends on the spectral absorption of the paints, on the type of paint used and the way it absorbs light, on the relative transparency or opaqueness of the paint, and on the type of surface on which the paint is applied. Furthermore, the particular way the artist applies the paint is important. If the artist chooses to apply the pigments in what is known as "broken color," where tiny strokes of different pigment colors produce a "confetti of different colored dots," he or she is using what we have referred to as the pointillist technique, where the color mixture produced is of an additive sort.

Because of the nature of pastel chalks and the texture of the surface to which they are applied, pastels also produce additive color mixtures. For example, if yellow and blue pastels are overlaid on textured paper, the two hues lie as separate specks of color and tend to act as paints do in the pointillist technique. The color impression in this case will approximate a gray, as in most additive mixtures, rather than produce a "subtractive" green. By smearing or blending the pastels with a fingertip, one does, of course, get a subtractive mixture.

The artist who paints in oils or acrylic has an immense number of pigments available. Their name and number are legion, and the average artist settles on from 12 to 20 different pigments. But there are wide individual differences: Gilbert Stuart did his portraits with only seven colors, whereas Ingres's palette contained 27 pigments. In any event, artists mix their pigments to achieve some of the hues, brightnesses, and saturations they are after. The general principle that is operative is subtractive mixture, just as in color photography and color printing. A simple example of subtractive color mixture was discussed at length in Chapter 8. The yellow pigment reflects the midspectral and long wavelengths and absorbs the short wavelengths, those that appear blue and violet. The blue-appearing pigment reflects the short and midspectral rays and absorbs the long wavelengths associated with yellow, orange, and red. Since the only rays not absorbed by either the yellow or blue pigments in the mixture are midspectral ones, we see the mixture as green.

This discussion is not intended to imply that artists can select a few seemingly appropriate pigments and sail merrily on. If the subtractive rule is that green is produced by a mixture of yellow and blue pigments, it does not follow that all pigments that *look* yellow or blue will work. Both the yellow- and blue-appearing pigments must also reflect midspectral light, those wavelengths responsible for evoking greenness. Thus a mixture of a lemon-yellow pigment with Prussian blue, both of which reflect light throughout the spectrum, produces a good green, whereas a mixture of ultramarine blue and chrome yellow makes for a dull green. Again, cadmium yellow mixed with cobalt blue produces a green that is inferior to that produced by mixing cadmium yellow with the bluish-green pigment called viridian.

In general, there are so many pigments which vary in their spectral absorbances that there are many ways to produce a given color. Furthermore, some pigment mixtures do not produce useful results. Although there are literally hundreds of books and many theories that are intended to help the novice, most are difficult to assimilate and put to ready use.* This should not be surprising when we consider the large variety of different pigments available, but it makes it difficult to state a few simple

* I leave aside here views of artists like Kandinsky, who see analogues between music and color and believe that through color the artist can release "inner necessities" and evoke "vibrations of the spirit."

principles for compounding their mixtures to achieve a desired result. Each painter has to learn afresh from personal experience and rule-of-thumb experiments how to mix and control particular paints.

One of the very few visual scientists who years ago concerned himself with problems of painting was H. E. Ives. He presented a helpful analysis of the subtractive color-mixture painting palette by comparing it with the results of additive color mixtures. Ives was even able to suggest, on the basis of an extended spectral analysis of pigments, three pigments with a high degree of permanence that would act as the basic yellow, cyan, and magenta paints. The three pigments he selected were extra pale cadmium yellow, Chinese blue, and a phosphomolybdotungstic acid lake of rhodamine 6G. Used in conjunction with a zinc white, Ives could produce a wide gamut of brilliant colors and demonstrated that he could adequately handle the vast majority of colors he needed for "naturalistic" painting. Maurice Grosser, the American painter, in his fascinating and delightful volume *Painter's Progress,* pays Ives's recommended palette high tribute. As an artist Grosser does, however, indicate ways in which he used a little "fudging," as he calls it, to improve on Ives's four-pigment palette. What Grosser did was to add a cadmium red to improve the reds and oranges.

It would be trite to say that there is more to painting than color. Since art is not my speciality, I will not belabor this point. But I can cite Grosser's summary remarks: "The only guide to color is to use it, to work with paints until one has learned to distinguish subtleties and relations visible only to an educated eye and until the painter can find instantly on the end of his brush the exact tone he has in mind, without ever stopping to think how it is done. This takes time and practice. No matter how good a sense of color the young painter is endowed with, its accurate expression is one of the last skills he acquires."

The artist is confronted by many problems other than the appropriate selection of a color palette and how to properly mix paints. Let us briefly review a few of them.

The problem of color constancy is one of the more important ones. We have seen that approximate color constancy operates in the real world. Over a wide range of different illuminants, the visual system compensates enough so that we tend to recognize most colored objects as essentially retaining their color identities. But consider the plein-air paintings of some of the impressionists, for example. What they are representing on canvas were their impressions of the moment, and this meant capturing, in different paintings, the subtle changes in light and color in landscapes, seascapes, and the surfaces of objects. These changes occur throughout the day from morning to evening, although many people tend to ignore them when they stress the approximate constancy of object colors. The subtle changes that the artist worked so assiduously to capture on canvas will, of course, be modified, and sometimes sharply, if the viewing illuminant for the painting is too far "off" from the original light. The plein-air painter, whether impressionist or representational, must be able to manipulate colors appropriately during the painting of the scene to adjust for the differences in the painting light and the ultimate gallery or home viewing illumination anticipated.

We know that hues change to some extent with illumination level and that color contrast effects are operative at all times. Since the total range of reflectances a painting covers is but a fraction of the range present in an original outdoor scene, the artist must have the perceptual and technical skills to exploit while painting so that the visual effects desired will occur within the restricted range of reflectances available from the canvas and within the restricted ranges of illumination in the home or gallery viewing situation.

In any painting the artist does, he confronts the "contrast problem". Whatever paint is applied to the canvas must be "adjusted," depending on the adjacent colors used. One thing is certain. Colors are not likely to appear on the canvas the way they do on the palette. As we saw in Chapter 13, contrast interactions are of a complex sort and their effects are determined by reciprocal spatial interactions in the visual system. Hence there will be interactions among all the painted elements on the canvas. Assimilation effects are often deliberately introduced in a painting, but they also occur without the painter's intention. The artist must very often deliberately introduce nonuniformities to achieve a colored field that is perceptually uniform, or in some cases may introduce a contrast shadow to enliven the painted surface.

Contrast effects must also be considered in hanging pictures side by side on gallery walls. The colors in each painting may affect the appearance of those in its neighbor, and vice versa. It is also important that the lightness or darkness of the gallery walls be considered relative to the lightness and darkness of the paintings themselves. Light walls will darken the colors in pictures (although the saturations of the colors may be enhanced) and dark walls will tend to lighten them.

Other issues that relate to the way artists seek to create the illusion of the third dimension in two-dimensional productions further complicate the problem of how colors are used, particularly for figurative and representational painting. For example, artists commonly use desaturated blues to create the illusion of distance in landscapes. Distant views are often seen in a blue haze because of the way light rays are scattered physically by the atmosphere. By appropriately using blues for the distant objects to represent this haze, along with perspective drawing and reduction of detail, the artist can achieve a strong three-dimensional appearance on a flat, two-dimensional canvas hung on a wall that is also two-dimensional.

What a visual scientist has to say about art, on the one hand, bears only on certain technical matters, and on the other hand provides an analysis based on an understanding of the visual system—of what the visual artist has been able to achieve in controlling our visual perceptions. What art and artists have to say about our world and the way we experience it—as they try to state it for us—is ultimately of greater importance in most value systems.

Background Readings

Albers, J. 1963. *Interactions of Color*. Yale University Press, New Haven, Conn.

Arnheim, R. 1974. *Art and Visual Perception*. A Psychology of the Creative Eye (new version). University of California Press, Berkeley, Calif.

Evans, R. M. 1948. *An Introduction to Color*. Wiley, New York.

Evans, R. M. 1959. *Eye, Film and Camera in Color Photography*. Wiley, New York.

Grosser, M. 1971. *Painter's Progress*. Potter, New York.

Hunt, R. W. G. 1975. *The Reproduction of Colour*. Photography, Printing and Television, 3rd. ed. Wiley, New York.

Ives, H. E. 1934. Thomas Young and the simplification of the artist's palette. *Proc. Phys. Soc. Lond. 46*: 16–34.

Jameson, D., and Hurvich, L. M. 1975. From contrast to assimilation: In art and in the eye. *Leonardo 8*: 125–131.

Judd, D. B., and Wyszecki, G. 1975. *Color In Business, Science and Industry*, 3rd ed. Wiley, New York.

Kowaliski, P. 1977. The Spectral Sensitivities of Color-Reproduction Systems. In F. W. Billmeyer, Jr., and G. Wyszecki (eds.), *AIC Color 77*. Hilger, Bristol.

MacAdam, D. L. 1951. Quality of color reproduction. *J. Soc. Mot. Pict. Telev. Eng. 56*: 487–512.

Maxwell, J. C. 1855. Experiments on colour, as perceived by the eye. With remarks on colour-blindness. *Trans. Roy. Soc. Edinb. 41*: 275–298.

Printing Color Negatives. 1978. Pamphlet No. E-66. Eastman Kodak Co., Rochester, N.Y.

Protter, E. 1971. *Painters on Painting*. Grosset & Dunlap, New York.

Yule, J. A. C. 1967. *Principles of Color Reproduction*. Wiley, New York.

Illustration Credits

Chapter 2

1 After F. L. Dimmick, 1948. In *Foundations of Psychology,* E. G. Boring, H. S. Langfeld, and H. P. Weld (eds.), Wiley, New York.

Chapter 3

1 After C. Rainwater, 1971. *Light and Color,* Golden Press, New York. Copyright © 1971 by Western Publishing Company, Inc.

2 After J. E. Kaufman, 1972. In *IES Lighting Handbook,* 5th Ed., J. E. Kaufman (ed.), Illuminating Engineering Society, New York.

4a After D. B. Judd, 1952. *Color in Business, Science and Industry,* Wiley, New York.

4b After J. A. C. Yule, 1967. *Principles of Color Reproduction,* Wiley, New York.

11 After C. Rainwater, 1971. *Light and Color,* Golden Press, New York. Copyright © 1971 by Western Publishing Company, Inc.

13 After G. Wyszecki and W. S. Stiles, 1967. *Color Science,* Wiley, New York.

Chapter 4

14 After L. T. Troland, 1930. In *The Principles of Psychophysiology,* Vol. 2, D. Van Nostrand, New York.

Chapter 5

2 From D. Jameson and L. M. Hurvich, 1955. *Journal of the Optical Society of America* 45: 546–552.

3–11 After D. Jameson and L. M. Hurvich, 1955. *Journal of the Optical Society of America* 45: 546–552.

12 After L. M. Hurvich and D. Jameson, 1953. *Journal of the Optical Society of America* 43: 485–494.

13 After G. Wagner and R. M. Boynton, 1972. *Journal of the Optical Society of America* 62: 1508–1515.

14, 15 After L. M. Hurvich and D. Jameson, 1957. *Psychological Review* 64: 384–404

Chapter 6

2 After L. M. Hurvich and D. Jameson, 1955. *Journal of the Optical Society of America* 45: 602–616.

3 After D. McL. Purdy, 1937. *American Journal of Psychology* 49: 313–315.

4 From L. M. Hurvich and D. Jameson, 1958. In *Visual Problems of Colour,* Vol. II, Chapter 22, pp. 691–723. Her Majesty's Stationery Office, London.

Chapter 7

2a After L. M. Hurvich and D. Jameson, 1955. *Journal of the Optical Society of America* 45: 602–616.

2b After L. A. Jones and E. M. Lowry, 1926. *Journal of the Optical Society of America* 13: 25–34.

2c   After D. Jameson and L. M. Hurvich, 1959. *Journal of the Optical Society of America 13*: 25–34.

3   After L. M. Hurvich and D. Jameson, 1956. *Journal of the Optical Society of America 46*: 416–421.

Chapter 8

2   After J. C. Maxwell, 1860. *Philosophical Transactions of the Royal Society of London 150*: 57–84.

4   After D. Jameson and L. M. Hurvich, 1955. *Journal of the Optical Society of America 45*: 546–552.

Chapter 9

1   From L. M. Hurvich and D. Jameson, 1957. *Psychological Review 64*: 384–404

2   After J. C. Maxwell, 1860. *Philosophical Transactions of the Royal Society of London 150*: 57–84.

3   From G. Wyszecki and W. S. Stiles, 1967. *Color Science*, Wiley, New York.

4   After D. B. Judd, 1966. *Proceedings of the National Academy of Sciences USA 55*: 1313–1330.

5   After W. D. Wright and F. H. G. Pitt, 1935. *Proceedings of the Physical Society (London) 47*: 205–217.

6   After W. D. Wright, 1972. In *Handbook of Sensory Physiology*, Vol. 7/4, D. Jameson and L. M. Hurvich (eds.), Springer-Verlag, Berlin.

Chapter 10

3   From S. L. Polyak, 1941. *The Retina*, University of Chicago Press, Chicago.

6   From W. H. Miller, 1979. In *Handbook of Sensory Physiology*, Vol. 7/6A, H. Autrum (ed.), Springer-Verlag, Berlin.

8   From D. Jameson, 1972. In *Handbook of Sensory Physiology*, Vol. 7/4, D. Jameson and L. M. Hurvich (eds.), Springer-Verlag, Berlin.

10   After P. K. Brown and G. Wald, 1964. *Science 144*: 45–52.

12   After J. E. Dowling and B. B. Boycott, 1966. *Proceedings of the Royal Society (London) B 166*: 80–111.

14   From S. W. Kuffler and J. G. Nicholls, 1976. *From Neuron to Brain*, Sinauer, Sunderland, Mass.

Chapter 11

2   After D. Jameson and L. M. Hurvich, 1968. *Journal of the Optical Society of America 58*: 429–430.

Chapter 12

1   After H. K. Hartline, 1938. *American Journal of Physiology 121*: 400–415.

2   After E. F. MacNichol Jr., and G. Svaetichin, 1958. *American Journal of Ophthalmology 46*: 26–40.

3   From G. Svaetichin et al., 1963. *Acta Científica Venezuela* Suppl. 1, 135–153.

4   From E. F. MacNichol Jr. et al., 1973. In *Colour 73*, The Second Congress of the International Color Association, Hilger, London.

5   From R. L. De Valois et al., 1966. *Journal of the Optical Society of America 56*: 966–977.

7, 8   After R. L. De Valois and K. K. De Valois, 1975. In *Handbook of Perception*, Vol. 5, E. C. Carterette and M. P. Friedman (eds.), Academic Press, New York.

Chapter 13

6, 7b   After L. M. Hurvich and D. Jameson, 1960. *Journal of General Physiology 43(6)* (Suppl.): 63–80.

8–11	From D. Jameson and L. M. Hurvich, 1961. *Journal of the Optical Society of America* 51: 46–53.
15a	After J. E. Dowling and F. S. Werblin, 1969. *Journal of Neurophysiology* 32: 315–338.
16	After L. M. Hurvich and D. Jameson, 1974. *American Psychologist* 29: 88–102.
17	After P. H. Lindsay and D. A. Norman, 1977. *Human Information Processing*, 2nd ed., Academic Press, New York.
18	After S. W. Kuffler, 1953. *Journal of Neurophysiology* 16: 37–68.
19	After L. M. Hurvich and D. Jameson, 1974. *American Psychologist* 29: 88–102.
20	After D. Jameson, 1975. *Color Vision*, John F. Shepard Memorial Lecture, University of Michigan.
21	After I. Abramov, 1972. In *Handbook of Sensory Physiology*, Vol. 7/2, M. G. F. Fuortes (ed.), Springer-Verlag, Berlin.
22	From D. H. Hubel and T. N. Wiesel, 1960. *Journal of Physiology (London)* 154: 572–580.

Chapter 14

| 6 | After R. L. De Valois and K. K. De Valois, 1975. In *Handbook of Perception*, Vol. 5, E. C. Carterette and M. P. Friedman (eds.), Academic Press, New York. |
| 9 | After C. von Campenhausen, 1968. *Zeitschrift für Vergleichende Physiologie* 60: 351–374. |

Chapter 15

1, 2	After D. Jameson, 1972. In *Handbook of Sensory Physiology*, Vol. 7/4, D. Jameson and L. M. Hurvich (eds.), Springer-Verlag, Berlin.
3–7	After D. Jameson and L. M. Hurvich, 1956. *Journal of the Optical Society of America* 46: 405–415.
8	From W. D. Wright, 1969. *The Measurement of Colour*, Van Nostrand Reinhold, New York.
10a	From R. A. Weale, 1951. *Journal of Physiology* 113: 115–122.
13a	After L. A. Riggs et al., 1953. *Journal of the Optical Society of America* 43: 495–501.
13b	After R. M. Pritchard et al., 1960. *Canadian Journal of Psychology* 14: 67–77.
14	After S. L. Polyak, 1941. *The Retina*, University of Chicago Press, Chicago.

Chapter 16

1	After L. M. Hurvich et al., 1968. *Perception and Psychophysics* 4: 65–68.
2, 3	After D. Jameson and L. M. Hurvich, 1956. *Journal of the Optical Society of America* 46: 1075–1089.
4	After I. Schmidt, 1955. *Journal of the Optical Society of America* 45: 514–522.
5, 7, 9–11	From D. Jameson and L. M. Hurvich, 1956. *Journal of the Optical Society of America* 46: 1075–1089.
12	After M. P. Willis and D. Farnsworth, 1952. Medical Research Laboratory Report, Bureau of Medical Surgery, U.S. Navy Department, Washington, D.C.
13, 14	From D. Jameson and L. M. Hurvich, 1956. *Journal of the Optical Society of America* 46: 1075–1089.

Chapter 17

2	After C. H. Graham and Y. Hsia, 1958. *Science* 157: 675–682.
3	After C. H. Graham and Y. Hsia, 1958. *Science* 157: 675–682. Deuteranopic data from F. H. G. Pitt, 1935. *Characteristics of Dichromatic Vision*, Her Majesty's Stationery Office, London.
6	After L. M. Hurvich and D. Jameson, 1955. *Journal of the Optical Society of America* 45: 602–616.
8	After R. G. Cameron, 1967. *Aerospace Medicine* 38: 51–59.
10	After L. M. Hurvich and D. Jameson, 1955. *Journal of the Optical Society of America* 45: 602–616.

Chapter 19

1   After J. F. Horner, 1876. *Amtlicher Bericht über die Verwaltung des Medizinalwesens des Kantons Zürich vom Jahr 1876,* 208–211.

Chapter 20

1   After D. B. Judd and G. Wyszecki, 1975. *Color in Business, Science and Industry,* 3rd ed., Wiley, New York.

2   From D. Nickerson, 1961. *Munsell Color System,* Intersociety Color Council. Rochester, N.Y.

3, 4   After D. B. Judd and G. Wyszecki, 1975. *Color in Business, Science and Industry,* 3rd ed., Wiley, New York.

5   After R. L. Kelly and D. B. Judd, 1976. *Color: Universal Language and Dictionary of Names,* National Bureau of Standards (U.S.), Washington, D.C.

6   After R. W. Burnham, 1952. *American Journal of Psychology* 15: 603–608.

13   After D. B. Judd and G. Wyszecki, 1975. *Color in Business, Science and Industry,* 3rd ed., Wiley, New York.

14   After D. Nickerson, 1979. Personal communication.

Color Plates

1-1   Photograph by E. S. Ross.

1-5   Courtesy of the Inmont Corporation, Clifton, N.J.

2-3   G. Braque, "Poster with Red Birds." © by ADAGP, Paris, 1981.

8-2   From T. N. Cornsweet, 1970. *Visual Perception,* Academic Press, New York.

13-2   V. Vasarely, "Arcturus." © by ADAGP, Paris, 1981 and by permission of the Hirshhorn Museum and Sculpture Garden, Smithsonian Institution.

13-3   From C. L. Musatti, 1957. *Problèmes de la Couleur,* Service d'Edition et de Vente des Publications de l'Education Nationale, Paris.

Author Index

Numbers in bold type refer to pages on which bibliographic entries occur. Numbers in regular type refer to references in the text.

Thompson, B., **179**
Thomson, L. C., 103, 121, 126
Thorpe, S., **148**
Trendelenburg, W., **98**
Triebel, W., **219**
Troland, L. T., **12, 25, 51**
Tschermak, A., **179**

Uttal, W. R., **24, 25**

Varner, F. D., **221**
Vasarely, V., 173, **179,** Plate 13-?
van Bussell, H. J. J., **12**
Verriest, G., **258, 262**
von Kries, J., 197, **220,** 242

Waardenburg, P. J., **269**
Wade, N. J., **194**
Wagner, G., **65**
Wald, G., **126, 220**
Walls, G. L., **126**
Walraven, P. L., **135**
Walsh, E. S., **23**
Wanscher, J. H., **12, 298**
Warburton, F. N., **88**
Weale, R. A., **220, 262**
Webster's Third New International Dictionary, 2, **12,** 271, **298**
Werblin, F. S., 167, **178**
Werner, J. S., **65**
Wiesel, T. N., **149, 178**
Willis, M. P., **240**

Wilson, E. B., **269**
Wilson, G., 241, 242, 244, 257, **258**
Witkovsky, P., **148**
Wooten, B. R., **65**
Wright, W. D., 103, **111,** 121, **126, 134, 220, 240, 258**
Wybar, K. C., **126**
Wyszecki, G., 37, **38, 111, 112, 126, 297, 313**

Yager, D., **126, 127, 148**
Yamanaka, T., **148**
Yarbus, A. L., **220**
Young, T., 120, **126,** 129, **134**
Yule, J. A. C., **38, 313**

Zeki, S. M., **149**

Subject Index

Camouflage, 1, 257
Cancellation technique. *See* Null method
Centroid color, 277
Chroma, in Munsell system, 275, 276
Chromatic response function. *See* Response
    function
Chromaticity coordinates, CIE, 286, 288
Chromaticity diagram, 290–297
  center of gravity analysis, 292
  confusion loci of color deficient dichromats,
    293–295
  specification of visual tolerances, use in,
    295–296
  stimulus, gamuts in, 291–292
  straight line rule, 290–292
CIE colorimetry system, 158, 282–297
  advanced colorimetry, 296
  Standard Observer spectral tristimulus val-
    ues, 282–283, 286
Colors(s). *See also* Hue; *Specific color*
  achromatic, 3n, 3, 6, 7, 9–11
  arithmetic, rules of, 108
  definition of, in opponent-color terms, 162
  light radiation and, 13, 28, 29, 39–50
  mutual exclusiveness between opponent
    pairs, 5–6, 11, 17–23
  names, 2–3, 277–279
  number of, 1–3
  pastel, 9, 309–310
  perceptual interrelations, and ordering of,
    1–11
  primary, 1n–2n
  wavelengths associated with, 39–41
Color adaptation, 195–219. *See also* Approxi-
    mate color constancy; Color constancy;
    von Kries Coefficient Law
  chromatic response function changes, 200–
    202
  constant non-uniform stimulation effects,
    215–217
  darkness condition for neutral state, 196
  electrophysiological evidence, 202–203
  hue coefficient function, 203–204
  light stimulus condition for neutral state,
    204–205
  neutral state, 41, 196, 201, 204, 205
  persistance of metameric color matches,
    206–208
  receptor sensitivity changes, 196–201, 206–
    208
  reflectance differences and hue changes
    with, 208–209
  saturation coefficient functions, 205
  selective bleaching, 219
  two-process interpretation, 212
  uniform stimulation effects, 213–215
Color blindness. *See* Color deficiencies
Color circle. *See* Hue circle
Color constancy, 195, 199, 209
Color deficiency, 21–23, 222–269

achromat, typical, 261–262
acquired, 21, 23, 244, 256
anomalous trichromats, 22n, 222–239
cone monochromacy, 259–261
confusion loci, 293–294
congenital achromatopsia, 261
deutan defects, 242
deuteranomalous, 225, 226–239
deuteranope, red-green confusers, 22, 241–
    257
diagnostic tests, 251–254
dichromats, 241–257
displaced color systems, 223–239
heredity, 263–268
incidence, 222, 267–268
monochromatism, 259–262
neuteranomalous, 231–235
neutral point, spectral, 243–245, 248
peripheral, in normals, 19–20
photopigment loss, 254–256
protan defects, 242
protanomalous, 231–235
protanope, red-green confusers, 22, 242n,
    254–255, 265, 293, 294
pseudoisochromacy, 261
reduced neural responsiveness, 232–239,
    242
rod monochromacy, 261–262
shifted color systems, 223–239
tetartanope, 254n
tritanomalous, 239
tritanope, yellow-blue confusers, 22, 242n,
    254–255, 265, 293, 294
unilateral defects, 23, 244
Color matching
  color adaptations, and, 110, 206–207
  color specification, 270–297
  complete, 99–111
  by deuteranopes, 245–247
  for diagnosis of color deficiencies, 227
  haploscopic, 245
  hue, 93–98
  metameric, 110, 206–208, 253–254
  by protanopes, 249
Color mixture, additive, 41, 48–50, 54–55, 67–
    69, 85–87, 89–123
  apparatus, 54–55, 89–92, 103–104
  chromaticity coordinates, 288–297
  CIE functions, 283–288
  complete matches, 99–111
  cone photopigments and, 119–125, 128–134
  equations, 107–111
  functions, 101–111
  Grassmann's Laws of, 108
  hue, 89–97
  material standards, preparation of, 273
  methods, 89–93
  pointillist, 93, 305, 306, 307, 309
  space dependent, 93
  time-weighted averaging, 90

uniform fields, 213–217
receptive field model, 169–177
structure, 114–118
synaptic connections, 123, 124, 166–167
Retinal noise, 196
Rhodopsin, 117–119
Rod monochromacy, 261–262
Rules of color arithmetic, 108

Saturation
broad-band light distribution and, 43–44
changes resulting from contrast effects, 151–152, 162
color zones and, 21n
desaturation, 7–11, 84n
in Munsell system, 275
size changes and, 162
Saturation coefficient, 79–86, 238
of anomalous trichromats, 238
for chromatic adaptation state, 204–205
Scina, R., 153
Scotopic vision, 118
Separation negative, 154, 301
Sex-linked trait, 264–266
Shadow, contrast effects, 153–156, 165
Size of stimulus object
color photography and, 304
visual response change and, 162
Small-field tritanopia, 162
Specific nerve energy, 16
Spectral energy distribution, 31–35
black body, 33
broad-band stimulus, 41, 43, 45
correlated color temperatures, 34
daylight, 32
fluorescent lamp, 34–35
gallium phosphide electroluminescent crystal, 34–35
helium neon laser, 35
incandescent lamps, tungsten, 33
line spectra, 34
mercury arc, 34, 41, 84
narrow-band stimulus, 43–44
ruby laser, 35
sunlight, 32
xenon arc, 34
Spectral luminosity function. See Luminosity function
Spectral radiation, 26–38
color appearance and, 39–50
chromatic and achromatic response functions and appearance of, 65–75
light level effects, 72–75
Newton's experiments, 39–41
relative energy distribution, 32–35
Spectral sensitivity. See Luminosity function
Spectral transmittance, 36
Spectroprojector, 31, 32
Spectroradiometer, 31–32

Spectrum, of radiant energy, 28–30
Stabilized retinal images, 215–218
Standard Observer, 282, 283n, 284–288
Stein, G., 110
Straight-line role, 290–292
Stuart, G., 310
Subjective color, 188–191
Subtractive color mixture, 97–98
Supersaturation, 187
Surface contrast, 162

Television, color reproduction, 306–308
Temporal contrast effect, 180–193. See Afterimage
Tetartanope, 254n
Threshold measures, 62
achromatic response, 62, 74
chromatic response and, 74
two-color technique, 218
Trichromatism, anomalous, 222–239. See also Deuteranomaly, Neuteranomaly, Protanomaly
Tristimulus values, CIE, 283–287
Tritanomaly, 239
Tritanope, 242n
confusion loci, 293, 294
Tritanopia, 254–255
Two-locus theory, of color deficiency heredity, 266–207

Value, in Munsell system, 275, 277, 278
Vasarely composition, 173
Veiling. See Saturation, desaturation
Visual colorimeter, 280–282
Visual experience
of colors, 1–11
neural organization and, 11–23
Visual field, zones, 20–21
Visual perimeter, 20
Visual purple. See Rhodopsin
Visual stimuli, inappropriate, inadequate, 14
cosmic rays, 15
drugs, 15
electric currents, 14
magnetic fields, 14
x-rays, 14
von Kries Coefficient Law, 197–199, 206–208, 242n. See also Approximate constancy, color constancy

Wavelength, 28
associated hues, 39–41
discrimination, 209–212, 248
neurophysiological responses specific to, 138–147
Weber's Law, 218
White (color)
desaturation of chromatic colors by, 9
hueless color, 3, 6

response function, 61–65
complementary wavelengths, 48–50, 55, 69–72, 74, 84–87, 292
White light, 41
Whiteness, 61–64, 67, 69–72. *See also* Blackness; Luminosity function; Saturation coefficient
of broad-band stimuli, 84–87
and "L"-type cells, 138
neural code, 168
and nonopponent cells, 144–145
temporal variation of, 180–182

Whiteness response measurement, 61–64

Yellow
color zones and, 20
normal response function, 54–61, 67
present at long wavelength spectrum extreme, 67
unitary hue, 3–6
wavelength and spectral-distribution functions that evoke, 39, 40, 45–46, 48–49, 67–69
Yellow-blue color, non-existent, 5–6, 11